**Integrated Sports Massage Therapy**

For Elsevier

Commissioning Editor: Claire Wilson
Development Editor: Clive Hewat, Fiona Conn
Project Manager: Sukanthi Sukumar
Designer: Stewart Larking
Illustration Manager: Gillian Richards
Illustrator: Jennifer Rose

Integrated Sports Massage Therapy

A Comprehensive Handbook

Anders Jelvéus DN, Leg. Naprapat, MTOM, LAc, CMT

International freelance educator in manual therapies; Founder of the
Swedish Health Institute, Los Angeles, CA, USA

With a contribution by

Kristjan Oddsson DN, Leg. Naprapat, PETE, Bachelor in Sport Science

Lecturer in Human Biology and Sports Medicine, GIH—Swedish School of Sport and
Health Sciences, Stockholm, Sweden

ELSEVIER
CHURCHILL
LIVINGSTONE

ELSEVIER
CHURCHILL
LIVINGSTONE

ISBN 978-0-443-10126-7
Reprinted 2011, 2012

British Library Cataloguing in Publication Data
A catalogue record for this book is available from the British Library

Library of Congress Cataloging in Publication Data
A catalog record for this book is available from the Library of Congress

Notices
Knowledge and best practice in this field are constantly changing. As new research and experience broaden our understanding, changes in research methods, professional practices, or medical treatment may become necessary.

Practitioners and researchers must always rely on their own experience and knowledge in evaluating and using any information, methods, compounds, or experiments described herein. In using such information or methods they should be mindful of their own safety and the safety of others, including parties for whom they have a professional responsibility.

With respect to any drug or pharmaceutical products identified, readers are advised to check the most current information provided (i) on procedures featured or (ii) by the manufacturer of each product to be administered, to verify the recommended dose or formula, the method and duration of administration, and contraindications. It is the responsibility of practitioners, relying on their own experience and knowledge of their patients, to make diagnoses, to determine dosages and the best treatment for each individual patient, and to take all appropriate safety precautions.

To the fullest extent of the law, neither the Publisher nor the authors, contributors, or editors, assume any liability for any injury and/or damage to persons or property as a matter of products liability, negligence or otherwise, or from any use or operation of any methods, products, instructions, or ideas contained in the material herein.

 your source for books, journals and multimedia in the health sciences

www.elsevierhealth.com

Working together to grow libraries in developing countries

www.elsevier.com | www.bookaid.org | www.sabre.org

ELSEVIER   BOOK AID International   Sabre Foundation

The Publisher's policy is to use paper manufactured from sustainable forests

Printed in China

Contents

Preface vii

Acknowledgments ix

1 An introduction to sports massage 1

2 Work postures, hand placements, and basic massage strokes 5

3 Sports massage applications 27

4 Examples of event-based sports massage treatments 35

5 Sports massage applications for different sports 61

6 Soft tissue stretching in sports massage 75

7 Applied stretches to common muscle groups 97

8 Positional release techniques applied in sports massage 119

9 Acupressure and Tui Na in sports massage 127

10 Myofascial release techniques and connective tissue massage 139

11 Myofascial pain syndrome—myofascial trigger points 161

12 Sports injuries 181
    Dr. Kristjan Oddsson

13 Taping for sports injuries 199
    Dr. Kristjan Oddsson

14 Soft tissue treatment techniques for maintenance and
    remedial sports massage 207

15 Self-massage and myofascial release techniques for the athlete 235

Index 247

Preface

The work of a sports massage therapist ranges from basic pre- and post-event massage applications to handling more complex scenarios, such as attempting to optimize the athlete's biomechanical and physiological performance, or contributing to sports injury rehabilitation treatment.

To accomplish this, it is necessary to integrate a variety of different techniques. I call this way of working Integrated Sports Massage Therapy, to highlight the fact that sports massage can combine almost any technique or method that may improve the athlete's level of performance and recovery.

This book is intended to illustrate a variety of sports massage therapy techniques, beginning with a brief presentation of its history, and physiological/psychological effects, followed by common massage strokes and a discussion of pre-, post-, and inter-event therapy applications. Since range of motion is an integral part of sports activity, assorted soft tissue stretching methods, and hands-on applications to common muscle groups are featured. There are also descriptions of related methods, such as osteopathic positional release techniques (Chaitow 1997) and Asian manual medicine systems like acupressure and Tui Na.

The concept of myofascial release, including Myers' myofascial lines (Myers 2002) and the common pain-producing dysfunction caused by myofascial trigger points, are outlined. Elisabeth Dicke's "Bindegewebsmassage" (Goats & Keir 1991; Ylinen & Cash 1993) is also covered, further demonstrating the possible neural reflexive reactions from manipulation of skin and subcutaneous tissues. Lymphatic drainage massage techniques are also presented, and different related treatment methods and commonly affected muscle sites in the body are discussed.

Sports injuries are common amongst athletes (Conn et al. 2003; Hootman et al. 2007) and so acute, overuse, and other common types of injury are discussed, along with basic athletic taping techniques for a selection of injuries and dysfunctions. Restorative, maintenance, and remedial sports massage is presented including lymphatic drainage massage techniques, where assorted treatment methods for commonly affected sites in the body are described.

The last chapter demonstrates a number of self-massage techniques utilizing the athlete's hands, tennis, exercise ball, and lacrosse balls, or tools like The Stick, myofascial roll, and trigger wheel.

My aim with this book is that the novice therapist can gain from it a basic understanding of the highly rewarding field of sports massage, and inspiration to study it further; while the more experienced sports massage therapist can pick up additional concepts or techniques to enhance their practice. It is my aspiration and hope that this book will serve as a valuable addition to other existing fine publications on sports massage.

References

Chaitow, L., 1997. Positional release techniques, second ed. Churchill Livingstone, Edinburgh.

Conn, J.M., et al., 2003. Sports and recreation related injury episodes in the US population, 1997–99. Inj. Prev. 9 (2), 117–123.

Goats, G.C., Keir, K.A., 1991. Connective tissue massage. Br. J. Sports Med. 25 (3), 131–133.

Hootman, J.M., et al., 2007. Epidemiology of collegiate injuries for 15 sports: summary and recommendations for injury prevention initiatives. J. Athl. Train. 42 (2), 311–319.

Myers, T.W., 2002. Anatomy trains. Churchill Livingstone, Edinburgh.

Ylinen, J., Cash, M., 1993. Idrottsmassage. ICA bokförlag, Västerås.

Acknowledgments

Producing a book is seldom the work of only one person. Many people have interacted with me over the years, directly or indirectly influencing this book. I want to extend my most profound gratitude for the support from everyone past or present who has enriched my life and generated inspiration; to my family: my wife and son for their love and encouragement, and my mother, father, and sister for their lifelong moral support to continuously venture into new territory.

I am obliged to my friend and colleague, Dr Kristjan Oddsson, for contributing two fine chapters, which serve as an invaluable part of this book. Warm thanks also to Matthew Raymond Cohen and Ian Olson for acting as models, and to Susan Valdez Cohen for her contribution as photographer.

Profound honor goes to Dr Leon Chaitow for his initial support, abounding generosity to fellow practitioners, and vast contribution through a continuous dedicated effort to broaden the scope and understanding of the field of manual medicine. Gratitude is also extended to those involved at Elsevier—Sarena Wolfaard, Claire Wilson (Commissioning Editors), Fiona Conn, Clive Hewat (Development Editors), Sukanthi Sukumar (Project Manager), Stewart Larking (Designer), Gillian Richards (Illustration Manager), Jennifer Rose (Illustrator)—for their abundant patience and support.

Dr Björn Jonsson Berg brought Naprapathy to Sweden in 1970. Together with Inger Berg, and a fine faculty, his substantial work generated the essence of what is today the Scandinavian College of Naprapathic Manual Medicine in Stockholm, Sweden, one of the foundation stones for my practice of manual medicine. The teaching staff at Emperor's College in Santa Monica presented the opportunity to further my ever-deepening interest in energetic and Asian medicine. I also owe gratitude to all the excellent teachers in Europe, USA, and Asia from whom I have been privileged to learn, and who have influenced much of the content of this book. Acknowledgment is additionally extended to Hans Axelson, founder of Axelsons Gymnastiska Institute in Scandinavia, for providing instruction and motivation during my first formal massage studies at his school in Stockholm, and to Maria Grove for offering my first long-term teaching opportunity in the USA, from which I learned so much.

I am grateful to Dr Pat E. Belcher, founder and developer of "The Stick"; Darryn Starwyn of East West Medicine, Custom Craftworks; and Pekka Koski at Lojer group in Finland, for supplying equipment or pictures of their respective products used in this book.

Finally, I would like to express tremendous gratitude to all my patients and students over the last 26 years. You are my greatest teachers.

An introduction to sports massage

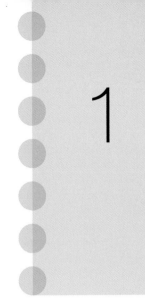

1

History

Various forms of massage from many cultures have existed since ancient times, and it is known that massage also was utilized in different athletic circumstances. The use of massage has been registered as early as 2200 BC in Egypt, and around 1400 BC in older Chinese cultures (Calvert 2002). In ancient Greece, Hippocrates (460–377 BC)—by many considered the "father of physical medicine,"—thought of massage as a vital therapy. Greek physicians at that time performed "anatripsis," meaning "to rub up," on athletes suffering from metabolic substance build-up in their muscles (Calvert 2002). Massages were also performed in Greek gymnasiums called "Esclapeion" where athletic training took place. The Greek physician Claudius Galenus (AD 129–201), a court physician to the Roman Emperor Markus Aurelius, wrote that the objective of massage is to soften the body before exercise (Calvert 2002). It is said that Galenus recommended that all exercise should be preceded by massage with oil (Calvert 2002). Massage was also used for the gladiators in Rome following exercise and fights, to relieve pain and serve as a revitalizing modality (Calvert 2002).

In India, where wrestling has always been a popular sport, massage has been used as a healing modality for wrestlers since ancient times. When regular people were in need of massage treatment they were often referred to specialists in tactile therapies; those therapists practicing massage were often wrestlers (Calvert 2002).

The "Swedish Movement Cure" was originally founded by fencing master and professor Per Henrik Ling (1776–1839). This was a concept of physical exercise, including nutrition, massage, and soft tissue stretching, all used as one unified concept. The techniques, likely influenced from Chinese, Indian, ancient Greek, and Roman sources, were used to generate overall health and treat specific pathological conditions (Taylor 1860). Ling initially developed a system of gymnastic exercises, i.e. "natural gymnastics," designed to produce medical benefits. In 1813 Ling founded the Royal Gymnastic Central Institute in Sweden, educating gymnastic instructors (Taylor 1860). The Institute still exists today in Stockholm as the "Swedish School of Sport and Health Sciences," educating aspiring physical education teachers and specialized sports coaches. With influences from the Swedish massage form, neighboring country Finland developed one of the first specific systems of sports massage at the beginning of the 1900s. The massage culture in Finland is strong, and the use of massage on athletes became a natural extension.

The Australian H. Joseph Fay described the use of massage on athletes at international events in 1916. In his book *Scientific massage for athletes* he described the use of massage to clear the muscles of toxic products, and to promote the growth of muscle and bone (Benjamin & Lamp 1996).

During the 1924 Olympic Games in Paris the Finnish runner Paavo Nurmi, nicknamed by the press "the flying Finn," won five gold medals, and he apparently ran the 1.5 km and 5 km races with only 30 min rest between the two events. Paavo Nurmi brought his own massage therapist to the games to receive daily massages in conjunction with the competitions.

© 2011, Elsevier Ltd.
DOI: 10.1016/B978-0-443-10126-7.00001-0

Almost five decades later, in 1972, the Finnish runner Lars Virén also won gold medals by breaking the world record in 10 000 m and an Olympic record in 5000 m, track and field, during the Olympic Games in Munich. Similar to Nurmi, Virén received daily massages (Benjamin & Lamp 1996). Coaches and athletes from other nations could once again observe a possible connection between massage and athletic performance, and an increased interest in sports massage started yet again to flourish.

In the United States, Jack Meagher, the American Massage Therapist Association (AMTA), Benny Vaughn, and many others have since the late 1970s helped to both repopularize and advance sports massage as a system.

The effects of sports massage

The perceived benefits from sports massage are many and there are numerous statements from active athletes about the different positive effects they experience from receiving sports massage. The demand for sports massage treatments remained steady when measured over a 10-year period, indicating a consistent use of this treatment modality (Galloway & Watt 2004).

To achieve maximum benefit, and to provide the right type of treatment for different athletic situations, it is important that sports massage therapy is performed with correct techniques at the right time. Since sports massage sessions can be very important in an athlete's active life, they should preferably be one of the athlete's regular routines included in their sports activities. Sports massage treatments are used to assist athletes optimally prepare for exercise or competition; they are also focused to help restore the athlete's body between heats, or shortly after strenuous exercise or competition; and they are used as an integrated modality for rehabilitation of sports injuries or specific physical dysfunctions. In professional sports, the sports massage therapist should, when possible, be part of the team surrounding and supporting the athlete. Ongoing communication and teamwork between the athlete, coach, trainer, and doctors will enhance the value of the sports massage treatments.

The observed positive effects of sports massage treatments seem, however, to be more difficult to prove through systematic research. Scientific evidence indicating beneficial effects of massage on athletes does exist, but in limited quantities. Petrissage strokes have been shown to enhance cycle ergometer pedaling performance unrelated to blood lactate, but parallel to improved recovery from muscle stiffness and perceived lower-limb fatigue (Ogai et al. 2008). Results also suggest that therapeutic massage may ease soreness and tenderness linked with delayed onset muscle soreness (DOMS) (Smith et al. 1994; Farr et al. 2002; Hilbert et al. 2003; Weerapong et al. 2005). It has been shown that manual massage of the forearm and hand after maximal exercise is related to better effects compared with nonmassage on post-exercise grip performance (Brooks et al. 2005). Musculotendinous massage with a duration of 10 and 30 seconds has shown to generate increased ROM through modified stretch perception, improved stretch tolerance, or increased compliance of the hamstring muscles, and it is further suggested that massage may be used as an alternative or a complement to static stretching for increasing ROM (Huang et al. 2010). On the other hand, more research is needed since the precise effects of different types of massage technique like petrissage, effleurage, friction, etc., and their application before or after exercise in relation to performance, recovery from injury, or injury prevention, are not yet fully clear (Weerapong et al. 2005). Quite a few studies do also indicate that massage on athletes has minute or even no added beneficial effect on athletic performance or recovery (Tiidus 1995; Drust et al. 2003; Hinds et al. 2004; Jönhagen et al. 2004; Robertson et al. 2004). It is suggested that no major physiological improvements are noted from massage treatments compared with rest. It is commonly accepted that blood lactate levels are reduced more efficiently during active recovery, since blood seems to circulate more effectively during active movements compared with receiving massage strokes at rest. Massage is considered to be indicated before physical performance, i.e. pre event massage, however, due to other benefits, like reduced muscle spasms and psychological stress (Goodwin et al. 2007). According to traditional scientific criteria, it is also suggested that massage is a valid modality in sports medicine (Goats 1994).

The different results from research may at first appear confusing. After all, should not the clear presence of perceived positive effects resulting from sports massage be fairly easy to measure? Factors that may strongly contribute to the different and sometimes completely opposite findings from sports massage research are many. Most studies on sports massage contain limitations in research methodology, inadequate therapist training, insufficient treatment time, over- or underworking the tested muscles, a small number of test subjects, etc. (Moraska 2005). Other limiting factors include inadequate outcome measures, and short-term follow-up (Ernst 2004). These and other limitations can make it difficult to draw definite conclusions from some research. There is also the reality that sometimes during specific circumstances, a standardized basic sports massage therapy may not always be the most effective tool to achieve the desired effects. The level of condition of an athlete, specific circumstances, type of sport, etc. all contribute to the different needs the body has at a specific moment in time. Combinations of effective sports massage techniques and other well-proven methods for recovery are perhaps a better standard. A good sports massage therapist must have a solid educational and experiential foundation, which includes a broad range of treatment techniques. This coupled with awareness and manual skill enables the therapist to better cater to the specific situational needs that arise. Given the popularity of sports massage among different athletes, it might be advisable to use specialized sports massage therapists as staff at major athletic events (Galloway & Watt 2004). The degree of massage therapist training has been shown to affect the efficiency of sports massage as a postevent recovery modality: greater reduction in muscle soreness was attained by therapists with 950 h of training as opposed to those with 700 or 450 h (Moraska 2007).

Another aspect of sports massage therapy is the likelihood it generates substantial psychological value for the athlete. It is suggested that effects from sports massage are foremost psychological rather than physiological (Hemmings et al. 2000). Sports massage may therefore serve as an additional mental/psychological "anchor" for the athlete. It was indicated that a 45% improvement in subsequent exercise performance resulted from a 20 min massage recovery period compared with passive recovery alone, without differences in cardiorespiratory and blood variables (Hemmings et al. 2000). These and additional findings have led to a hypothesis that an athlete's sense of initial recovery after a massage may originate from psychological effects through which massage could generate beneficial influences on recovery and subsequent performance levels (Hemmings et al. 2000).

It seems in reality to be quite difficult objectively to assess the true effects of sports massage treatments. The observed mental/emotional reactions in the body may be just as desirable as other more general physiological benefits sports massage is said to offer. Ultimately, it is what the athlete perceives as positive coupled with elevated sports performance that matters. The purpose of sports massage is after all to support the whole athlete (Taylor 1860) before, between, and after physical performance.

Today, with added experience and research, sports massage has become more specialized in relation to both the sports type and athletic situation. This is beneficial since it now is easier to more effectively complement the athlete's need at any given moment.

References

Benjamin, P., Lamp, S., 1996. Understanding sports massage. Human Kinetics, Champaign, IL.

Brooks, C.P., et al., 2005. The immediate effects of manual massage on power-grip performance after maximal exercise in healthy adults. J. Altern. Complement. Med. 11 (6), 1093–1101.

Calvert, R.N., 2002. The history of massage. Healing Arts Press, Rochester, VT.

Drust, B., et al., 2003. The effects of massage on intramuscular temperature in the vastus lateralis in humans. Int. J. Sports Med. 24 (6), 395–399.

Ernst, E., 2004. Manual therapies for pain control: chiropractic and massage. Clin. J. Pain 20, 8–12.

Farr, T., et al., 2002. The effects of therapeutic massage on delayed onset muscle soreness and muscle function following downhill walking. J. Sci. Med. Sport 5 (4), 297–306.

Galloway, S.D., Watt, J.M., 2004. Massage provision by physiotherapists at major athletics events between 1987 and 1998. Br. J. Sports Med. 38 (2), 235–236.

Goats, G.C., 1994. Massage—the scientific basis of an ancient art: part 2. Physiological and therapeutic effects. Br. J. Sports Med. 28 (3), 153–156.

Goodwin, J.E., et al., 2007. Effect of pre-performance lower-limb massage on thirty-meter sprint running. J. Strength Cond. Res. 21 (4), 1028–1031.

Hemmings, B., et al., 2000. Effects of massage on physiological restoration, perceived recovery, and repeated sports performance. Br. J. Sports Med. 34, 109–115.

Hilbert, J.E., et al., 2003. The effects of massage on delayed onset muscle soreness. Br. J. Sports Med. 37 (1), 72–75.

Hinds, T., et al., 2004. Effects of massage on limb and skin blood flow after quadriceps exercise. Med. Sci. Sports Exerc. 36 (8), 1308–1313.

Huang, S.Y., et al., 2010. Short-duration massage at the hamstrings musculotendinous junction induces greater range of motion. J. Strength Cond. Res. 24 (7), 1917–1924.

Jönhagen, S., et al., 2004. Sports massage after eccentric exercise. Am. J. Sports Med. 32 (6), 1499–1502.

Moraska, A., 2005. Sports massage. A comprehensive review. J. Sports Med. Phys. Fitness 45 (3), 370–380.

Moraska, A., 2007. Therapist education impacts the massage effect on postrace muscle recovery. Med. Sci. Sports Exerc. 39 (1), 34–37.

Ogai, R., et al., 2008. Effects of petrissage massage on fatigue and exercise performance following intensive cycle pedaling. Br. J. Sports Med. Apr 2. [Epub ahead of print].

Robertson, A., et al., 2004. Effects of leg massage on recovery from high intensity cycling exercise. Br. J. Sports Med. 38, 173–176.

Smith, L.L., et al., 1994. The effects of athletic massage on delayed onset muscle soreness, creatine kinase, and neutrophil count: a preliminary report. J. Orthop. Sports Phys. Ther. 19 (2), 93–99.

Taylor, G., 1860. An exposition of the Swedish Movement Cure. Fowler & Wells, New York.

Tiidus, P.M., 1995. Effleurage massage, muscle blood flow and long-term post-exercise strength recovery. Int. J. Sports Med. 16 (7), 478–483.

Weerapong, P., et al., 2005. The mechanisms of massage and effects on performance, muscle recovery and injury prevention. Sports Med. 35 (3), 235–256.

Work postures, hand placements, and basic massage strokes

2

As with any form of massage, working with sports massage requires correct work postures and hand placement. It is important to achieve the right amount of power through physical leverage without causing unnecessary stress on the therapist's body.

Sports massage work postures are generally sourced from the standard "fencing" (Fig. 2.1), and "horse" stance (Fig. 2.2), but must be constantly modified depending on the needs at hand. The stances must generate sufficient leveraged power whilst still feeling comfortable to the therapist.

To achieve more power, it may be beneficial to keep the table slightly lower than normal. Stress on the lower back and legs is minimized by bending the knees and gently leaning on the massage table. Some situations may even require working on the ground, for example preevent stretching of very tall

athletes like basketball players, and stances are then adjusted accordingly.

During a sports massage session, whether the treatment table is a portable massage table or a stationary hydraulic version, it must be strong, stable, and ideally be height-adjustable. An adjustable face cradle is also preferable (Fig. 2.3).

During remedial sports massage therapy, the preferred table height will commonly shift during the treatment, and it is more beneficial to use a hydraulic table (Fig. 2.4) than one of fixed height. A sports massage therapist must often improvise and use what is available at the moment, however, and if the table height cannot be changed during a treatment, the techniques have to be adapted accordingly. This can mean that when working with an increased table height, forearms and elbows are preferably used instead of the hands.

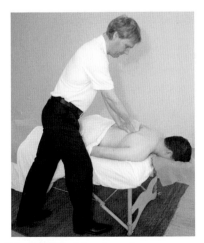

Figure 2.1 • Modified fencing stance

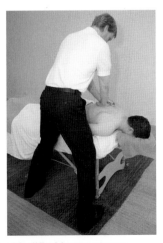

Figure 2.2 • Modified horse stance

© 2011, Elsevier Ltd.
DOI: 10.1016/B978-0-443-10126-7.00002-2

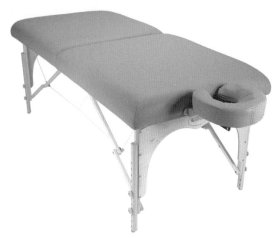

Figure 2.3 • Portable massage table • The Omni table by Custom Craftworks, USA

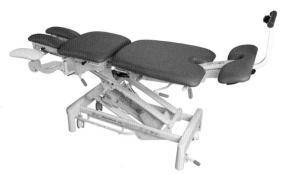

Figure 2.4 • Hydraulic treatment table • Manuthera 241 from Lojer Oy, Finland

Basic massage strokes

Integrated Sports Massage Therapy utilizes a wide range of techniques and massage strokes, but all of them share some common guidelines to achieve proper leverage (Figs 2.5–2.7). Since the goal is to achieve specific beneficial objectives for an athlete, any massage stroke that can accomplish this may be used. The following is a presentation of a few commonly used massage strokes; see Chapters 6, 9, 10, and 14 for additional strokes employed.

Effleurage strokes

The use of effleurage strokes generally aims to:

- improve circulation by moving venous blood and lymph toward the heart
- increase temperature in the worked tissues
- serve as a good method for a practitioner to palpate the soft tissues whilst massaging and thus

continuously facilitate instant adjustments and real-time planning of the treatment.

Effleurage strokes are performed along the venous flow toward the heart. This is especially valid in the extremities to avoid unnecessary stress on the venous valves and walls. Due to their perceived beneficial circulatory effects, it is common to both start and end a sports massage treatment with effleurage strokes to each tended body part. Although basic effleurage strokes are generally viewed as superficial, they can easily be executed with more depth. A faster effleurage is more stimulating whilst a slower application can generate more relaxing effects. Effleurage and friction strokes have shown to beneficially affect post-exercise grip performance after maximal exercise (Brooks et al. 2005).

In preevent massage, it is common to use effleurage strokes, without massage oil, especially when working on "long-term event" athletes. In this case, gliding strokes like effleurage can be applied over sweats, tights, or more commonly, a sheet covering the athlete (Fig. 2.8).

Regular superficial effleurage
(Figs 2.9; 2.10)

1. This stroke is applied with the whole hand but with the majority of the pressure on the palm heel.

2. There is an approximately 45-degree angle between the therapist's arms and the athlete's body. The angle of the wrists should also ideally be no more than 45 degrees.

3. As the tissue warms up, the depth of the stroke should increase in accordance with the athlete's needs.

Palm heel effleurage (Fig. 2.11)

1. Palm heel effleurage is slightly stronger than the regular superficial effleurage and employs additional focused pressure with the palm heel of the hands.

2. Due to the increased depth, this stroke is executed with a slower speed compared with regular effleurage.

Palm heel and fingertip effleurage
(Fig. 2.12)

1. Additional pressure is applied simultaneously with the fingertips; otherwise the execution is similar to palm heel effleurage.

2. This stroke is effective when simultaneous deeper palpation is required in an area.

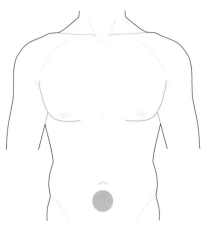

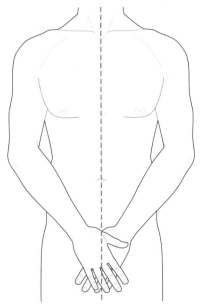

Figure 2.5 • Roughly 2 in below the navel is an area sometimes called "the center of movement." • It is where motion commonly is initiated in disciplines like dance and martial arts since it allows excellent control over the hips, access to the power generated by the lower extremities, and facilitates harmonizing movements between the lower and upper body. The sports massage therapist also initiates movement from this area to ensure the integration of hips and legs, attaining leveraged force during the massage treatment

Figure 2.6 • Hand placement • When the hands are placed in front of the midline of the body, body weight and power generated from the legs can more easily transfer to the arms and hands. When placed off-center, muscle power must compensate the loss of leverage, which leads to unnecessary energy expenditure. To maintain leveraged power, the therapist's midline should face the hands at all times

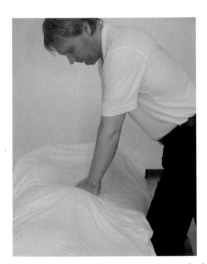

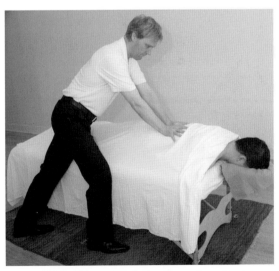

Figure 2.7 • Straight arms vs. bent arms during pushing • To achieve correct power transfer from the hips and legs during pushing strokes, and to minimize unnecessary use of muscle force, the arms should generally be kept straight but without locked joints

Figure 2.8 • Effleurage stroke through a sheet • Lock the sheet with one thigh or hip by leaning on the table

One-sided effleurage (Figs 2.13–2.15)

1. The hand furthest away from the table is placed superior to the other hand, i.e. when standing on the left side of the table, the left hand is placed superior to the right. The palm heel is fitted between the thumb and index finger of the inferior hand.

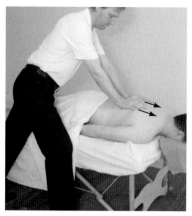

Figure 2.9 • Effleurage on the back

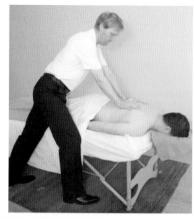

Figure 2.10 • Body posture

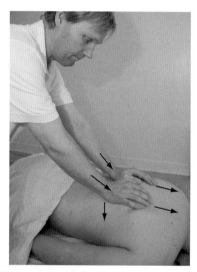

Figure 2.11 • Palm heel effleurage

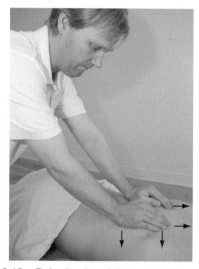

Figure 2.12 • Palm heel and fingertip effleurage

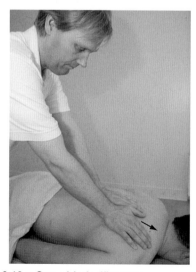

Figure 2.13 • One-sided effleurage

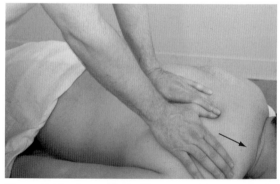

Figure 2.14 • One-sided effleurage with leveraged thumb pressure

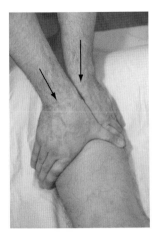

Figure 2.15 • One-sided effleurage modification

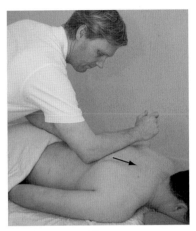

Figure 2.16 • Forearm effleurage

2. Pressure is applied with the whole hands but with the majority focused on the palm heel.

3. There is an approximately 45-degree angle between the therapist's arms and the athlete's body.

4. For added depth, the index and long finger of the inferior hand are placed on top of the thumb to apply extra pressure.

5. To increase pressure and depth during effleurage on legs and arms, the angle of the hands is increased to maximally 45 degrees (see Fig. 2.15).

Forearm effleurage (Fig. 2.16)

1. Forearm effleurage is used on larger areas with more muscle tissue with either one or both forearms.

2. The stroke is performed either simultaneously or alternately depending on preference or need.

3. The angle of the upper arm is placed in roughly 45 degrees flexion to avoid unnecessary stress on the sports massage therapist's shoulders.

Compression techniques

Compression techniques are perhaps the method most commonly viewed as a typical "sports massage stroke." The perceived purpose of this stroke is to stretch the muscle and connective tissue fibers in the area by spreading them against an underlying bone, dilate the local blood vessels from the created short-term ischemic effect, and create a pumping action for additional increased blood circulation. Compression techniques are normally executed in a steady frequency of one to three strokes per second. In contrast to effleurage strokes, compression

techniques are used in any direction. The strokes are easily administered over clothing or a sheet since no oil or lotion is used.

It is important to execute this stroke in a smooth fashion so as not to risk undesirable discomfort, muscle tension, or injury to the soft tissue. Pain and excess speed can trigger the myotatic reflex and thus increase muscle tension to unwanted levels. Therapeutic awareness is paramount during sports massage.

In areas where there is no direct underlying bone, the therapist's fingers are temporarily placed on the inferior part of the muscle whilst the palms are compressing the soft tissue from the superior aspect. This application works especially well on muscles like triceps surae.

Caution should be observed over the ribs and kidneys. The lower part of the kidneys lies somewhat more unprotected, and the 11th and 12th ribs are free floating, which consequently makes them more sensitive. This is especially valid if the stroke is applied in an incorrect and forceful manner. The ribs are generally more sensitive in areas where there are fewer muscles to stabilize and protect them.

Compression techniques must be executed in a systematic fashion to achieve maximal effect. The strokes are applied to one specific area of the body at a time, until signs of relaxation and increased circulation are observed.

Palm compression

Double-handed palm compression (Fig. 2.17)

1. One hand is placed on top of the other at a 90-degree angle.

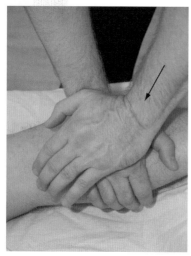

Figure 2.17 • Double-handed palm compression

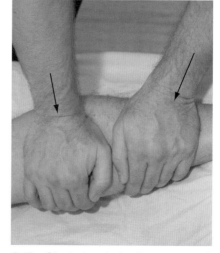

Figure 2.18 • Single-handed palm compression

2. As the therapist leans forward, the palm heel smoothly compresses the muscle toward an underlying bone until resistance is felt.

3. The pressure is subsequently released as the therapist leans away.

4. The stroke is repeated in a selected area until an effect is observed.

5. The stroke smoothly and systematically covers the entire length of the treated muscles.

Single-handed palm compression (Fig. 2.18)

1. This compression stroke is executed alternately with two hands.

2. The direction of the downward pressure is applied obliquely to eliminate unnecessary stress on the wrists. The amount of flexion in the wrists should ideally be 45 degrees, which eliminates much of the strain.

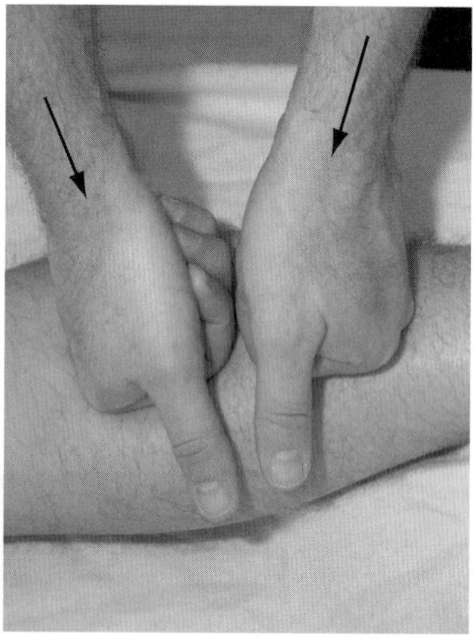

Fist compression (Fig. 2.19)

1. One of the main benefits of fist compressions is that the wrists are kept straight to minimize stress on the joints. The massage stroke is executed with the thumbs facing anterior to maximize the biomechanical benefits.

2. Fist compressions are initiated with the main pressure placed on the second and third knuckles (index and long finger) and their proximal phalanges.

Figure 2.19 • Fist compression

3. As the pressure increases, a slight radial deviation is applied to smoothly roll the pressure toward the fifth finger. This slight roll enables a smoother transition between the hands, and feels more comfortable to the athlete. The fists are kept fairly loose to create an even contact surface.

Thumb compression (Fig. 2.20)

1. One thumb is placed on its side to avoid unnecessary stress on its joints. The thumb will merely function as a passive tool.

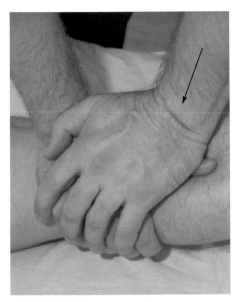

Figure 2.20 • Thumb compression

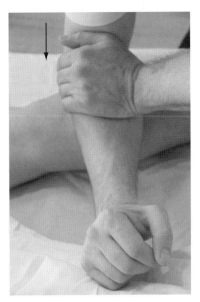

Figure 2.21 • Elbow compression

2. The heel of the palm of the other hand performs the actual stroke by compressing muscle and connective tissue toward underlying bones through the thumb.

3. Thumb compressions are normally used in smaller areas where regular palm or fist compressions may be difficult to use, or between muscle bellies and larger fascias. The stretch effect increases if additional lateral force is applied at the end section of the stroke.

Elbow compression (Fig. 2.21)

1. This stroke is mostly used over areas with denser muscle tissue and/or when the intent is to affect more deeply situated muscles.

2. Different parts of the elbow can be used to make the stroke more or less specific.

3. Added horizontal pressure, as the muscle warms up, will also increase the stretch effect in the treated soft tissue.

Forearm compression (Fig. 2.22)

1. Forearm compressions are beneficial to use on thigh, arm, and larger back areas.

2. A slight additional rolling motion with the forearm gives this stroke a softer quality.

Broadening (Figs 2.23; 2.24)

The broadening stroke is a combination of muscular compression and a lateral gliding pressure that

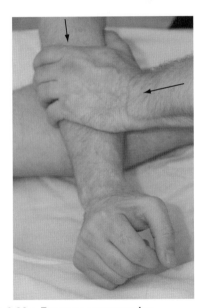

Figure 2.22 • Forearm compression

generates a stronger manual stretch. Broadening is normally performed in three different ways:

- heel of the palm of the hands
- thenar eminence
- elbows.

1. For larger muscles, the palm heels are placed in the middle of the muscle belly/group with the palmar side of the wrists facing and almost touching each other.

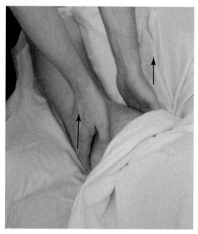

Figure 2.23 • Palm heel broadening, start

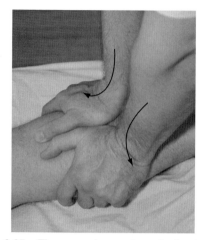

Figure 2.25 • Thenar eminence broadening

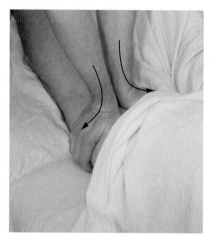

Figure 2.24 • Palm heel broadening, finish

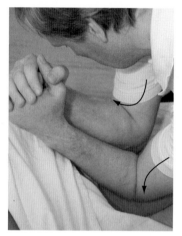

Figure 2.26 • Elbow broadening

2. Body weight is applied by leaning over the hands, allowing the palms to slowly push and glide laterally on the muscle bellies.

3. The fingertips gently lift the treated muscle between each pushing motion. Care is taken not to hyperextend wrists during this stroke.

4. For smaller muscle groups, the thenar eminence of the hand is used instead of the palm heel (Fig. 2.25).

5. For more developed and massive muscles, two elbows can replace the hands (Fig. 2.26). The hands are held together and the part of the elbows inferior to the olecranon serves as the contact point.

When the broadening stroke is applied over a sheet or towel, as commonly used during a pre- or postevent massage, it is important initially to slacken the fabric to enable transfer of the desired stretch effect to the soft tissue.

Petrissage

Petrissage strokes belong to the "kneading" category. Their perceived effects are to stretch soft tissue, and increase blood circulation locally in the muscle. Petrissage has been shown to improve cycle ergometer pedaling performance in relation to improved recovery from muscle stiffness and experienced lower-limb fatigue (Ogai et al. 2008). Research also indicates that petrissage can create a reduction in alpha motor neuron activity, and thus have a relaxing effect (Sullivan et al. 1991). The stroke pushes, squeezes, and/or grasps the massaged soft tissue. Although generally executed at a tempo of one stroke per second, the speed and frequency can vary depending on the desired outcome of the massage.

Sliding on the skin is minimized to achieve optimal soft tissue stretch. Massage oil or lotion is thus applied conservatively.

Palm heel petrissage

1. The soft tissue is massaged in a semicircle with the palm heel and the base of the thenar muscle group.
2. Power and rhythm are developed by alternately shifting the body weight between the left and right hand.
3. The tissue is first pushed upward with the palm of the hand, directly followed by an obliquely directed stretch executed with the base of the thenar eminence (Fig. 2.27).
4. The stroke is either performed as a reinforced one-hand palm heel petrissage (Fig. 2.28), or a two-handed petrissage. During reinforced petrissage, one hand grasps the wrist of the massaging hand. The amount of applied force can be increased here without stressing the wrist.

Lifting petrissage

1. This stroke both kneads the muscle and lifts it off the bone. (Fig. 2.29).
2. Lifting petrissage can only be used on muscles with a graspable edge, and though generally executed with both hands alternately, a one-handed application is sometimes useful.
3. The muscle is grasped between the therapist's thumb and remaining four fingers. During the downward phase, the skin web between thumb and index finger as well as the radial side of the index finger are included.
4. Elbows are bent and hands kept in front of the midline of the therapist's body.
5. The therapist massages the muscle by first dropping the body weight through bending the knees. Moving the hips laterally and finally lifting the muscle by straightening the knees completes the stroke. The process is repeated toward the other side, back and forth.

Forearm petrissage

1. Forearm petrissage (Fig. 2.30) is useful on larger muscles.
2. To add more power to this stroke, the forearm and hand are moved from a semisupinated toward a pronated position during the semicircular execution of this stroke.

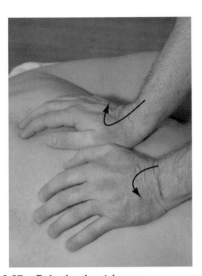

Figure 2.27 • Palm heel petrissage

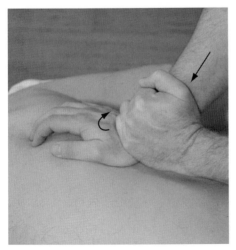

Figure 2.28 • Reinforced palm heel petrissage

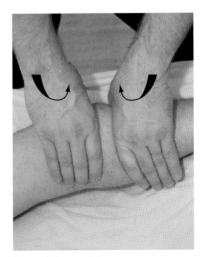

Figure 2.29 • Lifting petrissage

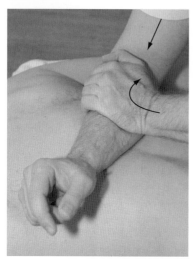

Figure 2.30 • Forearm petrissage

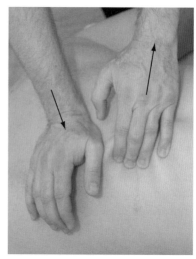

Figure 2.31 • S-stroke of the erector spinae muscle

S-stroke petrissage

Among the petrissage strokes, S-stroke has the strongest stretch effect on muscle and connective tissue. It is, when needed, used on any muscle with a "graspable" edge. Examples are erector spinae, quadriceps femoris, trapezius, latissimus dorsi, ischiocrural/hamstring, and gastrocnemius muscle groups.

The strokes are initially executed mildly and their intensity is amplified gradually. For very tight and dense muscles, the therapist can gain more strength by firstly pulling the muscle to its end point and secondly pushing the other edge of the muscle into a stretch. For muscles with more than one head, each muscle belly is treated separately. S-strokes are performed with straightened arms to ensure leveraged power from the hips. If oil is previously applied on the skin, application over a sheet ensures a good grip of the tissue.

Regular S-stroke petrissage

1. One edge of the muscle is pushed with the heel of the palm of the hand, and the other edge is pulled with the fingertips. This creates an S-shape with the focal stretch-point in the center of the stroke (Fig. 2.31).
2. At the end point, the stretch is held for 1 or 2 s.
3. Once the muscle has been stretched in one direction, the hands will smoothly switch the pushing and pulling action to the opposite direction.
4. The stroke is repeated until the desired effect is attained.

Modified S-stroke petrissage

1. In some instances both hands may not have enough room to correctly execute the regular S-stroke petrissage. The muscle is thus lifted with only three fingers, normally fingers III–V (Fig. 2.32).
2. The hypothenar edge of the other hand will accordingly push the muscle into a stretch. The stroke is otherwise performed as a regular S-stroke.

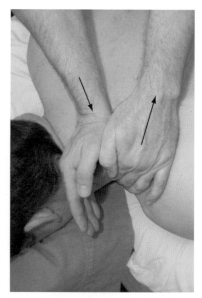

Figure 2.32 • Modified S-stroke of the descending part of the trapezius muscle

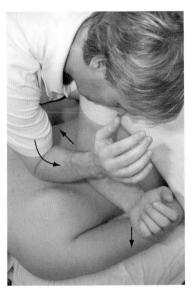

Figure 2.33 • Modified S-stroke/elbow

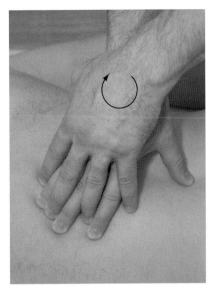

Figure 2.34 • 8-finger frictions

Modified S-stroke/elbow (Fig. 2.33)

1. The elbows can occasionally serve as effective tools for S-strokes.
2. One edge of the muscle is gradually pushed by one elbow with the inferior part of the olecranon process, whilst simultaneously slowly flexing the elbow joint.
3. The other elbow pulls the opposite edge of the muscle with the superior part of the olecranon by concurrently slowly extending the elbow joint.
4. The therapist's body is here placed directly over the elbows to ensure control and power.

Frictions

Frictions are massage strokes intended to increase local blood circulation, and have a slightly more focused stretch effect in the treated tissue. Frictions are generally performed with fingertips, palms, fists, or elbows. It is important to minimize sliding on the skin (with the exception of V-frictions), and instead move the skin with the stroke to effectively treat the underlying tissue.

8-finger frictions (Fig. 2.34)

1. One hand is placed on top of the other as the fingertips are interlocked.
2. The thumb is used as an anchor merely to determine the angle of the hands in relation to the athlete's body. A more horizontal angle produces an added superficial stroke, and an increased vertical angle will generate a stroke reaching deeper into the tissue. For more depth, a 45-degree angle of the hands is needed.
3. The elbows are kept to the side of the body as the hips and legs move the body and hands in a circular motion.
4. Using the fingertips to actively push/pull the soft tissue will enhance the 8-finger frictions further (Fig. 2.35). The distal phalanges are slightly flexed

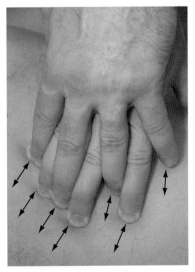

Figure 2.35 • Detail picture of fingertip action

at the beginning of the stroke, pushing the muscle out further by straightening the fingertips during the first half of the circle. After being straightened, the phalanges are once again flexed during the second half of the circle, thus pulling the soft tissue into stretch from the other direction.

4-finger frictions (Fig. 2.36)

Both hands are used separately to perform circular 4-finger frictions. This stroke is beneficial to use on muscles on rounder shapes like the arms, legs, and neck.

1. The muscle is massaged with the fingertips in circular motions with each hand.
2. The movement is generated from the hips, rhythmically rocking the body back and forth.
3. The fingertips are used to push and pull the muscle fibers into stretch during the massage.
4. The thumbs of each hand are used as an anchor. For added strength, each thumb is positioned on the opposite side of the treated body part, allowing the hands to squeeze together during the massage. The main force is thereby acquired from the leveraged hands and not the arms.

One-finger friction

1. This type of friction is executed with a reinforced long finger and/or index finger. Placing the index finger or long finger of the same hand on top of the nail of the other finger reinforces the stroke.

One-finger circular frictions can be very effective when used for smaller, harder to reach areas (Fig. 2.37).

2. Thumb friction (Figs 2.38; 2.39) is another example of one-finger friction. Thumbs should normally not be used on larger areas, but can serve as an excellent tool for focused work. It is important not to stress the thumbs extensively during massage treatments since they are vital for the normal function of the hands. For deep tissue work, the thumbs should always be braced.

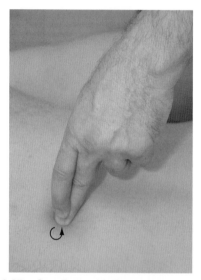

Figure 2.37 • One-finger friction

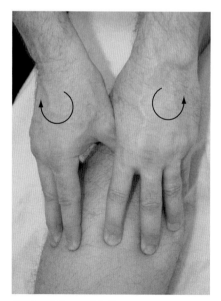

Figure 2.36 • 4-finger frictions

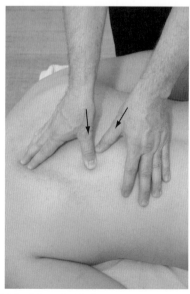

Figure 2.38 • Thumb friction

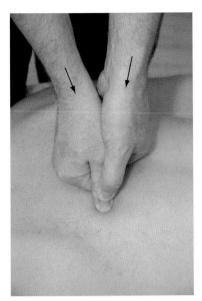

Figure 2.39 • Thumb friction modification

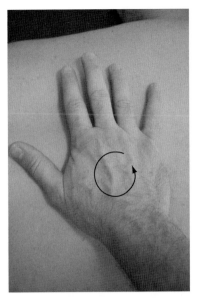

Figure 2.41 • Palm frictions

Fist frictions (Fig. 2.40)

1. The fists are kept loose and massage in a circular motion.
2. Wrists are relaxed to ensure smooth motion.
To achieve slightly more depth in the stroke, the therapist utilizes the body weight by leaning forward.

Palm frictions

Here the palms work in a circular motion. This stroke is less specific, and can be used more briskly to generate increased blood circulation and temperature.

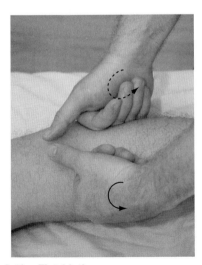

Figure 2.40 • Fist frictions

To achieve more depth in the stroke, the pressure is focused on the palm heel (Fig. 2.41).

V-frictions

V-frictions were created by the author at the beginning of his massage career out of a sheer need for a more variable stroke that yet retained a great palpatory quality. V-frictions are normally executed alternately with four fingers of each hand while the thumbs act as anchors. V-frictions are generally used in all directions, but particularly in a 45-degree angle across the soft tissue fibers. Some caution should be observed when executing against the venous flow in the extremities: in this case, the strokes are shortened to a maximum of 1–2 in to decrease potential stress on the veins. The fingers constantly monitor tension and other changes of state in the tissues. By constantly observing reactions from the muscle tissue, the pressure can rapidly be adapted by each finger to ensure maximum effect without unpleasant pain sensations. The movement is generated from the hips.

Regular V-frictions (Figs 2.42; 2.43)

1. The hands act as an extension of the hips and legs. The thumbs serve as anchors, and the wrists are relaxed.
2. With the movement starting from the therapist's hips, the four fingers are pushed at a 45-degree angle in relation to each other to enhance the stretch effect in the soft tissue.

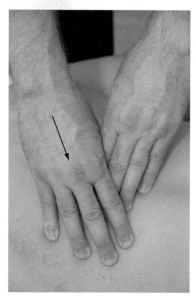

Figure 2.42 • Regular V-frictions, start

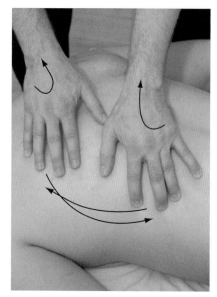

Figure 2.44 • Reversed V-frictions, start

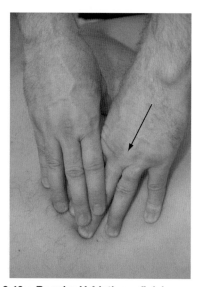

Figure 2.43 • Regular V-frictions, finish

3. One hand alternately keeps the tension in the tissue as the other glides under the first hand to stretch the muscle in the other direction.

4. The depth of this stroke, controlled by the thumbs, is determined by the angle of the hands in relation to the body.

5. The fingers are slightly flexed to maintain depth in the stroke.

Reversed V-frictions (Fig. 2.44)

1. This stroke massages the soft tissue by pulling it in semicircles toward the therapist's midline.

2. The fingertips are bent to hook into the massaged soft tissue.

3. The other hand alternately massages in a mirrored fashion, but overlaps the area of the stroke of the previous hand, which is keeping tension in the tissue.

4. To increase the depth of this stroke, the therapist leans backward and alternately moves the body from side to side to utilize momentum effectively.

Cross-fiber frictions (Fig. 2.45)

This stroke is perceived to effectively generate a local hyperemia and stretch effect in the treated muscle tissue. It was popularized in the west by therapists like Jack Meagher (Meagher 1990), and is a stroke still used by many sports massage therapists.

1. The thumb or other fingertip massages the muscle or tendon transverse to the fiber direction (Burke 2003; Cash 1996) (Figs 2.45 & 2.46). It is important not to slide on the skin but instead move the skin to effectively treat the underlying tissue (Johnson 1995).

2. The stroke is initially executed slowly to minimize activation of the myotatic/stretch reflex, and increases in intensity as the tensed tissue softens. The more force that is applied to this stroke, the slower the pace of its execution.

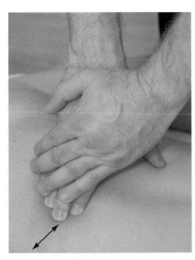

Figure 2.45 • Cross-fiber frictions

3. It is imperative that the therapist carefully monitors and adjusts to the changing state in the treated soft tissue to avoid unpleasant sensations for the athlete.

Transverse frictions (see Fig. 2.46)

The British orthopedic doctor, James Cyriax, empirically developed this technique as one of his many great contributions to manual medicine. Deep transverse frictions are specifically used for breaking up, stretching and/or restructuring connective tissue adhesions in muscles, tendons, and ligaments stemming from acute trauma and/or mechanical overload.

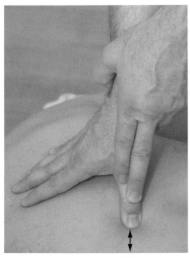

Figure 2.46 • Deep transverse frictions

As an untreated or poorly rehabilitated soft tissue injury heals, adhesions or fibrosis from growing scar tissue often form. The adhesion generally restricts normal movement, and a common result is local pain sensation with additional tearing at the outer edges of the scar as the soft tissue is forcibly lengthened beyond the restricted ROM. The scar can thereby gradually grow, with an increased risk of more severe future soft tissue tears.

Deep transverse frictions are useful for tending to milder soft tissue injuries as early as one to two days after the moment of injury, as well as for treating old, chronic scarring. The beginning of the treatment is mild, normally lasting only 1 min, with increased time and intensity as the days progress. The treatment is generally combined with active, passive, or non-weight-bearing movements. Deep transverse frictions should not be painful since, correctly performed, they have an analgesic effect that may last up to 24 h (Edwardsson 2001). Complete treatment results may take up to 6 weeks but are lasting. Chronic adhesions are treated more aggressively. This can be a very valuable technique during remedial sports massage.

Deep transverse frictions

1. One or two fingers are placed directly over the adhesion or lesion. The muscle belly is kept relaxed.
2. The soft tissue is gently pushed and pulled transverse to the direction of the treated muscle, tendon, or ligament fibers. It is important not to slide on the skin but instead move the skin to successfully treat the underlying tissue.
3. For larger tendons, a broader contact surface is applied to effectively spread and stretch the tissue.
4. Chronic adhesions are treated for 15–20 min/treatment, whereas recent injuries start in 1 min intervals.
5. Cryotherapy can be applied after each treatment to reduce an inflammatory response.

Stripping

Stripping utilizes a continual longitudinal pressure to the treated tissue, gliding from origin to insertion, or insertion to origin of the muscle. In the extremities, if using a broader contact point, like an elbow, the stroke is almost always applied in a direction towards the heart to avoid unnecessary stress on the venous

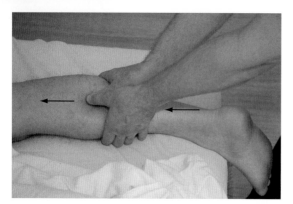

Figure 2.47 • Stripping

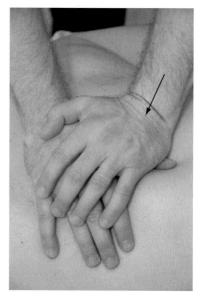

Figure 2.48 • Thumb edging

valves and walls. Stripping is often executed using reinforced thumbs, fingertips, or an elbow. It can be applied by the sports therapist in event based or remedial massage, or utilized during athletic self-massage (see Chapter 15). This stroke is executed deep or superficially over the muscles, all depending on the situational need.

1. The therapist places both thumbs together beginning at one end of the treated muscle (Fig. 2.47).
2. The therapist utilizes the body weight to lean forward, making the stroke slowly glide along the muscle, or between muscle bellies. This gives the stroke either a "milking" or separating character.
3. The stroke is repeated along the muscle until tissue softening is noted. If the intent is to stimulate a hypotonic muscle, a faster pace is used.

Edging

Edging focuses on effectively stretching muscle and connective tissue by pushing it away from its attachments. It can only be used where a muscle has a clear edge, like erector spinae, gastrocnemius, etc.

Edging is normally performed with the thumbs, palm heel, or elbows. Both sides of the muscle should be edged to achieve a maximum stretch effect from the stroke. The edging stroke can also serve as an excellent preparation stroke for the S-stroke petrissage. It is important to avoid sliding over the muscle belly to maximally stretch the tissue.

Thumb edging (Fig. 2.48)

1. The side of one thumb is placed along the edge of the muscle. The thumb is only used as a tool while

the other hand's palm heel presses the thumb obliquely down and away from the bone to create an effective stretch in the soft tissue.

2. The end position of the stroke is held for about 2 s before the stretch is slowly released.
3. The stroke is repeated up and down the edge of the muscle until a desired reduction in muscle tension is achieved.
4. The stroke can thereafter be used on the other edge of the same muscle.

Palm heel edging (Fig. 2.49)

1. Used on more prominent muscles, this stroke is executed by pushing the muscle obliquely down and away from the bone with the palm heel.
2. The other palm heel follows up by alternately pushing the muscle right beside the first hand.
3. The muscle is successively stretched along the edge and the procedure is repeated on the opposite edge of the same muscle.

Elbow edging (Fig. 2.50)

1. The elbow is normally only used for well developed muscles. Both the inferior and superior part of the olecranon process can be used. When the inferior part of olecranon is used, the elbow position at the start of the stroke is

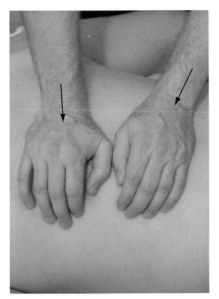

Figure 2.49 • Palm heel edging

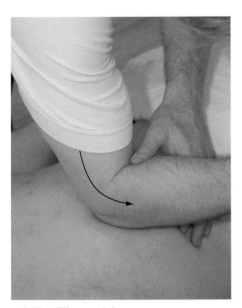

Figure 2.50 • Elbow edging

semiextended. As the pressure is increased the elbow is slowly flexed to add the stretch effect.

2. When using the superior part of the olecranon the situation is reversed. The elbow position is initially semiflexed, and as the stroke progresses the elbow is slowly extended to achieve the desired stretch effect.

Tapotement

Tapotement strokes are used to invigorate the nervous system and, according to Asian medicine, increase the energy flow in the channels. It is very important not to use too much force in these strokes since it can be easy to inflict injury on the treated tissue. When contact is made with the skin, the power of the stroke should be pulled away from the body.

The wrists are always relaxed to ensure speed and avoid early fatigue. Tapotement strokes are normally used toward the end of the massage if the desired result is to help the client toward more mental alertness. These strokes can therefore be used in pre-, inter-, and some postevent sports massage treatments. Due to the risk of injury, however, it is not recommended to use strong tapotement strokes during a postevent massage following long-term sports events.

Hacking (Fig. 2.51)

1. Performed with the ulnar side of the 5th phalanges. The fingers are separated to create a springing contact surface.
2. The wrists are relaxed, and the fingers contact the skin alternately in a rapid fashion of about four strokes per second.

Double-handed hacking (Fig. 2.52)

1. The palms are placed together, wrists extended, and the fingers spread apart.

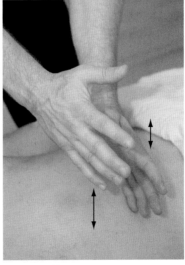

Figure 2.51 • Hacking

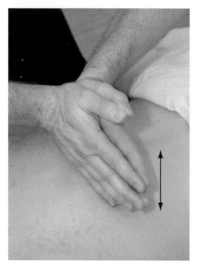

Figure 2.52 • Double-handed hacking

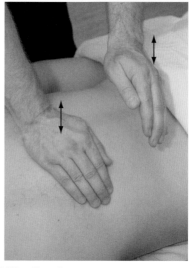

Figure 2.54 • Cupping

2. The ulnar surface of the 5th phalanges will contact the skin as the wrists and forearms are passively turned from the movement of the hands.

3. An audible clapping noise should be heard during contact as the stroke is executed at a pace of about two strokes per second.

Slapping (Fig. 2.53)

This tapotement stroke is performed with flat palms of the hands that alternately contact the skin.

Cupping (Fig. 2.54)

Cupping is performed like slapping tapotement, but with cupped hands. This softens the impact of the stroke.

Pounding (Fig. 2.55)

Pounding is performed with the ulnar side of loosely made fists. It is the most powerful of all the tapotement strokes and is accordingly used with caution. Pounding is normally used on areas with larger muscles, like the gluteal region and legs.

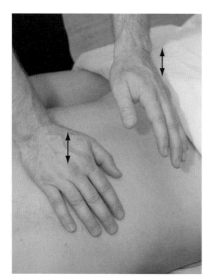

Figure 2.53 • Slapping

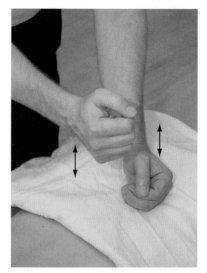

Figure 2.55 • Pounding

Ischemic muscle pressure

Ischemic muscle pressure is well suited to taut bands or "knots" in muscle tissue, and as one element of myofascial trigger point treatment. The applied pressure is thought to induce a state of local ischemia in the muscle, which as the pressure is released, reverts to local hyperemia. The increased blood flow is considered to aid in normalizing the metabolic state of the muscle. There may also exist an added local stretch effect in the soft tissue as the pressure spreads muscle and connective tissue fibers apart. A reinforced thumb tip is a common application for this stroke, but a reinforced index, long finger, or even the tip of an elbow are used, depending on the density of the treated soft tissue. To decrease stress on the fingers during treatment, tools such as "Neuromuscular T-bars," and similar pressure devices are available.

Ischemic muscle pressure (Fig. 2.56)

1. The treated muscle is slowly compressed until the client starts perceiving a mild identical pain, i.e. the same pain as in the original complaint.
2. The pressure, remaining at the same level, is held until the pain gradually decreases, and finally disappears. This should happen within 20 s maximum.
3. The pressure is further increased from this point until pain is perceived again.
4. The procedure is repeated a total of three to five cycles.
5. After the last cycle, the pressure is slowly released over a 10 s interval.
6. If the triggered pain does not release within 20 s, the applied pressure is too great. In this case the compression is slowly eased until the pain sensation is relieved, and the treatment procedure can start over from this point.

Some form of soft tissue stretch, like S-stroke petrissage or a more specific therapeutic muscle stretch, generally follows the treatment to consolidate the result.

Jostling/oscillation (Fig. 2.57)

Jostling is a commonly used stroke in sports massage. By rhythmically moving individual muscles, joints, or entire sections of an athlete's body, the aim is to increase neuromuscular feedback. This is perceived to generally have a relaxing effect on the muscles, but may also increase muscle tone if performed at a fast pace. By executing jostling on the legs while the athlete is prone, less mobile areas of the body are easily detected. This makes it a very useful tool for assessment during the initial phase of the sports massage treatment. Jostling works well in pre-, post- and interevent massage.

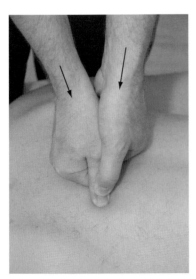

Figure 2.56 • Ischemic muscle pressure

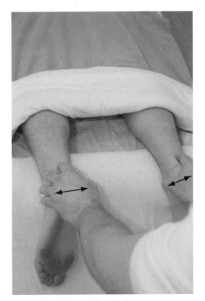

Figure 2.57 • Jostling of both legs

Vibrations

Vibrations applied in sports massage are often used to create small shaking movements as joints are moved through the full range of motion. The purpose is to create neural feedback between muscle tissue and the nervous system. This can be beneficial during sports injury rehabilitation but has additional value when an increased muscle tone is desired.

Skin strokes

Skin strokes are used to enhance nerve and blood circulation (Chaitow & DeLany 2003). This is accomplished by stretching the skin and "breaking up" or stretching adhesions/fibrosis between the skin and its underlying fascia. A number of skin strokes can accomplish this.

Skin rolling

The skin is alternately grasped between the index fingers/thumb and long fingers/thumb (Fig. 2.58). This will create a pinching effect of the skin as the index and long fingers alternately "walk" along the skin with the thumbs sliding close behind. The intensity is determined by the narrowness of the created skin fold.

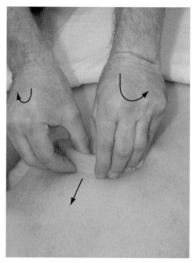

Figure 2.59 • Skin bend

Skin bend

1. Both hands grasp a skin fold between the thumbs and remaining four fingers (Fig. 2.59).
2. The skin is bent and stretched by pushing the thumbs forward. The stroke is repeated over the entire treated area.

Skin push

1. The hands are placed close together with palms down on the athlete's skin (Fig. 2.60).

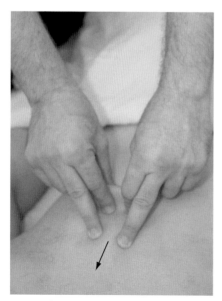

Figure 2.58 • Skin rolling

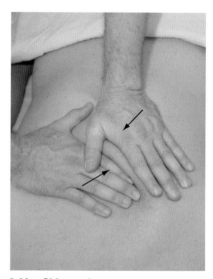

Figure 2.60 • Skin push

2. One hand pushes the skin over the fingers of the other hand as the therapist leans forward. The trapped skin is then stretched as the therapist leans backward. The therapist should work in a rhythmic manner all over the treated area. This stroke is wider and not so specific as the skin roll, and a firm force is generally applied without producing unpleasant pain.

Skin lift

1. Skin lifts are generally executed over a sheet to get a better grip of the skin. They can be used only when a fold can actually be grasped.

2. The procedure starts at the sacrum and continues up along the spine.

3. The skin is grasped between the thumbs and flexed index fingers of both hands, creating a fold, which is further lifted off the spine (Fig. 2.61). This may create a popping sound as the skin is released.

4. This stroke may produce pain but should not feel too uncomfortable to the athlete.

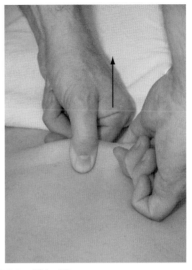

Figure 2.61 • Skin lift

After this treatment, the athlete may notice improved flexibility in the lower back, thanks to reduced restriction.

References

Brooks, C.P., et al., 2005. The immediate effects of manual massage on power-grip performance after maximal exercise in healthy adults. J. Altern. Complement. Med. 11 (6), 1093–1101.

Burke, E., 2003. Massage for cyclists. Vitesse Press, College Park, MD.

Cash, M., 1996. Sports and remedial massage therapy. Ebury Press, London.

Chaitow, L., DeLany, J., 2003. Modern neuromuscular techniques. Churchill Livingstone, Edinburgh.

Edwardsson, S., 2001. Advanced exam in orthopedic medicine. Ortopedmedicinska kliniken, Malmö AB, Sweden.

Huang, S.Y., et al., 2010. Short-duration massage at the hamstrings musculotendinous junction induces greater range of motion. J. Strength Cond. Res. 24 (7), 1917–1924.

Johnson, J., 1995. The healing art of sports massage. Rodale Press, Emmaus, PA.

Meagher, J., 1990. Sports massage. Station Hill Press, New York.

Ogai, R., et al., 2008. Effects of petrissage massage on fatigue and exercise performance following intensive cycle pedaling. Br. J. Sports Med. Apr 2. [Epub ahead of print].

Sullivan, S.J., et al., 1991. Effects of massage on alpha motoneuron excitability. Phys. Ther. 71 (8), 555–560.

Sports massage applications

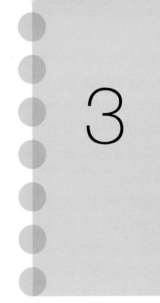

3

Massage is considered to assist athletes to achieve enhanced performance levels and possibly reduce the risk of injury (Weerapong et al. 2005). Massage strokes generating mechanical pressure on muscles do either increase or decrease neural excitability through neurological mechanisms (Weerapong et al. 2005). This may allow the sports massage therapist to facilitate regulation of the muscle tone, either relaxing overly tensed muscles or stimulating relaxed muscles to enable faster muscle contractions. Other effects of massage include relaxation through increased parasympathetic activity and changes in cortisol levels (Weerapong et al. 2005). Psychological mechanisms like reduced anxiety and a better frame of mind also contribute to perceived relaxation (Hemmings et al. 2000; Weerapong et al. 2005).

The manifestation of massage on athletes can often vary depending on country of origin, massage history, sporting habits, cultural values, etc. Sports massage used in Nordic countries like Sweden and Finland was initially not very different from a "regular" classic muscle massage. Some distinctions were, however, that a sports massage treatment could be more area specific for a particular sport, with additional focus on treatment depth and intensity. Since athletes commonly possess an elevated pain tolerance cultivated from endless hours of pushing their bodies through perceived performance limitations, Nordic sports massage was mostly implemented as a very strong and painful treatment as a result.

Sports massage continues steadily to evolve and is today divided into specific categories. Increased knowledge of sports physiology combined with empirical treatment experience has refined massage applications to be more specific in regard to the occasion and/or category of an event, environmental conditions, and sports-specific needs. These added requirements produced four basic differentiations (Archer 2007; Benjamin & Lamp 1996):

Event-based sports massage:

- preevent massage
- interevent massage
- postevent massage.

Sports therapy massage:

- maintenance and remedial massage.

Preevent massage

Preevent massage is utilized prior to competition or training to support enhanced sport performance and to increase the "mechanical efficiency" (Meagher & Broughton 1990) of the athlete's body. It is not intended to replace already existing warm-up routines since preevent massage has not demonstrated the capability to elevate the athlete's blood circulation, core temperature, or ROM, or to prime the nervous system for upcoming sports-related movements, to the same extent as active warm-up routines produce (Archer 2007). Preevent sports massage does, however, serve as one important aspect of an athlete's preparatory measures for upcoming sport activity. Research also suggests that massage can increase flexibility of muscles without a change in power, and may consequently serve as an alternative to static stretching during athletic warm-up (McKechnie et al. 2007). Other objectives of preevent sports massage are to increase blood circulation (Gillespie 2003) and local temperature in the treated tissues through

DOI: 10.1016/B978-0-443-10126-7.00003-4

Box 3.1

Highlights of preevent sports massage

- Used to prepare athlete for event, support enhanced sport performance, and to increase the "mechanical efficiency" of the athlete's body.
- Preevent massage is primarily conducted reasonably close to the actual event, normally 1 h or less, and has a maximal duration of 10–20 min.
- Preevent massage is performed rather superficially at a speed generally faster than the athlete's resting heart rate, on performance-specific muscle groups.
- The preevent massage should start with the most active muscle groups, followed by the less active areas.
- Preevent massage does not contain structural integration or other deep tissue techniques.
- Preevent massage often contains gentle stretching of important muscle groups and fascial structures to facilitate the desired ROM.

mechanical and circulatory stimulation which may increase pliability of connective tissue in structures such as fascia, muscles, tendons, joint capsules, and ligaments (Archer 2007). This combined with therapeutic stretching techniques will also facilitate a desired ROM (Box 3.1).

Preevent massage is primarily conducted reasonably close to the actual event, normally 1 h or less (Meagher & Broughton 1990; Benjamin & Lamp 1996; Archer 2007), but some therapists occasionally use it from several hours up to a couple of days before major sports activity (Ylinen & Cash 1993; Cash 1996). Certain variations in preevent massage applications will depend on how close the treatment is administered prior to a competitive or training event. As a general rule, if the sports event starts within 1 h, the massage is performed with increased speed and less depth on performance-specific muscle groups of the athlete's body. This to ensure the desired effects occur where they are most relevant, and to keep the athlete stimulated to minimize the risk of reducing mental and physical "peak performance." Although preevent sports massage is foremost intended as a more general preparatory measure for the athlete, the treatment focus is on muscles and fascial structures primarily stressed in each sport. The preevent massage should start on the most active muscle groups, followed by

treatment of less active areas. If the massage has to end earlier than planned for some unforeseen reason, the most important muscle groups and fascial structures have thus already received treatment.

It is often common not to use any emollients such as oils, creams, gels, etc., during preevent massage, especially when treating endurance athletes or during elevated environmental temperatures. This is particularly valid for mineral-based products since they are believed not to be absorbed through the skin to the same degree as natural vegetable-based products. Some people are concerned that certain emollients may block the pores and thus reduce the athlete's ability to expel heat during intense sports activity. Another more practical reason is that the athletes are commonly fully dressed to stay warm during the sport preparation, and it is easier and above all more time efficient, to perform the preevent massage over a sheet (Fig. 3.1) or, if circumstances permit, directly on the clothing.

In short-duration sport events requiring rapid reaction times and muscle contractions, the muscle tone needs to remain slightly elevated. Here, a fast-paced superficial preevent massage is desirable since a deeper and slower massage may cause unwanted levels of relaxation. A slow-paced more relaxing massage may, however, be in order in specific circumstances: if the athlete is too nervous and tense, a more soothing massage can lower the muscle tone to desired levels and facilitate recovery of the required mental focus. Asking athletes about

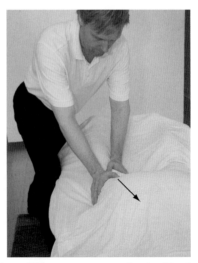

Figure 3.1 • Effleurage over a sheet • The therapist secures the sheet to the table with one thigh

their needs and habits prior to massage will clear up any possible confusion. Initiating unnecessary talk during the treatment is generally avoided during a preevent massage since it may disrupt the mental preparation routine athletes often have.

Event-based sports massage does generally not contain structural integration or other deep tissue techniques since the possible new movement patterns they produce can disrupt the neuromuscular conditioning the athlete has previously optimized. This can easily lead to reduced sports performance. This type of work is instead used during maintenance and remedial massage since it allows enough time for the athlete to recondition their nervous system to the new circumstances. As a general rule, sports massage is never static, but instead constantly adjusting to the athlete's current needs and type of sport event they participate in.

See Box 3.2 for a list of suggested items to bring to event massage.

Pace

Preevent massage strokes are normally executed in a pace faster than one stroke per second, whilst still remaining smooth. They should generally be faster than the athlete's resting heart rate since this tends to have an invigorating effect, whereas a stroke rate slower than the resting heart beat may instead have a more sedative effect. The normal duration of a preevent massage, performed close to an event, is a maximum of 10–20 min to avoid undesired levels of mental relaxation and to decrease the risk of potential muscle cramps during the sports activity.

Even though many different massage strokes can be utilized for preevent sports massage, it is easier for the less experienced sports massage therapist to at first choose from a selected group of strokes with more general effects (see Chapter 4). Supplementary strokes are used when their beneficial effects are relevant to the treatment goals.

Muscle stretching

Gentle stretching of important muscle groups and fascial structures is also included in the preevent massage. The stretches can be used:

- toward the end of the treatment
- as part of the massage technique (see Chapter 6, Thai massage), or
- as a combination of both.

Therapeutic stretching applied in preevent massage is merely aimed at facilitating the ROM considered "normal" for each athlete and the type of sport they participate in. Tensed and shortened soft tissue can compress blood and lymphatic vessels, which may lead to decreased physical performance and muscle

---

Box 3.2

Suggested items to bring to event massage

1. One portable sports massage table (Fig. 3.2).
2. A fitted plastic sheet to protect the table surface.
3. Four cutout tennis balls for protection of wooden massage table legs (see Fig. 3.2).
4. Bolster or a bodyCushion system, and a pillow.
5. At least two thermal blankets: one placed on the massage table under a sheet, and the other to cover the athlete.
6. Enough sets of sheets for the treatments.
7. One warm blanket for the athlete.
8. Massage emollients for inter- or postevent massage.
9. Alcohol gel for hand sanitation between clients.
10. Rubbing alcohol for cleaning the table surface and headrest.
11. Paper towels.
12. Garbage bag.
13. Latex gloves as a protective barrier if blood or body fluids other than sweat are present.
14. Bleach solution (1 part bleach to 10 parts water). Used to clean hands and table if blood from the athlete is present.
15. Ice chest with small bags of crushed ice and/or cups of ice for possible hyperthermia treatment, pain relief, and as an additional part of cramp release treatment.
16. First aid kit.
17. Elastic ACE bandages.
18. Sunscreen/sunblock.
19. Insect spray.
20. A hat for the therapist.
21. Sunglasses.
22. Ample water for the therapist.
23. Ample food and snacks for the therapist.
24. Layered clothing for the therapist.

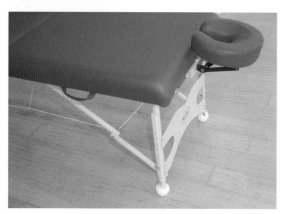

Figure 3.2 • Portable massage table with leg protectors

cramps during sports activity through reduced circulation and metabolic limitations. There is a wide range of different stretching techniques that may be utilized, some of which are described in more detail in Chapters 6 and 7.

Interevent massage

Sports massage treatments are also beneficial between different heats in a competition or if the sports contest ranges over several days. The interevent massage is aimed at addressing areas of excessive tension (Archer 2007), and supporting the athlete's short-term recovery and preparation for the next event (Benjamin & Lamp 1996). It is focused on the most important muscle groups for each particular sport, and additionally serves as one aspect of the athlete's complete interevent routine (Archer 2007). The treatment works on the previously stressed areas and sections majorly active in the upcoming event. Since the interevent massage is used after a previous athletic activity but also before a new event, it can be described as a combination of pre- and postevent massage with a reversed application order. Depending on the length of time between the heats, the massage can be performed in different ways. Interevent massage is generally 10–15 min in duration and should be rather light and comfortable for the athlete. This also means that an interevent treatment must have an invigorating effect on the athlete if the upcoming event is imminent (Benjamin & Lamp 1996; Archer 2007). In sports like boxing, the interevent massage may only last 20 s to a maximum of 1 min between rounds. If, on the other hand, there is several hours up to

one day between the events, the massage treatment can last for 1–1.5 h with more specific and relaxing objectives (Benjamin & Lamp 1996). Sliding strokes like effleurage are well suited to begin with since they have perceived beneficial circulatory effects on both blood and lymph, but additionally as they serve as an excellent palpation tool during the initial stage of the treatment. Interevent massage strokes are otherwise generally the same as used in pre- and postevent massage (Box 3.3).

Postevent massage

After sports activity, it is beneficial to support the athlete in the recovery process. It has been shown that massage intervention significantly increases amateur boxers' perception of recovery compared with passive rest intervention (Hemmings et al. 2000). Postexercise massage has been demonstrated to reduce the severity of muscle soreness, while massage seemed to have no effect on muscle functional loss (Farr et al. 2002). Research has also indicated that massage can reduce delayed onset muscle soreness after exercise (Smith et al. 1994; Hemmings 2001; Hilbert et al. 2003; Weerapong et al. 2005). This is especially valid if the massage is conducted 2 h or more after the event since this seems to disrupt the body's inflammatory process by reducing neutrophil accumulation (Archer 2007). Massage therapy has additionally been shown to facilitate the recovery process between two high-intensity, intermittent cycling exercise sessions separated by

Box 3.4

Highlights of postevent massage

- The therapist ensures the athlete has performed a minimum 20 min cool-down routine after ending an intense longer sports event.
- The therapist repeatedly monitors the athlete's coherency levels after long-term sports events.
- Signs of hypo- or hyperthermia are monitored.
- The athlete must hydrate before and during the massage after an intense long-term event or sports activity in hot weather.
- The athlete is covered with an extra blanket during the massage to prevent further hypothermia.
- No deep tissue massage is utilized, especially after long-term sports events.
- The massage is normally limited to a maximum of 15 min.
- Cramp release is often part of postevent sports massage.
- Light to moderate muscle stretching is normally included in the massage.

24 h (Lane & Wenger 2004). Athletes that complete long-term endurance events benefit from conducting a 20 min cool-down routine before receiving post-event sports massage therapy. This includes walking, ample hydration, and gentle stretching. The cool-down routine supports the body's process of normalizing heart rate, body temperature, blood circulation, and muscle function values. After intense long-term sport activity, the body continues to clear excessive heat produced by the previous muscle work and increased cell metabolism. As a result, the body will initially continue to expel heat when the athlete stops working. This combined with exercise-induced fluid loss makes it easy for the athlete to feel cold and begin shivering, even during warm temperatures. The shivering arises from small rapid muscle contractions aimed at generating more heat to warm the body as the athlete's blood volume is lowered from fluid loss. To prevent further hypothermia during the treatment, the therapist should cover the athlete with a warm blanket and give instructions to hydrate continuously (Box 3.4).

Coherency

During postevent massage of long-term sports event athletes, it is crucial to continuously monitor athletes' mental coherency. It is not uncommon

for exhausted participants to go into shock when relaxing on a massage table, resulting from either hyper- or hypothermia, especially if the heart rate still remains high when the massage treatment is begun. Fluid deficiency during the race combined with the rapid change to complete rest can lead to a gradual loss of consciousness. The loss of fluid decreases the blood volume and it is not uncommon with a sudden drop in blood pressure as the body still moves blood to the surface to release heat. This happens more easily if the athlete has not performed the mandatory minimum 20 min cool-down routine, including rehydration, after completing the race. It is therefore today often common to premonitor the athlete's pulse rate to ensure it is below at least 100 bpm before they can receive a postevent massage. A pulse that continuously remains high may indicate a more severe dehydration and/or hyperthermia. Asking the athlete simple questions during the massage, while observing the reaction time and quality of speech can be a good way to establish if coherency is present or not, since slurred speech and delayed answers can be a sign of beginning loss of consciousness. Exercise in hot weather may induce hyperthermia, i.e. heat exhaustion or heat stroke, which in the worst-case scenario can lead to fatality if not treated correctly. A medical professional must immediately be contacted for further assistance if the athlete's consciousness decreases below coherent levels. It is crucial for the sports massage therapist to be prepared to quickly assess and respond to heat-related illness symptoms in order to minimize possible severe complications (Eichner 1998; Binkley et al. 2002).

Caution should be taken if there is blood, vomit, or any body fluid other than sweat on the athlete. After long-term events like a marathon, for example, it is not uncommon for athletes to bleed from the nipples (if not previously taped), groin area, etc., or vomit from exhaustion. Mountain and road bikers may have fallen off during the race and received bleeding "road rash" from the fall. To protect against HIV, hepatitis B and C, and other blood- or fluid-transmitted diseases, the therapist must wear latex/rubber gloves as a safety barrier, and use bleach solution immediately to disinfect the hands, massage table, and any other surface that has been in contact with the fluids (Benjamin & Lamp 1996). If the athlete bleeds it is highly recommended to have them treated and "cleaned up" by a medical professional before the postevent massage commences.

Treatment

The execution of a postevent massage treatment will vary depending on the duration of the activity and what condition the athlete is in. After long-term sports events like a marathon or triathlon race, it is very important not to massage deep into the muscle. The muscles are mostly very fatigued and tensed due to the extreme conditions during the competition, and it is more than likely there already exist injuries to the soft tissues inflicted through the struggle to finish the race. Any deeper stroke can easily injure the soft tissue further and should not be used until the muscle has recovered to a more normal state. Postevent massage often includes the use of emollients and is commonly based on sliding strokes like effleurage in the beginning phase, to more effectively move blood and lymph from the tired muscles. Massage strokes like scrubbing, light compression, petrissage, broadening, and jostling/oscillation techniques are also normally included.

The postevent treatment also usually includes light therapeutic stretching of the muscles involved, to normalize their length and facilitate relaxation. This may help decompress smaller blood vessels to increase blood circulation in the area. The postevent massage should generally not last longer than 10–15 min, particularly after long-term endurance events. If the athlete stays longer than 15 min in these circumstances, there may be an increased risk of muscle cramps and/or other potentially more serious problems. Cramp release is often a component of postevent massage and is described in greater detail in Chapters 4 and 12.

Maintenance and remedial massage

In the period between training and competition the goal is to work more directly with the soft tissues in a more problem-solving manner. The massage can range from a thorough full body massage, which aims to generally support the athlete's recovery process, to working on specific areas of the body to facilitate both rehabilitation and healing after injury. The strokes used in remedial massage have a wide range, and are often executed more deeply into the muscles and fascial structures, providing there is no acute injury in the area. It is important to stay informed of the athlete's habits and training routines in order to more fully understand their specific problems and needs. It is beneficial for the sports massage therapist to be integrated with the team surrounding and supporting semi- or fully professional athletes. Ongoing communication and teamwork between the athlete, coach, trainer, and team doctors will increase the value of the sports massage treatments. Maintenance and remedial sports massage is described in Chapter 14.

Examples of cautions and contraindications for sports massage

Conditioned athletes are generally healthy but sports massage is commonly conducted on a wide range of individuals, particularly during event-based massage, so athletes may present different conditions and/or be more or less physically fit. Caution must also be taken with athletes suffering from hypertension, diabetes mellitus, heart conditions, cancer, kidney disease, etc. (Benjamin & Lamp 1996; Archer 2007). The list can be extensive and sports massage should as a general rule only be utilized when it is perceived to produce beneficial effects. Sports massage is contraindicated during special circumstances and some important contraindications are:

- Feverish infections or other types of fever.
- Directly on acute inflammations.
- Directly or near open wounds or burns.
- Deep massage directly on varicose veins.
- Phlebothrombosis.
- Directly on cardiovascular inflammations.
- Severe skin diseases/problems.
- Tuberculosis or other bacterial infection.
- Acute bone fractures.
- Acute ruptures in muscles, tendons, or ligaments. The condition should first be diagnosed, treated, and approved by the treating medical doctor for sports massage treatment.
- Pregnancy, especially the first three months and close to labor. Consult the treating medical doctor.
- Cancer diseases, unless the treatment is cleared by the treating physician in writing.
- Any type of physical or psychological disorder that can become worse by receiving a sports massage.

References

Archer, P., 2007. Therapeutic massage in athletics. Lippincott Williams & Wilkins, Baltimore, MD.

Benjamin, P.J., Lamp, S.P., 1996. Understanding sports massage, vol. 2. Human Kinetics, Champaign, IL.

Binkley, H.M., et al., 2002. National Athletic Trainers' Association Position Statement: exertional heat illnesses. J. Athl. Train. 37 (3), 329–343.

Cash, M., 1996. Sport & remedial massage therapy. Ebury Press, London.

Eichner, E.R., 1998. Treatment of suspected heat illness. Int. J. Sports Med. 19 (Suppl 2), S150–S153.

Farr, T., et al., 2002. The effects of therapeutic massage on delayed onset muscle soreness and muscle function following downhill walking. J. Sci. Med. Sport 5 (4), 297–306.

Gillespie, S., 2003. WTA tour sports massage therapy. Med. Sci. Tennis 2 (8), 17.

Hemmings, B., 2001. Physiological, psychological and performance effects of massage therapy in sport: a review of the literature. Phys. Ther. Sport. 4 (2), 165–170.

Hemmings, B., et al., 2000. Effects of massage on physiological restoration, perceived recovery, and repeated sports performance. Br. J. Sports Med. 34, 109–115.

Hilbert, J.E., et al., 2003. The effects of massage on delayed onset muscle soreness. Br. J. Sports Med. 37 (1), 72–75.

Lane, K.N., Wenger, H.A., 2004. Effect of selected recovery conditions on performance of repeated bouts of intermittent cycling separated by 24 hours. J. Strength Cond. Res. 18 (4), 855–860.

McKechnie, G., et al., 2007. Acute effects of two massage techniques on ankle joint flexibility and power of the plantar flexors. J. Sports Sci. Med. (6), 498–504.

Meagher, J., Broughton, P., 1990. Sports massage. Station Hill Press, Barrytown, NY.

Smith, L.L., et al., 1994. The effects of athletic massage on delayed onset muscle soreness, creatine kinase, and neutrophil count: a preliminary report. J. Orthop. Sports Phys. Ther. 19 (2), 93–99.

Ylinen, J., Cash, M., 1993. Idrottsmassage. ICA bokförlag, Västerås.

Weerapong, P., et al., 2005. The mechanisms of massage and effects on performance, muscle recovery and injury prevention. Sports Med. 35 (3), 235–256.

Examples of event-based sports massage treatments

4

The following examples of applied pre-, inter-, and postevent massage treatments are basic suggestions, which can be helpful for the novice sports massage therapist. It is important to realize, however, that a large number of options exist in real treatment situations since a good sports massage therapist continuously needs to adapt to existing scenarios including the requirements of each athlete treated during competition or training events.

Preevent sports massage treatment

Since preevent sports massage is aimed at preparing the athlete for a more or less imminent upcoming event (Meagher & Broughton 1990; Ylinen & Cash 1993; Benjamin & Lamp 1996; Cash 1996; Hemmings 2001; Archer 2007), the standard treatment duration close to a competition or training session is ideally around 15–20 min. Preevent massage is thought to stimulate increased blood circulation through activation of autonomic vascular reflexes (Gillespie 2003). The speed of the massage strokes is, as previously mentioned, also faster compared with a regular massage treatment, preferably more rapid than the athlete's resting heart rate, to ensure that the athlete stays alert and maintains their "mental peak" prior to the competition.

The following example will describe a preevent treatment of a long distance runner. In this case, the main areas treated areas are the feet, legs, hips/gluteal area, lower back, neck, and shoulders (Fig. 4.1). The massage always starts with a focus on the most frequently used areas for each athlete, which for most sports are the legs.

The time distribution for each sports massage treatment must be planned in advance to ensure treatment of all necessary areas of the athlete's body. As the following example illustrates, it is easy to see the actual time limitations imposed for each area. Every applied massage stroke must therefore be highly effective with regards to execution of technique, timing, and focal intent. It may be easier for the less experienced sports massage therapist at first to choose from a limited group of strokes with more general effects, initially keeping the treatment very basic by perhaps employing only four to five different strokes, using them systematically and thoroughly to ensure a real effect in the treated tissues. Supplementary strokes are added later, when the therapist is more confident about the treatment and the strokes' beneficial effects are relevant to the treatment goals.

Examples of some common massage strokes used during preevent massage

- effleurage
- scrubbing
- jostling/oscillation
- compression techniques – palm, fist, elbow
- broadening – palm heel, thenar eminence
- petrissage – palm
- frictions – transverse and circular
- edging
- rubbing – thenar, hypothenar
- rolling
- light tapotement.

© 2011, Elsevier Ltd.
DOI: 10.1016/B978-0-443-10126-7.00004-6

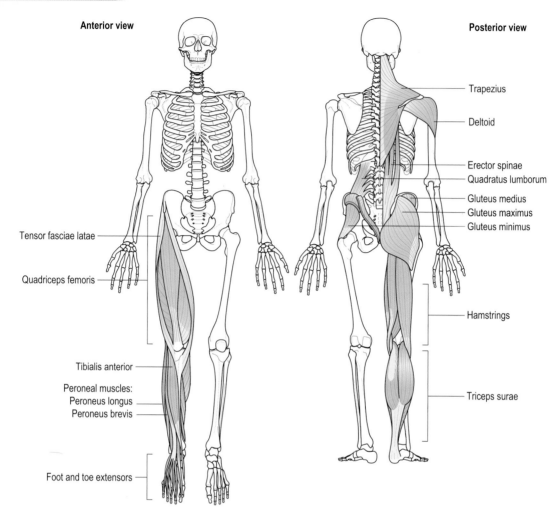

Anterior view

Posterior view

Trapezius

Deltoid

Erector spinae
Quadratus lumborum

Gluteus medius
Gluteus maximus
Gluteus minimus

Tensor fasciae latae

Quadriceps femoris

Hamstrings

Tibialis anterior

Peroneal muscles:
Peroneus longus
Peroneus brevis

Triceps surae

Foot and toe extensors

Figure 4.1 • Primary massaged areas for middle- to long-distance runners

Example of time distribution of a preevent sports massage treatment

- Back of left leg including the foot — 3 min
- Back of left gluteal area, hip, and lower back — 2 min
- Back of right leg including the foot — 3 min
- Back of right gluteal area, hip, and lower back — 2 min
- Upper back and shoulder area — 2 min
- Front of left leg — 2 min
- Front of right leg — 2 min
- Gentle stretches and ROM movements — 4 min

Total: 20 min

Suggestion for a general preevent sports massage treatment

1. **Jostling of both legs.** The therapist grabs both heels and rocks them side to side (Fig. 4.2). This movement will transfer to the rest of the body. The therapist looks for areas of restricted movements as the whole body moves from the jostling. It is easy for the therapist to notice areas in need of additional treatment.

2. **Palm scrubbing** of the posterior aspect of the right leg, gluteal area, and lower back (Fig. 4.3). Palm scrubbing generates heat and is ideal to use in preevent massage when

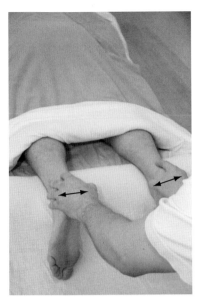

Figure 4.2 • Jostling of both legs

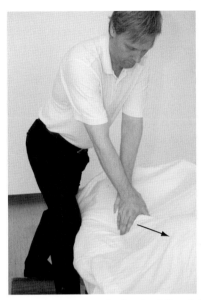

Figure 4.4 • Effleurage of the back of the right leg

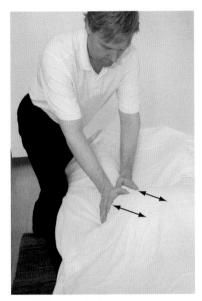

Figure 4.3 • Palm scrubbing

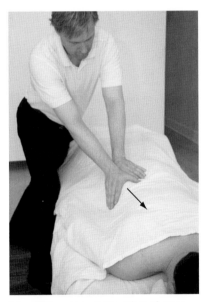

Figure 4.5 • Effleurage of the gluteal area and lower back

environmental temperatures are lower, or if the athlete feels cold.

3. **Effleurage of the back of the right leg.** The athlete is lying prone with a bolster under the feet. Use a sheet to cover the athlete's body and/or an added blanket if the temperature is cooler. It is many times easier to work through a sheet since it creates a smooth and even surface to massage on. This stroke starts superficially with the whole surface of the palms and is gradually deepened, by increasing the angle of the hands, as the tissue warms up (Fig. 4.4).

4. **Effleurage of the right gluteal and lower back area** including gluteus maximus, medius, minimus, quadratus lumborum, and erector spinae muscles (Fig. 4.5).

5. **Fist compressions of the right gluteal and lower back muscles.** The stroke is initially light, and deepens slightly as the tissue warms up (Fig. 4.6).

6. **Fist and palm compressions of the ischiocrural/hamstring muscle group.** The muscles are massaged from origin to insertion and special attention is placed on abnormally tight areas (Fig. 4.7).

7. **Broadening of the ischiocrural/hamstring muscle group.** Palmar or thenar broadening is used depending on the size of the thigh (Fig. 4.8).

8. **Broadening of right calf.** Thenar or palm broadening is used (Fig. 4.9).

9. **Rhythmic lock and stretch of the soleus and tibialis posterior muscles.** The right knee is flexed and foot passively plantar

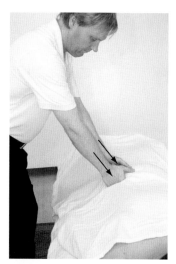

Figure 4.6 • Fist compressions of the right gluteal and lower back muscles

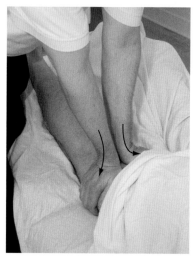

Figure 4.8 • Broadening of the ischiocrural/hamstring muscle group

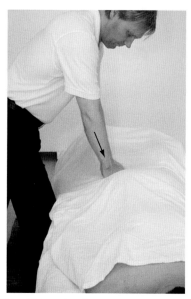

Figure 4.7 • Fist and palm compressions of the ischiocrural/hamstring muscle group

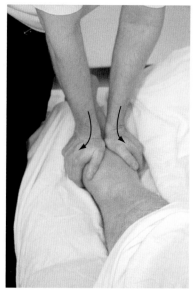

Figure 4.9 • Broadening of right calf

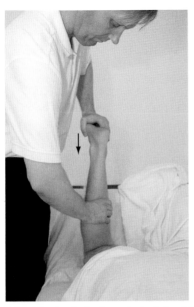

Figure 4.10 • Rhythmic lock and stretch of the soleus and tibialis posterior muscles

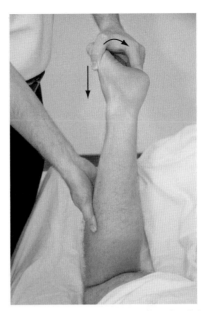

Figure 4.11 • Rhythmic lock and stretch of the peroneal muscles

flexed. The calf muscle is grasped on the lateral aspect as the therapist uses the elbow to perform dorsal flexion of the athlete's ankle. The athlete remains relaxed as the muscles systematically are compressed and stretched along the length of the treated muscles (Fig. 4.10). This massage and stretch also includes the calcaneus tendon.

10. **Rhythmic lock and stretch of the peroneal muscles.** The right knee is flexed and foot passively plantar flexed and inverted. The peroneal muscles are locked with one thumb, as the foot is dorsal flexed. The inversion should be approximately 50% of maximal movement to avoid pinching in the ankle joint. The athlete remains relaxed as the muscles systematically are compressed and stretched along the length of the treated muscles (Fig. 4.11).

11. **Edging of the right calf muscle.** The side of one thumb or tip of both thumbs is edging each belly of the gastrocnemius muscle (Fig. 4.12).

12. **Fist and thumb compressions of the right foot** (Fig. 4.13).

13. **Effleurage of the right leg and gluteal area** (Fig. 4.14).

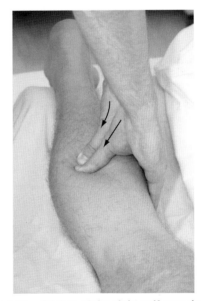

Figure 4.12 • Edging of the right calf muscle

Repeat sequence 2–13 on the left leg,

14. **Effleurage of the back** (Fig. 4.15).

15. **Palm and thumb compressions of the shoulder and neck area** (Fig. 4.16). The athlete lies prone.

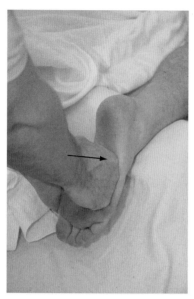

Figure 4.13 • Fist and thumb compressions of the right foot

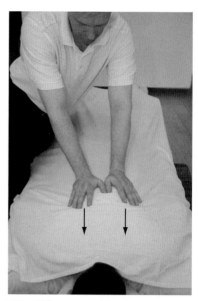

Figure 4.15 • Effleurage of the back

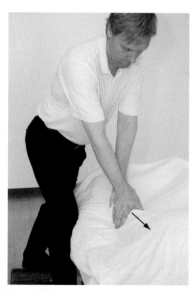

Figure 4.14 • Effleurage of the right leg and gluteal area

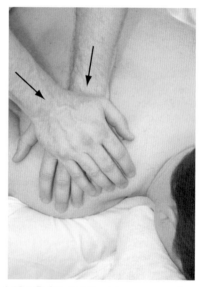

Figure 4.16 • Palm and thumb compressions of the shoulder and neck area

16. Scrubbing of the right leg (Fig. 4.17).
17. **Effleurage of the right leg.** The therapist gradually increases the depth slightly as the tissue warms up by increasing the angle of the hands (Fig. 4.18).

18. **Fist and palm compressions of the right thigh.** The entire anterior and lateral aspects of the thigh are massaged (Fig. 4.19).
19. **Palm broadening of the right thigh.** The tips of the fingers initially lift the medial and lateral

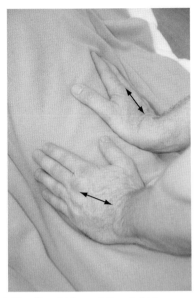

Figure 4.17 • Scrubbing of the right leg

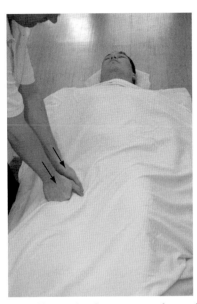

Figure 4.19 • Fist and palm compressions of the right thigh

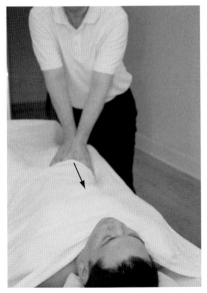

Figure 4.18 • Effleurage of the right leg

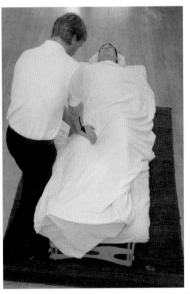

Figure 4.20 • Palm broadening of the right thigh

aspects of the muscles, followed by a laterally sliding compression by the heels of the hands (Fig. 4.20).

20. **Hypothenar rubbing of right quadriceps muscle.** The rubbing stroke starts slowly, and the speed is gradually increased as the tissue warms up (Fig. 4.21).

21. **Palm compressions of the right tibialis anterior and peroneal muscles.** The compressions span the whole length of the anterior and lateral compartments, while a slight lateral (for tibialis anterior) and posterior (for the peroneal muscle group) direction is added to the compressions to enhance the stretch effect (Fig. 4.22).

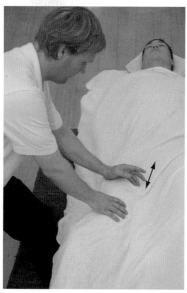

Figure 4.21 • Hypothenar rubbing of right quadriceps muscle

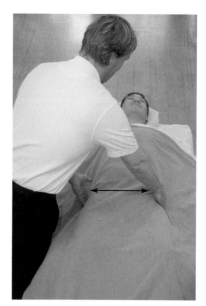

Figure 4.23 • Jostling of the hip and both legs

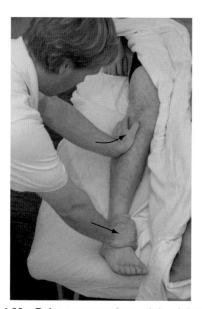

Figure 4.22 • Palm compressions of the right tibialis anterior and peroneal muscles

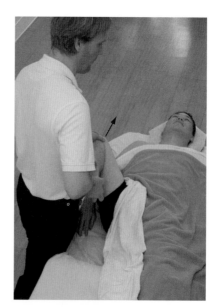

Figure 4.24 • ROM stretch of the right hip joint

Repeat sequence 16–21 on the left leg.

22. Jostling of the hip and both legs (Fig. 4.23).
23. ROM stretch of the right hip joint (Fig. 4.24).
24. Stretch of right ischiocrural/hamstring muscles (Fig. 4.25).

25. Stretch of right gastrocnemius and soleus muscles (Fig. 4.26).
26. Stretch of right quadriceps and iliopsoas muscles, athlete positioned on side (Fig. 4.27).
27. ROM stretch of the left hip joint (Fig. 4.28).

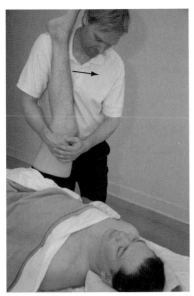

Figure 4.25 • Stretch of right ischiocrural/hamstring muscles

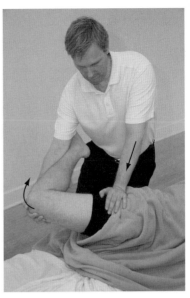

Figure 4.27 • Athlete on side, stretch of right quadriceps and iliopsoas muscles

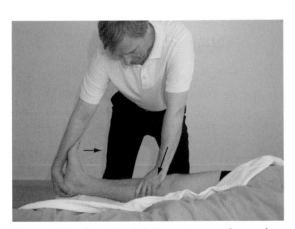

Figure 4.26 • Stretch of right gastrocnemius and soleus muscles

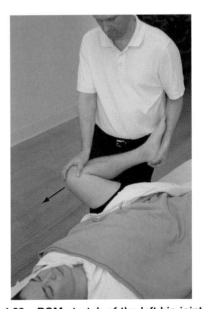

Figure 4.28 • ROM stretch of the left hip joint

28. Stretch of left hamstring muscles (ischiocrural muscles) (Fig. 4.29).
29. Stretch of left gastrocnemius and soleus muscles (Fig. 4.30).
30. Stretch of left quadriceps and iliopsoas muscles with additional hip lock by the therapist, athlete positioned on side (Fig. 4.31).
31. Palm compression of shoulder area, athlete positioned supine (Fig. 4.32).
32. Circular finger frictions of neck area (Fig. 4.33).

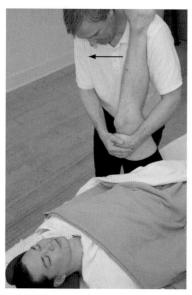

Figure 4.29 • Stretch of left ischiocrural/hamstring muscles

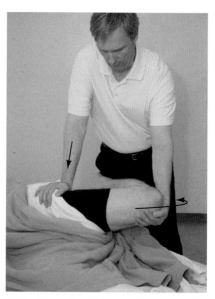

Figure 4.31 • Stretch of left quadriceps and iliopsoas muscles with additional hip lock by the therapist

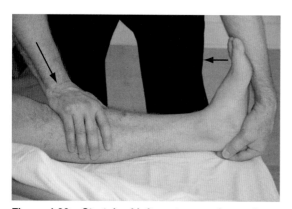

Figure 4.30 • Stretch of left gastrocnemius and soleus muscles

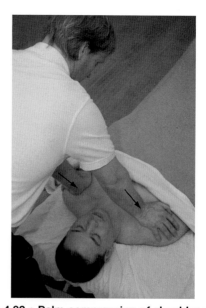

Figure 4.32 • Palm compression of shoulder area

Interevent sports massage

As explained in Chapter 3, interevent massage treatments are most commonly utilized between heats, rounds, etc., and specifically focus on areas with problems and/or excessive tension caused by the sport activity (Archer 2007). Interevent massage is also perceived to assist the athlete's recovery process (Benjamin & Lamp 1996; Lane & Wenger 2004; Brooks et al. 2005; Archer 2007), and incorporate preparatory support to the athlete for the upcoming event (Benjamin & Lamp 1996;

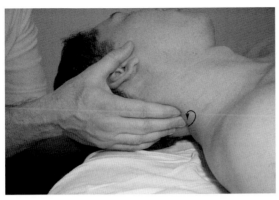

Figure 4.33 • Circular finger frictions of neck area

Example of time distribution of an interevent sports massage treatment

• Back of left leg including the foot	3 min
• Back of left gluteal area, hip, and lower back	1 min
• Back of right leg including the foot	3 min
• Back of right gluteal area, hip, and lower back	1 min
• Upper back and shoulder area	1 min
• Front of left leg	2 min
• Front of right leg	2 min
• Gentle stretches and ROM movements	2 min
Total:	**15 min**

Hemmings 2001; Archer 2007). This means that an interevent treatment must also be invigorating to the athlete if the following event is impending (Benjamin & Lamp 1996). The treatment is focused on areas previously stressed during the competition, and that will be majorly active in the upcoming competition.

Interevent massage is generally 10–15 min in duration (Benjamin & Lamp 1996), (or even 1 min or less for boxing and similar sports), and should be rather light and comfortable for the athlete (Benjamin & Lamp 1996; Archer 2007). Deep tissue and general invasive techniques are also avoided (Benjamin & Lamp 1996).

It is advisable to firstly ask the athlete about existing problem areas to be able to best address the athlete's needs. Sliding strokes like effleurage work very well during the initial stage for their perceived circulatory and palpatory qualities. Interevent massage strokes are otherwise normally the same as used in pre- and postevent massage. The effleurage stroke is beneficially modified during the treatment by placing more pressure on the finger tips, reinforcing one hand with the other, and/or changing the angle of treatment in relation to the muscle fiber direction. The general treatment direction of effleurage, however, is always along the venous flow, toward the heart. Depending on what areas the athlete initially needs to have tended, the treatment commences either in a prone or supine position.

The following interevent massage example is of a track and field 1500 m runner. It will start in the prone position since the athlete in this case has excessive tension in the left ischiocrural/hamstring muscles.

Suggestion for a general interevent sports massage treatment

33. Effleurage of the posterior aspect of the left leg (Figs 4.34 & 4.35). The athlete is lying prone with a bolster under the feet. Use a sheet to cover the athlete's body and/or an additional blanket if the temperature is cooler. The therapist locks the sheet against the table with one thigh (see Fig. 4.34). The stroke starts superficially, at a slow to moderate speed, with the whole surface of the palms, and is slightly deepened by increasing

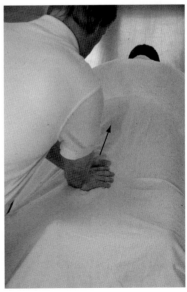

Figure 4.34 • Effleurage of the posterior aspect of the left leg

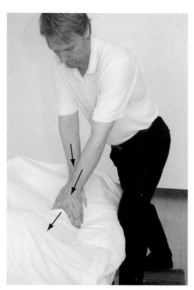

Figure 4.35 • Effleurage of the posterior aspect of the left leg

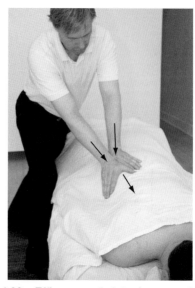

Figure 4.36 • Effleurage of gluteal area and lower back

the angle of the hands as the tissue softens (see Fig. 4.35). The hands constantly palpate for excessive muscle and/or fascial tension. Moving the pressure toward the palm heels or slightly flexed fingers tips reinforces the effleurage strokes over areas of excess tension. The pressure and angles are slightly altered to constantly modify the treatment effect. The tensed areas are massaged until the tissue begins to soften.

34. **Effleurage of gluteal area and lower back.** The effleurage is smoothly continued on the left gluteal and lower back area including gluteus maximus, medius, and minimus, quadratus lumborum, and erector spinae muscles (Fig. 4.36).

35. **Palm heel petrissage of selected tensed areas of the left leg.** The therapist employs palm heel petrissage on selected tension-ridden areas and gently utilizes the body weight to controllably enhance the stretch effect. The sheet is slackened to ensure that the full movement of the stroke has effect in the tissue (Fig. 4.37).

36. **S-stroke petrissage of selected tensed areas of the left leg.** The fingertips pull one side of the tensed muscle while the palm heel of the other hand pushes the other side of the tissue. The stretch should be mild and is held for 4–5 s before the stroke shifts in the other direction (Fig. 4.38).

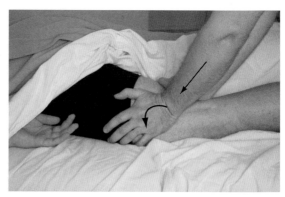

Figure 4.37 • Palm heel petrissage of selected tensed areas of the left leg

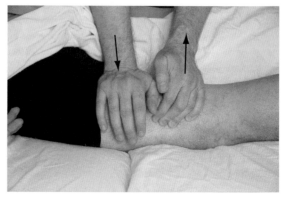

Figure 4.38 • S-stroke petrissage of selected tensed areas of the left leg

37. **Rhythmic lock and stretch of the ischiocrural/ hamstring muscles.** The therapist grips the athlete's left ankle, and passively flexes the knee of the left leg to relax the hamstring muscles. The fist or palm of the other hand locks the superior area of the excessively tensed muscle with a pressure directed obliquely anterior/superior toward the ischial tuberosity. With the palm heel, or second and third knuckle steadily fixating the muscle, the therapist slowly lowers the leg until a mild stretch is felt (Fig. 4.39), and this position is held for 2–6 s. The procedure is repeated as the therapist gradually locks the muscle further inferior to the original start position.

38. **Fist compressions of the left gluteal and lower back muscles.** The stroke is initially light, and deepens slightly as the soft tissues begin to relax (Fig. 4.40).

39. **Fist and palm compressions of the ischiocrural/hamstring muscle group.** The muscles are massaged from origin to insertion and special attention is paid to abnormally tight areas (Fig. 4.41).

40. **Broadening of the ischiocrural/hamstring muscle group** (Fig. 4.42).

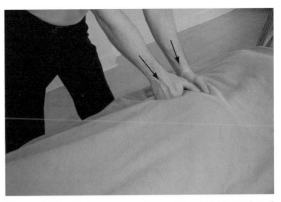

Figure 4.40 • Fist compressions of the left gluteal and lower back muscles

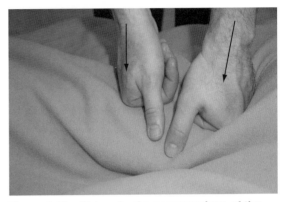

Figure 4.41 • Fist and palm compressions of the ischiocrural/hamstring muscle group

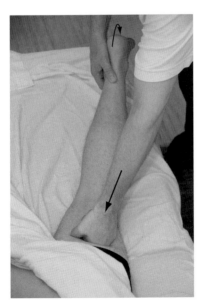

Figure 4.39 • Rhythmic lock and stretch of the ischiocrural/hamstring muscles

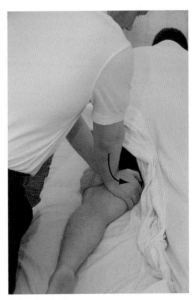

Figure 4.42 • Broadening of the ischiocrural/ hamstring muscle group

41. **Alternating palm compressions of the left calf muscles.** The medial and lateral head of the muscle are treated separately (Fig. 4.43).

42. **Broadening of the left calf muscles.** Thenar broadening is used in this example, but palmar broadening may be necessary when treating larger calf muscles (Fig. 4.44).

43. **Lock and stretch of the soleus, tibialis posterior, and peroneal muscles.** The left knee is flexed and the foot passively plantar flexed by the therapist. The muscles are grasped and "locked" on both the lateral and medial aspects of the lower leg as the therapist consequently uses the elbow to perform dorsal flexion of the athlete's ankle. The athlete remains relaxed as the muscles gradually are massaged and stretched along their length (Fig. 4.45). This lock and stretch also includes the calcaneus tendon.

44. **Edging of the left calf muscle.** The side of one thumb, pressed by the palm heel of the other hand, is separately edging both bellies of the gastrocnemius muscle (Fig. 4.46).

45. **Fist compressions of the left foot.** The therapist uses a loose fist of one hand to gently perform compression techniques of the left

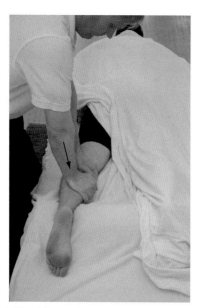

Figure 4.43 • Alternating palm compressions of the left calf muscles

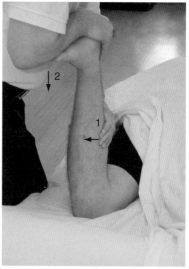

Figure 4.45 • Lock and stretch of the soleus, tibialis posterior, and peroneal muscles

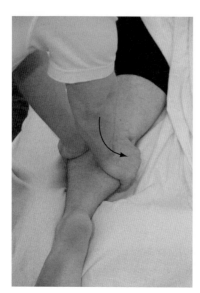

Figure 4.44 • Broadening of the left calf muscles

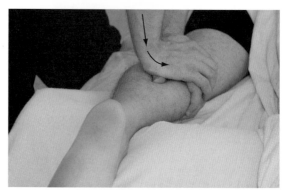

Figure 4.46 • Edging of the left calf muscle

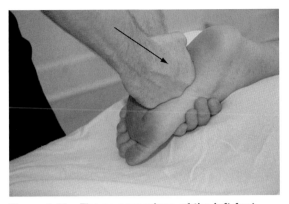

Figure 4.47 • Fist compressions of the left foot

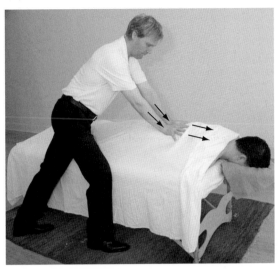

Figure 4.49 • Effleurage of the back

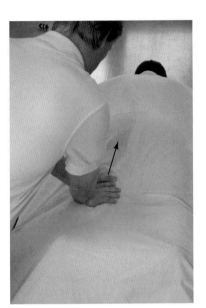

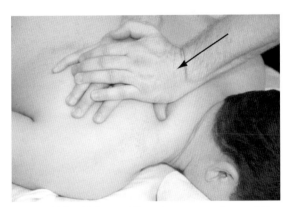

Figure 4.50 • Palm and thumb compressions of the shoulder and neck area

Figure 4.48 • Effleurage of the left leg and gluteal area

foot while the other hand supports the dorsal side of the foot (Fig. 4.47).

46. Effleurage of the left leg and gluteal area (Fig. 4.48).

Repeat sequence 33–46 on the right leg.

47. Effleurage of the back (Fig. 4.49).

48. Palm and thumb compressions of the shoulder and neck area (Fig. 4.50).

The athlete lies supine.

49. Effleurage of the right leg. The athlete is lying supine with a bolster under the knees. The stroke starts superficially, at a slow to moderate speed with the whole surface of the palms, and is slightly deepened as the tissue softens, by increasing the angle of the hands (Fig. 4.51). The hands constantly palpate for excessive muscle and/or fascial tension. The therapist gradually increases the depth slightly by increasing the angle of the hands (see Fig. 4.51), as the soft tissue relaxes. Extra time is spent on the modifications of the effleurage stroke before the more preevent compression techniques begin.

50. Fist and palm compressions of the right thigh. The entire anterior and lateral aspects of the thigh are massaged (Fig. 4.52).

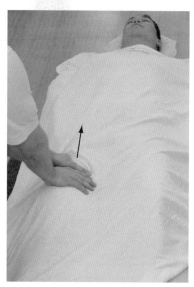

Figure 4.51 • Effleurage of the right leg

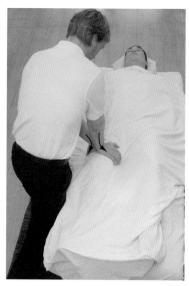

Figure 4.53 • Palm broadening of the right thigh

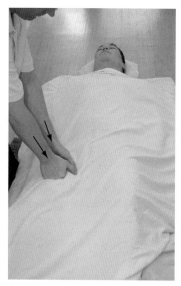

Figure 4.52 • Fist and palm compressions of the right thigh

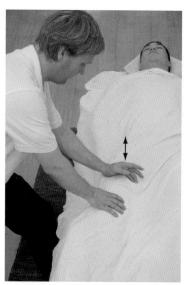

Figure 4.54 • Hypothenar rubbing of right quadriceps muscle

51. **Palm broadening of the right thigh** (Fig. 4.53). The tips of the fingers initially lift the medial and lateral aspects of the muscles followed by a laterally sliding compression by the heels of the hands.

52. **Hypothenar rubbing of right quadriceps muscle** (Fig. 4.54). The rubbing stroke starts

slowly, and the speed is gradually increased as the tissue warms up.

53. **Palm compressions of the right tibialis anterior and peroneal muscles.** The compressions span the whole length of the anterior and lateral compartment of the lower leg, while a slight lateral (for tibialis anterior) and posterior

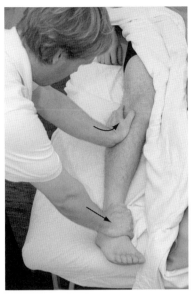

Figure 4.55 • Palm compressions of the right tibialis anterior and peroneal muscles

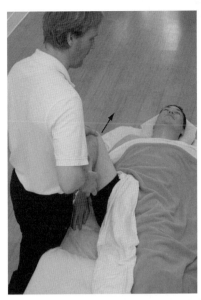

Figure 4.57 • ROM stretch of the right hip joint

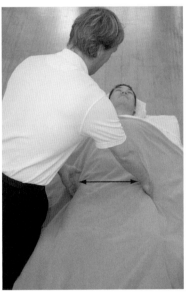

Figure 4.56 • Jostling of the hip and both legs

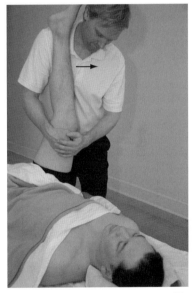

Figure 4.58 • Stretch of right ischiocrural/ hamstring muscles

(for the peroneal muscle group) direction is added to enhance the stretch effect (Fig. 4.55).

Repeat sequence 49–53 on the left leg.

54. Jostling of the hip and both legs (Fig. 4.56).
55. ROM stretch of the right hip joint (Fig. 4.57).

56. Stretch of right ischiocrural/hamstring muscles (Fig. 4.58).
57. Stretch of right gastrocnemius and soleus muscles (Fig. 4.59).
58. Stretch of right quadriceps and iliopsoas muscles, athlete positioned on side (Fig. 4.60).

Repeat sequence 54–58 on the left leg.

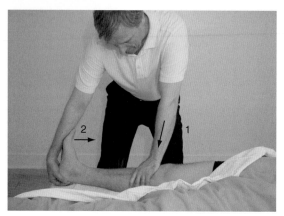

Figure 4.59 • Stretch of right gastrocnemius and soleus muscles

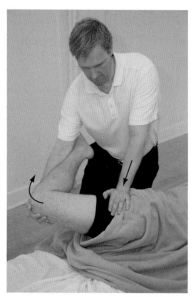

Figure 4.60 • Athlete on side, stretch of right quadriceps and iliopsoas muscles

Postevent sports massage treatment

Postevent massage treatments will vary depending on the length and type of sports event that has taken place. After ending duration sports like marathon, triathlon, road biking, etc., it is important that at least lower- to mid-level athletes have completed a minimum 20 min cool-down routine before the postevent session can commence. For this group of athletes it is

also crucial for the therapist to repeatedly monitor their coherency levels, and watch for signs of added hypo- or hyperthermia. Higher-level amateurs and professional athletes have generally perfected their own routines and know very well how their body responds before, during, and after the sport event and massage treatment.

Example of time distribution of a postevent sports massage treatment

• Back of left leg including the foot	2 min
• Back of left gluteal area, hip, and lower back	1 min
• Back of right leg including the foot	2 min
• Back of right gluteal area, hip, and lower back	1 min
• Upper back and shoulder area	1 min
• Front of left leg	2 min
• Front of right leg	2 min
• Cramp release, gentle stretches, and ROM movements	3 min
Total:	**14 min**

The therapist should ensure the athlete hydrates before and during the massage after an intense endurance event, or during hot environmental situations, to decrease the risk of muscle cramps or other more serious conditions. During postevent massage it is frequently advantageous to cover the athlete with an extra blanket to reduce the risk of additional hypothermia. As in pre-, and interevent sports massage, there is no deep tissue massage applied in the treatment. This is especially important after long-term sports events due to the fragile and hypertensile state of the soft tissue.

The massage is usually limited to a maximum of 15 min, particularly for more extreme endurance athletes. As previously mentioned, cramp release is often part of a postevent sports massage. Light therapeutic stretching is often additionally utilized to facilitate normalization of length of muscles and fascial structures. The following example of a postevent massage is of a midlevel marathon runner. The treatment of this type of athlete may be more eventful than for those undergoing other less physically draining sport situations. An emollient is often used unless the athlete is treated over a sheet and blanket.

Suggestion for a general postevent sports massage treatment

59. Observation. The therapist observes the athlete as they walk toward the massage table for signs of hyper- or hypothermia, coherency level, and possible existing muscle cramps and/or injuries. To assess basic coherency level, the therapist may ask the athlete how the race progressed, and how they enjoyed it. Slurred speech and delayed response time might be a sign of reduced coherency.

60. Alternate palm scrubbing of the posterior aspect of the right leg, gluteal area, and lower back. The athlete lies prone with a bolster under the feet. A sheet with an additional blanket is used to cover the athlete's body. The therapist locks the sheet and blanket against the table with one thigh. The stroke is performed with brisk alternating superficial movements with the whole surface of the palms (Fig. 4.61). This is an ideal massage stroke to initiate a postevent sports massage treatment for a hypothermic athlete.

61. Jostling of both legs. The therapist grasps both of the athlete's heels and rocks the legs side to side (Fig. 4.62). This movement will transfer

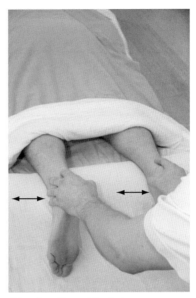

Figure 4.62 • Jostling of both legs

to the rest of the body and besides having a relaxing effect, reveals areas of tight and restricted movement.

62. Effleurage of the back of the right leg. The strokes start superficially from the ankle with the whole surface of the palms, and move repeatedly all the way up to the ischial tuberosity (Fig. 4.63). These initial effleurage strokes are performed thoroughly and systematically at a slow to moderate pace to ensure adequate circulatory effect.

63. Continued effleurage of the right gluteal and lower back area including gluteus maximus, medius, and minimus, quadratus lumborum, and the erector spinae muscles (Fig. 4.64).

64. Light fist compressions of the right gluteal and lower back muscles (Fig. 4.65). The strokes are performed rhythmically with light pressure.

65. Light fist and palm compressions on the ischiocrural/hamstring muscle group (Fig. 4.66). The muscles are gently but systematically massaged, covering origin to insertion, and special attention is placed on abnormally tensed areas.

66. Gentle palmar broadening of the ischiocrural/hamstring muscle group, including the posterior aspect of the adductor magnus muscle (Fig. 4.67).

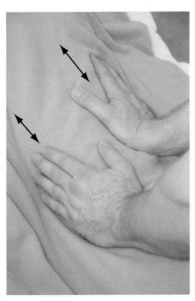

Figure 4.61 • Alternate palm scrubbing of the posterior aspect of right leg, gluteal area, and lower back

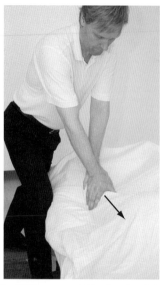

Figure 4.63 • Effleurage of the back of the right leg

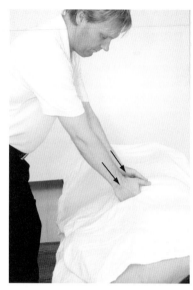

Figure 4.65 • Light fist compressions of the right gluteal and lower back muscles. The strokes are performed rhythmically with light pressure

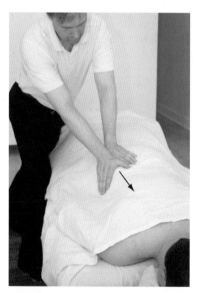

Figure 4.64 • Continued effleurage of the right gluteal and lower back area including gluteus maximus, medius, and minimus, quadratus lumborum, and the erector spinae muscles

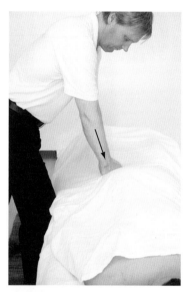

Figure 4.66 • Light fist and palm compressions on the ischiocrural/hamstring muscle group

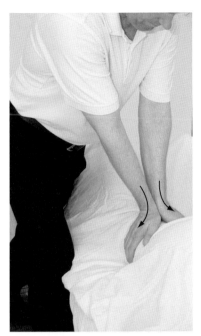

Figure 4.67 • Gentle palmar broadening of the ischiocrural/hamstring muscle group, including the posterior aspect of the adductor magnus muscle

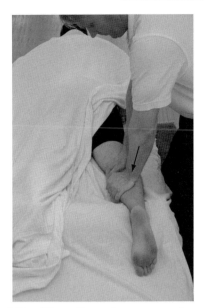

Figure 4.68 • Alternating palm compressions of the right calf muscles

67. **Alternating palm compressions of the right calf muscles.** The medial and lateral heads of the gastrocnemius muscle are treated separately (Fig. 4.68). At this point, the therapist can ask the athlete additional questions in order to monitor the coherence level. The therapist may also suggest the athlete continues to hydrate as the massage progresses.

68. **Broadening of the right calf muscles.** Thenar or palm broadening is used depending on the muscle size (Fig. 4.69).

69. **The right ischiocrural/hamstring muscle group suddenly cramps.** Fibrillation of the local muscle area is often initially detected before an actual cramp onset. A simple manual approximation of the muscle belly may prevent the cramp if administered immediately upon detection of the fibrillation. When an actual cramp develops, the muscle is firstly approximated; in this case the athlete's knee is flexed by the therapist. The therapist places one thigh under the athlete's shin, as the muscle is additionally manually approximated. Approximation will reduce

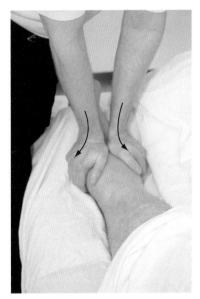

Figure 4.69 • Broadening of the right calf muscles

activation of the muscle spindles in the cramping muscle, and is believed to assist in deactivating a muscle cramp. For larger muscle areas like this, one fist may compress the cramping area simultaneously as the palm of the other hand, together with the fist, approximates the whole muscle belly (Fig. 4.70).

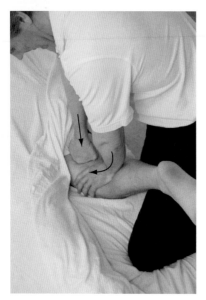

Figure 4.70 • The right ischiocrural/hamstring muscle group suddenly cramps

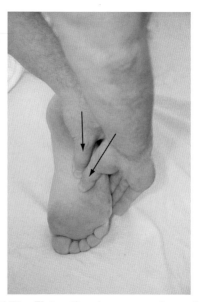

Figure 4.71 • Fist or thumb compressions of the right foot

The athlete is asked to press the shin against the therapist's leg, thus activating the antagonistic muscle group. This activates reciprocal inhibition of the cramping muscle, which facilitates deactivation of the muscle cramp. This contraction lasts for approximately 4 s, with the muscle further compressed and approximated as the contraction ceases. These alternating actions continue until the cramp is released, which normally takes three to four repetitions, but if the athlete is too dehydrated and depleted, no manual treatment may release the cramp. When this situation occurs, and normal coherency is present, the athlete is simply asked to get off the massage table and return after 20 min of walking with ample hydration. As the athlete starts to "walk" and thus initiate contractions in multiple muscles, the cramp tends to release within a few seconds.

If the athlete's coherency is additionally decreased, a medical professional needs to assess the situation since intravenous fluid administration might be necessary. If the athlete is too dehydrated and/or depleted, muscle cramps also tend to spread. A released cramp in the ischiocrural/hamstring muscle group may restart in the gastrocnemius, a gluteal, lower back, or even an antagonistic muscle like the quadriceps femoris. If the ongoing cramping initiates in more than one area, it is also time to have the athlete get

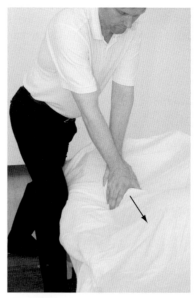

Figure 4.72 • Effleurage of the right leg and gluteal area

off the table or receive attention from a medical professional. Cramps spreading to the abdominal region might be a sign of more severe dehydration or hyperthermia.

70. **Fist or thumb compressions of the right foot** (Fig. 4.71).

71. **Effleurage of the right leg and gluteal area** (Fig. 4.72).

Repeat sequence 60–71 on the left leg (cramp release is omitted unless cramp is present).

The athlete lies supine.

72. Palm scrubbing of the right leg (Fig. 4.73).

73. Effleurage of the right leg. The strokes start superficially from the ankle with the whole surface of the palms (Fig. 4.74), and move repeatedly all the way up to the hip area. The effleurage strokes are performed thoroughly and systematically at a slow to moderate pace to ensure adequate circulatory effect.

74. Gentle fist and palm compressions of the right thigh. The entire anterior and lateral aspects of the thigh are massaged (Fig. 4.75).

75. Palm broadening of the right thigh. The tips of the fingers initially lift the medial and lateral aspects of the muscles followed by a laterally sliding compression by the heels of the hands from a central point of the muscle (Fig. 4.76).

76. Palm compressions of the lower leg. The compressions span the whole length of the anterior and lateral compartment, with a slight

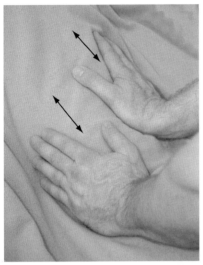

Figure 4.73 • Palm scrubbing of the right leg

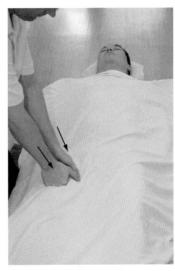

Figure 4.75 • Gentle fist and palm compressions of the right thigh

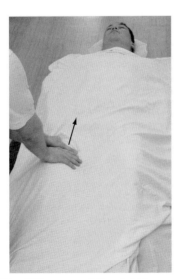

Figure 4.74 • Effleurage of the right leg

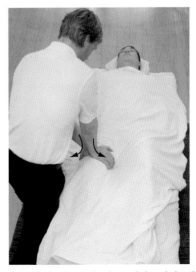

Figure 4.76 • Palm broadening of the right thigh

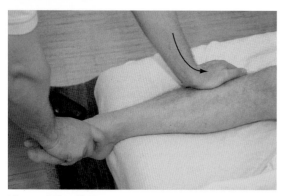

Figure 4.77 • Palm compressions of the lower leg

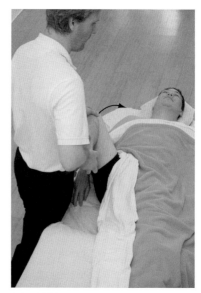

Figure 4.79 • ROM stretch of the right hip joint

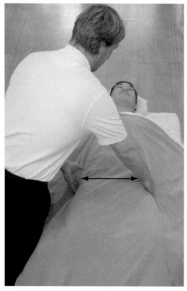

Figure 4.78 • Jostling of the shoulders, pelvis, hips, and legs

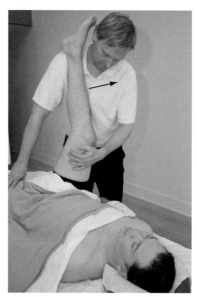

Figure 4.80 • Gentle stretch of right ischiocrural/ hamstring muscles

lateral (for tibialis anterior) and posterior (for the peroneal muscle group) direction added to the compression to enhance the stretch effect (Fig. 4.77).

77. Jostling of the shoulders, pelvis, hips, and legs (Fig. 4.78).

78. ROM stretch of the right hip joint (Fig. 4.79).

79. Gentle stretch of right ischiocrural/hamstring muscles (Fig. 4.80).

80. Stretch of right gastrocnemius and soleus muscles (Fig. 4.81).

81. Stretch of right quadriceps and iliopsoas muscles. The athlete is positioned on the side (Fig. 4.82).

Repeat 72–80 on the left leg.

82. Palm compression of shoulder area. The athlete lies supine. The anterior and lateral aspects of the shoulder regions are alternately compressed with the palms (Fig. 4.83).

83. Circular finger frictions and mild traction of neck area (Fig. 4.84).

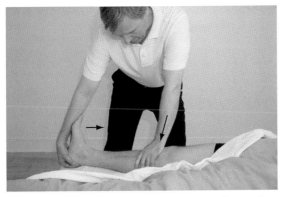

Figure 4.81 • Stretch of right gastrocnemius and soleus muscles

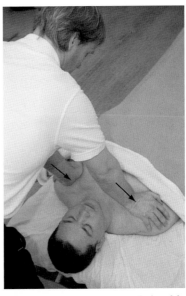

Figure 4.83 • Palm compression of shoulder area

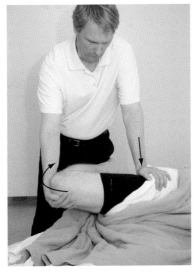

Figure 4.82 • Stretch of right quadriceps and iliopsoas muscles

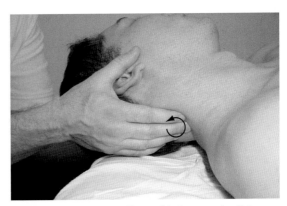

Figure 4.84 • Circular finger frictions and mild traction of neck area

References

Archer, P., 2007. Therapeutic massage in athletics, vol. 5. Lippincott Williams & Wilkins, Baltimore, MD.

Benjamin, P.J., Lamp, S.P., 1996. Understanding sports massage, vol. 4. Human Kinetics, Champaign, IL.

Brooks, C.P., et al., 2005. The immediate effects of manual massage on power-grip performance after maximal exercise in healthy adults. J. Altern. Complement. Med. 11 (6), 1093–1101.

Cash, M., 1996. Sports & remedial massage therapy. Ebury Press, London.

Gillespie, S., 2003. WTA tour sports massage therapy. Med. Sci. Tennis 2 (8), 17.

Hemmings, B., 2001. Physiological, psychological and performance effects of massage therapy in sport: a review of the literature. Phys. Ther. Sport 4 (2), 165–170.

Lane, K.N., Wenger, H.A., 2004. Effect of selected recovery conditions on performance of repeated bouts of intermittent cycling separated by 24 hours. J. Strength Cond. Res. 18 (4), 855–860.

Meagher, J., Broughton, P., 1990. Sports massage. Station Hill Press, Barrytown, NY.

Ylinen, J., Cash, M., 1993. Idrottsmassage. ICA bokförlag, Västerås.

Sports massage applications for different sports

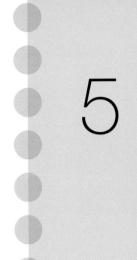

5

Event-based sports massage is utilized in a wide range of sports scenarios. Even though the execution of pre-, post-, and interevent massage may share basic principles and fundamentally similar treatment concepts, regardless of sport, different sports can have specific stress areas that may benefit from additional treatment focus. Most sports do use the legs to propel the athlete, however, and so initial attention is more often than not given to different areas of the lower extremities.

It is indicated that muscle stiffness is a risk factor for more severe symptoms of muscle damage after eccentric exercise (McHugh et al. 1999). Research further suggests that increased hamstring flexibility reduces overuse injuries in the lower extremities (Hartig & Henderson 1999), and this may be one reason why today there is a positive trend toward the use of sports massage to benefit athletic recovery and performance (Moraska 2005).

The following examples are suggestions for a few sports-specific treatment areas, based on the principle of suggested higher stress areas, and muscle and/or joint involvement for each stated sport. This is intended to serve as a basic outline for the novice sports massage therapist to more quickly enable assessment of necessary areas, but in many cases the treatments will certainly need to be further tailored to each athlete.

Runners

Most sports include some form of running, but for the devoted runner, areas like legs, hips, and lower back are placed under particular stress. It is suggested it is important for running athletes to have adequate

plantar flexion during the push off phase in the running stride (Alter 2004). Shortened hamstrings and/or iliopsoas muscles may additionally shorten the athlete's stride and need treatment consideration.

Suggested areas to massage on runners (Meagher & Broughton 1990; Alter 2004) (Fig. 5.1)

1. **Feet.** The feet are important, particularly for long-distance runners, due to the duration of stress.
2. **Ankles and lower legs.** The muscles affecting the ankles are treated, with special treatment focus on the triceps surae, peroneal, and tibialis anterior muscles (Fig. 5.2).
3. **Thighs.** Quadriceps femoris, adductors, and the hamstring muscle group.
4. **Hips and gluteal area.** The gluteal muscles, particularly gluteus medius and minimus, and piriformis. Additionally the TFL and iliopsoas muscle should be attended to.
5. **Lower back.** Quadratus lumborum and the lower erector spinae muscle.
6. **Neck and shoulders.** Trapezius, levator scapulae, splenii, and erector spinae.

Swimming

Swimmers generally have great overall flexibility, particularly in areas like the ankles and shoulders. Their elevated ROM makes it necessary to

DOI: 10.1016/B978-0-443-10126-7.00005-8

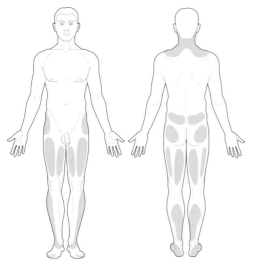

Figure 5.1 • Suggested areas to massage for runners

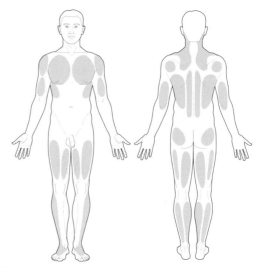

Figure 5.3 • Suggested areas to massage for swimmers

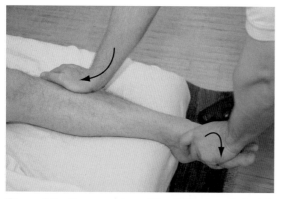

Figure 5.2 • Compression with mild lock and stretch of the tibialis anterior muscle

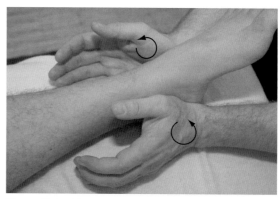

Figure 5.4 • Alternate bilateral palm frictions of the ankles

have sufficient muscle strength around the joints to prevent overuse injuries and unnecessary joint stress.

It is suggested that flexibility of the spine is important in swimming (Alter 2004), enabling the body to twist and produce correct power transference.

Suggested areas to massage for swimmers (Fig. 5.3)

1. Ankles and calves. Triceps surae, peroneal, and tibialis anterior muscles (Fig. 5.4).

2. Knees and thighs. Quadriceps femoris, adductors, and hamstring muscles.

3. Gluteal area and the hip joint. Gluteus maximus, medius, and minimus muscles.

4. Spine. Erector spinae, quadratus lumborum, latissimus dorsi, rhomboids, and trapezius muscles.

5. Shoulders. Infraspinatus, teres major and minor, latissimus dorsi, subscapularis, deltoid, pectoralis major and minor, and serratus anterior muscles.

6. Arms. Triceps brachii, biceps brachii, and brachialis muscles.

Wrestling

Suggested areas to massage for wrestlers (Fig. 5.5)

1. **Ankles and calves.** Triceps surae, peroneal, tibialis posterior, and tibialis anterior muscles.

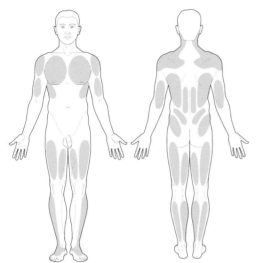

Figure 5.5 • Suggested areas to massage for wrestlers

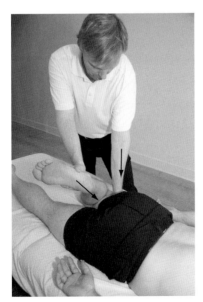

Figure 5.6 • Lock and stretch massage of the vastus lateralis muscle

2. **Knees and thighs.** Quadriceps femoris, adductors, and hamstring muscles (Fig. 5.6).
3. **Gluteal and hip area.** Gluteus maximus, medius and minimus, TFL, and iliopsoas muscles.
4. **Lower back.** Quadratus lumborum, erector spinae, and lower latissimus dorsi muscles.
5. **Shoulders.** Latissimus dorsi, teres major and minor, infraspinatus, subscapularis, deltoid, serratus anterior, and pectoralis major muscles.
6. **Neck.** Splenius capitis, splenius cervicis, trapezius, levator scapulae (Fig. 5.7), and suboccipital muscle group.
7. **Arms.** Biceps and triceps brachii muscles.

Olympic weight lifting

Olympic weight lifting requires good flexibility in the ankles, knees, spine, and shoulders to generate the correct technique and necessary power (Alter 2004).

Suggested areas to massage for weight lifters (Meagher & Broughton 1990; Alter 2004) (Fig. 5.8)

1. **Feet.**
2. **Ankles and calves.** Triceps surae, peroneal, tibialis posterior, and tibialis anterior muscles.
3. **Knees and thighs.** Quadriceps femoris, adductors, and hamstring muscles (Fig. 5.9).
4. **Gluteal and hip area.** Gluteus maximus, medius and minimus, TFL, and iliopsoas muscles.

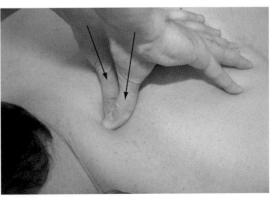

Figure 5.7 • Braced thumb compression of the levator scapulae muscle

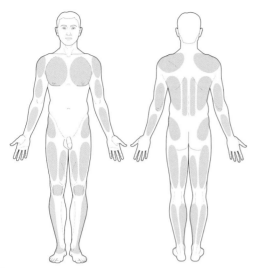

Figure 5.8 • Suggested areas to massage for Olympic weight lifters

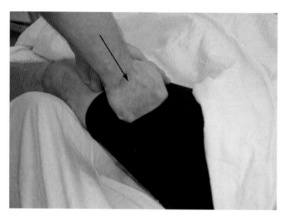

Figure 5.9 • Fist compressions of the quadriceps femoris muscle

5. **Lower back.** Quadratus lumborum, erector spinae, and lower latissimus dorsi muscles.
6. **Spine.** Erector spinae, quadratus lumborum, latissimus dorsi, rhomboids, and trapezius muscles.
7. **Shoulders.** Latissimus dorsi, teres major and minor, infraspinatus, subscapularis, deltoid, serratus anterior, and pectoralis major muscles.
8. **Arms.** Biceps and triceps brachii muscles. Flexor and extensor muscles of the forearm.

Platform and springboard diving

It is suggested that competitive platform and springboard diving places frequent stress on the wrist, shoulder, and lumbar spine (Rubin 1999).

Suggested areas to massage for platform and springboard divers (Fig. 5.10)

1. **Ankles and calves.** Triceps surae, peroneal, tibialis posterior, and tibialis anterior muscles.
2. **Thighs.** Quadriceps femoris, adductors, and hamstring muscles.
3. **Lower back.** Quadratus lumborum, erector spinae, and lower latissimus dorsi muscles.
4. **Spine.** Erector spinae, latissimus dorsi, rhomboids, and trapezius muscles.
5. **Neck.** Splenius capitis, splenius cervicis, trapezius, levator scapulae, and suboccipital muscle group.
6. **Shoulders.** Teres major and minor, infraspinatus, subscapularis, serratus anterior, and pectoralis major muscles.
7. **Arms, wrists, and hands.** Triceps brachii, biceps brachii, flexor and extensor muscles of the forearm, and the muscles of the hands.

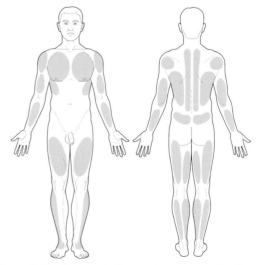

Figure 5.10 • Suggested areas to massage for divers

Golf

The major stress on the body is presented during the actual swing in golf. The movement is repetitive and one sided, which generates an uneven stress on the body. The focus is on the hips, spine, shoulders, and arms.

Suggested areas to massage for golfers (Fig. 5.11)

1. **Ankles and calves.** Triceps surae, peroneal, and tibialis anterior muscles.
2. **Knees and thighs.** Quadriceps femoris, adductors, and hamstring muscles.
3. **Hips.** Gluteus medius and minimus, TFL, and iliopsoas muscles.
4. **Spine.** Erector spinae (Fig. 5.12), quadratus lumborum, latissimus dorsi, rhomboids, and trapezius muscles.
5. **Shoulders.** Teres major and minor, infraspinatus, subscapularis, deltoid, serratus anterior, and pectoralis major muscles.
6. **Neck.** Splenius capitis and cervicis, trapezius, levator scapulae, and suboccipital muscle group.
7. **Forearms.** Flexor and extensor muscles.
8. **Hands.** Muscles in the palms of the hands.

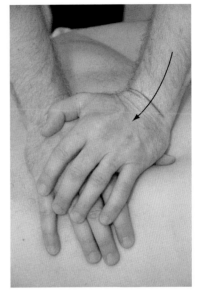

Figure 5.12 • Thumb edging of the erector spinae muscle

Dance

Suggested areas to massage for dancers (Fig. 5.13)

1. **Feet.** Plantar aspect.
2. **Ankle and calves.** Triceps surae, peroneal, and tibialis anterior muscles (Fig. 5.14).

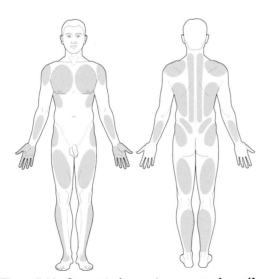

Figure 5.11 • Suggested areas to massage for golfers

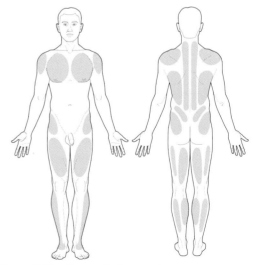

Figure 5.13 • Suggested areas to massage for dancers

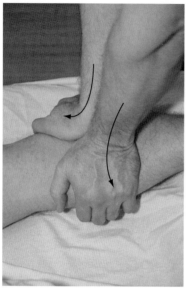

Figure 5.14 • Broadening of the gastrocnemius muscle

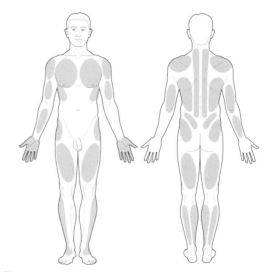

Figure 5.15 • Suggested areas to massage for tennis players

3. **Knees and thighs.** Quadriceps femoris, adductors, and hamstring muscles.
4. **Hips.** Gluteus maximus, medius and minimus, piriformis, gemelli, obturators, quadratus femoris, TFL, and iliopsoas muscles.
5. **Spine.** Erector spinae, quadratus lumborum, latissimus dorsi, rhomboids, and trapezius muscles.
6. **Shoulders.** Latissimus dorsi, teres major and minor, infraspinatus, subscapularis, deltoid, serratus anterior, and pectoralis major muscles.
7. **Neck.** Trapezius, levator scapulae, splenius capitis and cervicis, and suboccipital muscle group.

Tennis

Tennis is an explosive sport that places great stress on joints like ankles, knees, hips, spine, shoulders, elbows, and wrists. Besides focusing on the muscles considered prime movers, attention is also placed on stabilizing muscles such as serratus anterior and lower trapezius (Kibler et al. 2007).

Suggested areas to massage for tennis players (Fig. 5.15)

1. **Feet.** Plantar aspect.
2. **Ankles and calves.** Triceps surae, peroneal, and tibialis anterior muscles (Fig. 5.16).

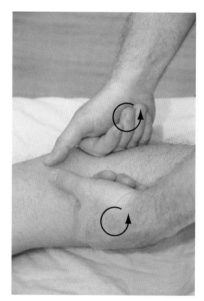

Figure 5.16 • Fist frictions of the triceps surae group

3. **Legs, including knees and thighs.** Quadriceps femoris, adductors, and hamstring muscles.
4. **Gluteal and hip area.** Gluteus maximus, medius and minimus, piriformis, TFL, and iliopsoas muscles (Fig. 5.17).
5. **Spine.** Erector spinae, quadratus lumborum, latissimus dorsi, rhomboids, and trapezius muscles.

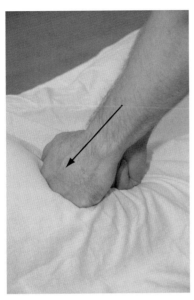

Figure 5.17 • Fist compressions of the gluteal muscles

6. **Shoulder.** Latissimus dorsi, teres major and minor, infraspinatus, subscapularis, deltoid, serratus anterior, and pectoralis major muscles.
7. **Arms.** Biceps and triceps brachii muscles. Flexor and extensor muscles of the forearm.
8. **Forearm.** Flexor and extensor muscles.
9. **Hand.** Muscles in the palm of the hands.

Skiing

Downhill skiing may generate stress on areas like the legs, knees, hips, and back, but injuries additionally include the head, shoulders, arms, wrists, and hands.

Suggested areas to massage for downhill skiing and snowboarding (Fig. 5.18)

1. **Legs, including knees and thighs.** Quadriceps femoris, adductors, and hamstring muscles.
2. **Gluteal and hip area.** Gluteus maximus, medius and minimus, piriformis, TFL, and iliopsoas muscles.
3. **Spine.** Erector spinae, quadratus lumborum, latissimus dorsi, rhomboids, and trapezius muscles.

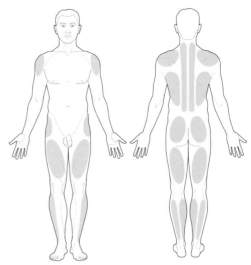

Figure 5.18 • Suggested areas to massage for downhill skiers

Suggested areas to massage for cross-country skiers (Fig. 5.19)

1. **Ankles and calves.** Triceps surae, peroneal, and tibialis anterior muscles (Fig. 5.20).
2. **Legs, including knees and thighs.** Quadriceps femoris, adductors, and hamstring muscles.
3. **Gluteal and hip area.** Gluteus maximus, medius and minimus, piriformis, TFL, and iliopsoas muscles.

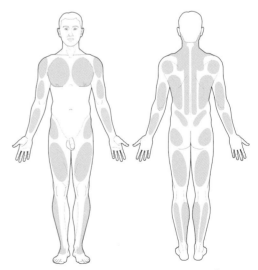

Figure 5.19 • Suggested areas to massage for cross-country skiers

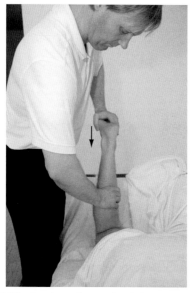

Figure 5.20 • Lock and stretch of the soleus muscle

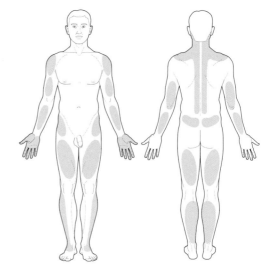

Figure 5.21 • Suggested areas to massage for cyclists

4. **Spine, with focus on the lower back.** Erector spinae, quadratus lumborum, latissimus dorsi, rhomboids, and trapezius muscles.
5. **Shoulder.** Latissimus dorsi, teres major and minor, infraspinatus, subscapularis, deltoid, serratus anterior, and pectoralis major muscles.
6. **Arms.** Biceps and triceps brachii muscles. Flexor and extensor muscles of the forearm.

Cycling

Great areas of stress for cyclists are the legs, hips, back, and neck. Mountain bikers may additionally further stress the arms, wrists, and hands due to the different riding style and rougher terrain conditions.

Suggested areas to massage for cyclists (Fig. 5.21)

1. **Ankles and calves.** Triceps surae, peroneal (Fig. 5.22), and tibialis anterior muscles.
2. **Legs, including knees and thighs.** Quadriceps femoris, adductors, hamstring, TFL, and iliopsoas muscles.
3. **Spine, with focus on the lower back.** Erector spinae, quadratus lumborum, latissimus dorsi, rhomboids, and trapezius muscles.

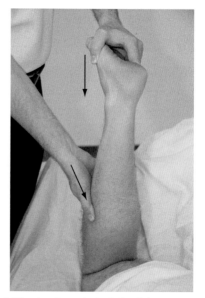

Figure 5.22 • Lock and stretch of the peroneal muscle group

4. **Shoulder.** Latissimus dorsi, teres major and minor, infraspinatus, subscapularis, deltoid, serratus anterior, and pectoralis major muscles.
5. **Neck.** Trapezius, levator scapulae, splenius capitis and cervicis, and suboccipital muscle group.
6. **Arms and hands.** Biceps, triceps brachii, and flexor and extensor muscles of the forearm, including the palmar muscles of the hands.

Baseball

Baseball may place great stress on the legs, hips, back, and shoulders, and baseball pitchers have more stress on the spine, throwing arm's shoulder, and elbow.

Suggested areas to massage for baseball players (Fig. 5.23)

1. **Ankles and calves.** Triceps surae, peroneal, and tibialis anterior muscles.
2. **Legs, including knees and thighs.** Quadriceps femoris, adductors, hamstring (Fig. 5.24), and TFL muscles.
3. **Gluteal and hip area.** Gluteus maximus, medius and minimus, piriformis, TFL, and iliopsoas muscles.
4. **Spine.** Erector spinae, quadratus lumborum, latissimus dorsi, rhomboids, and trapezius muscles.
5. **Abdomen.** Abdominal oblique muscles.
6. **Shoulder.** Teres major and minor, infraspinatus, subscapularis, deltoid, serratus anterior, and pectoralis major muscles.
7. **Arms and hands.** Biceps, triceps brachii, and flexor and extensor muscles of the forearm, including the palmar muscles of the hands.

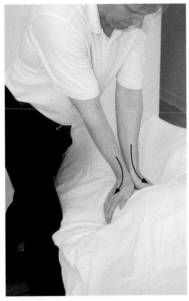

Figure 5.24 • Palm broadening of the hamstring muscles

Basketball

Suggested areas to massage for basketball players (Fig. 5.25)

1. **Feet.** Plantar aspect of the feet (Fig. 5.26).
2. **Ankles and calves.** Triceps surae, peroneal, and tibialis anterior muscles.

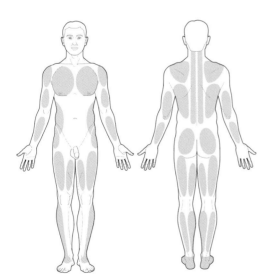

Figure 5.23 • Suggested areas to massage for baseball players

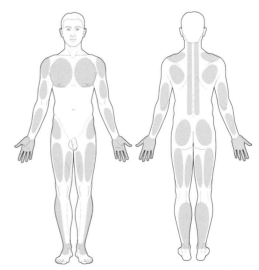

Figure 5.25 • Suggested areas to massage for basketball players

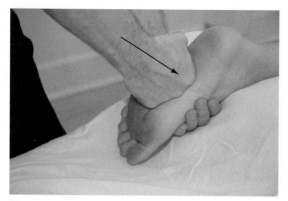

Figure 5.26 • Fist compression of the foot

3. **Legs, including knees and thighs.** Quadriceps femoris, adductors, and hamstring muscles.
4. **Gluteal and hip area.** Gluteus maximus, medius and minimus, piriformis, and TFL muscles.
5. **Spine.** Erector spinae, quadratus lumborum, latissimus dorsi, rhomboids, and trapezius muscles.
6. **Shoulder.** Teres major and minor, infraspinatus, subscapularis, deltoid, and pectoralis major and minor muscles.
7. **Arms and hands.** Triceps brachii, biceps brachii, flexor and extensor muscles of the forearms, hands.

Ice hockey

Ice hockey is both a sport with very intense activity periods and substantial physical contact. Major stress areas are the legs (particularly the adductors), hips, lower back, neck, and shoulder area. It is suggested that therapeutically strengthening the adductor muscle group seems to be an effective way to prevent adductor strains in professional ice hockey players (Tyler et al. 2002). It is suggested that an ice hockey player may be roughly 17 times more likely to sustain an adductor muscle strain if the adductor strength is less than 80% of the abductor strength (Tyler et al. 2001).

Suggested areas to massage for ice hockey players (Fig. 5.27)

1. **Feet.** Plantar aspect of the feet.
2. **Ankles and calves.** Triceps surae, peroneal, and tibialis anterior muscles.
3. **Legs, including knees and thighs.** Quadriceps femoris, adductors, and hamstring muscles.

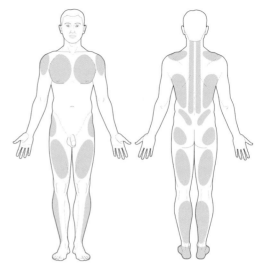

Figure 5.27 • Suggested areas to massage for ice hockey players

4. **Gluteal and hip area.** Gluteus maximus, medius and minimus, piriformis, and TFL muscles (Fig. 5.28).
5. **Spine.** Erector spinae, quadratus lumborum, latissimus dorsi, rhomboids, and trapezius muscles.
6. **Shoulder.** Teres major and minor, infraspinatus, subscapularis, deltoid, and pectoralis major and minor muscles.

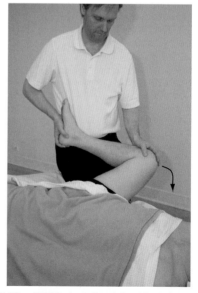

Figure 5.28 • ROM stretch of the hip joint

Soccer

Soccer players' major stress areas are the legs, i.e. ankles, knees, quadriceps, hamstring, and adductor muscles. It is suggested that 6 weeks' strength training emphasizing the hamstring muscles helps prevention of ACL injuries (Cross & Worell 1999). Hamstring strengthening exercises may additionally reduce the frequency and severity of hamstring injuries sustained during training or competition (Holocomb et al. 2007). Muscle strains in soccer additionally frequently affect players with muscle tightness (Ekstrand & Gillquist 1983).

Suggested areas to massage for soccer players (Fig. 5.29)

1. **Feet.** Plantar aspect of the feet.
2. **Ankles and calves.** Triceps surae, peroneal, and tibialis anterior muscles.
3. **Legs, including knees and thighs.** Quadriceps femoris, adductors, and hamstring muscles (Fig. 5.30).
4. **Gluteal and hip area.** Gluteus maximus, medius and minimus, piriformis, and TFL muscles.
5. **Spine, with focus on the lower back.** Erector spinae, quadratus lumborum, latissimus dorsi, rhomboids, and trapezius muscles.
6. **Shoulder.** Infraspinatus, teres minor, subscapularis, deltoid, and pectoralis major and minor muscles.

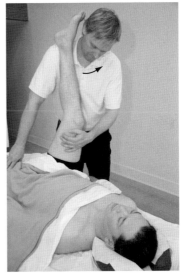

Figure 5.30 • Hamstring stretch

Football and rugby

Suggested areas to massage for football and rugby players (Fig. 5.31)

1. **Ankles and calves.** Triceps surae, peroneal, and tibialis anterior muscles (Fig. 5.32).

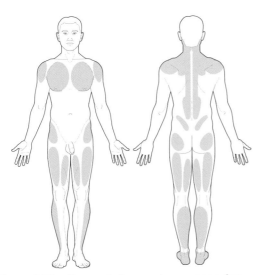

Figure 5.29 • Suggested areas to massage for soccer players

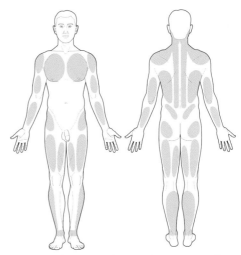

Figure 5.31 • Suggested areas to massage for football and rugby players

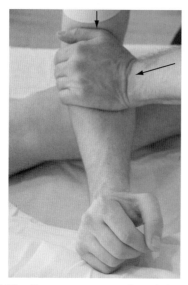

Figure 5.32 • Forearm compression of the gastrocnemius muscle

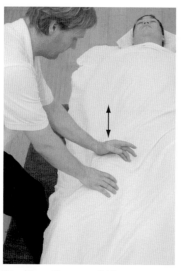

Figure 5.33 • Hypothenar rubbing of the quadriceps femoris muscle

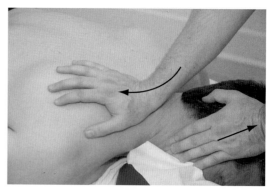

Figure 5.34 • Lower neck release

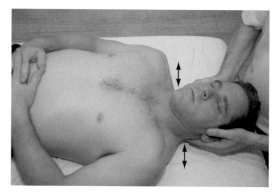

Figure 5.35 • General neck release

2. **Legs, including knees and thighs.** Quadriceps femoris (Fig. 5.33), adductors, and hamstring muscles.
3. **Gluteal and hip area.** Gluteus maximus, medius and minimus, piriformis, and TFL muscles.
4. **Spine.** Erector spinae, quadratus lumborum, latissimus dorsi, rhomboids, and trapezius muscles.
5. **Shoulder.** Infraspinatus, teres minor, deltoid, and pectoralis major and minor muscles.
6. **Neck.** Trapezius, levator scapulae, splenius capitis and cervicis, and suboccipital muscle group (Figs 5.34; 5.35). One hand fixates the athlete's head in a position of lateral flexion and ipsilateral rotation, whilst the other hand performs gentle circular petrissage with the palm heel. The therapist places the fingertips at the C7 level, posterior to the athlete's transverse processes. The therapist then gently and rhythmically slides the neck from side to side, increasing the lateral flexion in the neck. The movement works upward, segment by segment, until the entire neck is treated and relaxation is observed.
7. **Arms and hands.** Biceps, triceps brachii, flexor and extensor muscles of the forearm, and the palmar aspect of the hands.

References

Alter, M., 2004. Science of flexibility, third ed. Human Kinetics, Champaign, IL.

Cross, K.M., Worell, T.W., 1999. Effects of a static stretching program on the incidence of lower extremity musculotendinous strains. J. Athl. Train. 34 (1), 11–14.

Ekstrand, J., Gillquist, J., 1983. The avoidability of soccer injuries. Int. J. Sports Med. 4 (2), 124–128.

Hartig, D.E., Henderson, J.M., 1999. Increasing hamstring flexibility decreases lower extremity overuse injuries in military basic trainees. Am. J. Sports Med. 27 (2), 173–176.

Holocomb, W.R., et al., 2007. Effect of hamstring-emphasized resistance training on hamstring:quadriceps strength ratios. J. Strength Cond. Res. 21 (1), 41–47.

Kibler, W.B., et al., 2007. Muscle activation in coupled scapulohumeral motions in the high performance tennis serve. Br. J. Sports Med. 41, 745–749.

McHugh, M.P., et al., 1999. The role of passive muscle stiffness in symptoms of exercise-induced muscle damage. Am. J. Sports Med. 27 (5), 594–599.

Meagher, J., Broughton, P., 1990. Sports massage. Station Hill Press, Barrytown, NY.

Moraska, A., 2005. Sports massage. A comprehensive review. J. Sports Med. Phys. Fitness 45 (3), 370–380.

Rubin, B.D., 1999. The basics of competitive diving and its injuries. Clin. Sports Med. 18 (2), 293–303.

Tyler, T.F., et al., 2001. The association of hip strength and flexibility with the incidence of adductor muscle strains in professional ice hockey players. Am. J. Sports Med. 29 (2), 124–128.

Tyler, T.F., et al., 2002. The effectiveness of a preseason exercise program to prevent adductor muscle strains in professional ice hockey players. Am. J. Sports Med. 30 (5), 680–683.

Soft tissue stretching in sports massage

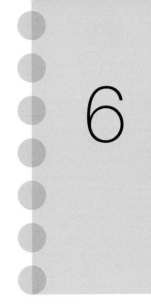

6

Therapeutic muscle stretching can be described as a voluntary lengthening of muscle and connective tissue with the overall goal of increasing general flexibility and/or range of motion (ROM) about the affected joint(s). Stretching and flexibility are concepts perceived to be deeply integrated with sports-related performance. Each type of sport has its own demands, and every athlete has their own personal flexibility requirements as one of the components for optimal athletic performance. Even though stretching is often viewed as the means to increase mobility, flexibility can be achieved in a variety of ways where muscle stretching is one common method.

It has been indicated that chronic static stretching exercises by themselves can improve specific exercise performance (Kokkonen et al. 2007), but it is also suggested that relatively extensive static stretching decreases power performance (Yamaguchi et al. 2006), and both static and proprioceptive neuromuscular facilitation stretching have been seen to cause similar deficits in strength, power output, and muscle activation at both slow and fast velocities (Marek et al. 2005). One study indicated that the loss of force after static stretching is not related to time, but even a short duration of static stretching caused loss of force (Brandenburg 2006). Trained athletes, however, seem to be less susceptible to a stretching-induced force deficit compared with untrained nonathletic individuals (Egan et al. 2006), especially if incorporating adequate warm-up and dynamic sport-specific actions, with a minimum of 5 minutes of recovery, before sport activity commences (Chaouachi et al. 2010). Another study proposes that static stretching has no negative effect on maximal eccentric isokinetic torque or power production, nor does it change

the degree of muscle activation (Cramer et al. 2007), and that moderate static stretching does not have a negative effect on performance in all muscle groups (Winke et al. 2010). It has also been indicated that utilizing CRAC, static, or active control techniques during stretching can increase and retain ROM prior to physical activity (Ford & McChesney 2007) and create some gains in muscular performance (Ferreira et al. 2007). CRAC has also shown to be a useful modality for improving postural stability, either alone or in combination with other warm-up routines (Ryan et al. 2010).

Even though some research has indicated that stretching techniques used as a specific modality during warm-up, within 15 min of athletic activity, can be helpful as a means of decreasing the risk of muscle injuries (Woods et al. 2007), it is rarely used alone as an instrument for improved performance or injury prevention. In some instances, stretching exercises can even cause certain types of strain injury, even when performed slowly (Askling et al. 2007). A combination of general and sports-specific strength, coordination, warm-up, and stretching exercises may create better, more consistent results. The general consensus today is that dynamic stretching exercises are preferred over static stretch methods prior to sports performance (Needham et al. 2009; Sekir et al. 2010; Fletcher & Monte-Colombo 2010).

Flexibility

The literal description of the word "flexibility" is "ability to bend," (McKean 2005) and the term "flexible" applies to "whatever can be bent without

DOI: 10.1016/B978-0-443-10126-7.00006-X

breaking" (McKean 2005). The exact definition of normal flexibility is somewhat disputed, but a generally adopted definition is that flexibility is the amount of ROM in or around a joint or group of joints (Alter 2004). Measurement of ROM in a joint is called goniometry, and it can be assessed in either linear (cm/in) or angular (degrees) units (Alter 2004). To better understand and assess an athlete's "true" ROM in various joints, flexibility is divided into a few subcategories, some more frequently used than others.

Static flexibility

Alter (2004) describes static flexibility as the amount of ROM about a joint with no emphasis on speed. It is considered by some to be difficult to obtain accurate objective readings of static flexibility since either the stretch subject or tester assesses the amount subjectively (Alter 2004).

Static passive flexibility is described by Kurz (1991) as the ability to assume and maintain extended positions by using one's body weight without assistance from additional external measures (Fig. 6.1).

Static active flexibility is described as the capability to execute and hold extended positions using only muscle power (Kurz 1991); i.e. agonistic and synergistic muscles will move the affected joint(s) and thus stretch the antagonistic muscles. Static active flexibility assessment can also be a useful tool to measure muscle strength vs. soft tissue flexibility ratios, which may be valuable from a perspective of potential injury prevention. Great flexibility about a joint without sufficient active stabilization from strong conditioned muscles may create imbalances, potentially leading to an elevated injury risk during sports activity.

When the adductor muscle group is assessed, the muscles generating hip abduction will bring the leg as

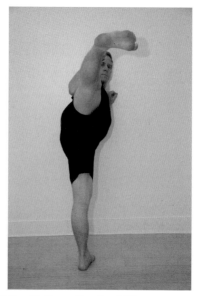

Figure 6.2 • Static active flexibility

far into hip abduction as possible whilst maintaining the knee joint extended (Fig. 6.2).

Dynamic flexibility

Dynamic flexibility can be defined as the ability to perform a range of joint movement during physical activity at either "normal or rapid speed" (Alter 2004) (Fig. 6.3). It is also described as the ability to execute dynamic movements in the joints at full

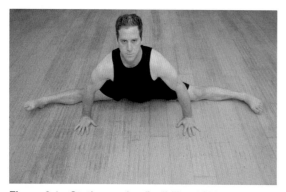

Figure 6.1 • Static passive flexibility, "Chinese splits"

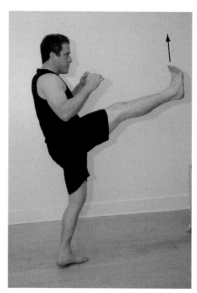

Figure 6.3 • Fast dynamic flexibility

ROM (Kurz 1991). Dynamic flexibility may often create an increase in ROM over static flexibility, since the momentum and weight of the body part (lever) can create additional stretch in the tissue. Slower dynamic movements, like controllably lifting the leg out in a stretch, are also called "functional flexibility" (Alter 2004).

Ballistic flexibility (Fig. 6.4)

Ballistic flexibility is measurement of ROM during faster and more forceful movements, which can be referred to as "bouncing, rebounding, and rhythmic motion" (Alter 2004).

Stretching

Static stretching

Static stretching (Fig. 6.5) is probably the form of muscle stretching most well known to the general public. It is sometimes referred to as "yoga type" stretching, and albeit not fully correct, this term makes the stretch easier to relate to. Yoga often involves poses which additionally trigger contractions in other muscle groups, thus stimulating supplementary relaxation through reflexes such as reciprocal inhibition (Box 6.1). Static stretching has been

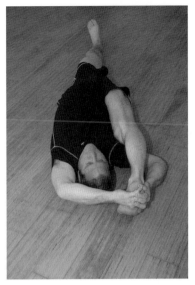

Figure 6.5 • Static stretching • A static stretch involves slowly stretching a muscle or muscle group to the end point, which is where a good stretch is felt, and the stretched target muscle begins to contract as the stretch/myotatic reflex (see Box 6.3) is triggered. The muscle stretch is held in this position while slow and relaxed breathing is continued

Box 6.1

Reciprocal inhibition/innervation
When one muscle contracts, the antagonistic muscle will relax; e.g. if the biceps brachii muscle contracts, the triceps brachii muscle will relax via the reflex named reciprocal inhibition. This is controlled by inhibitory neurons located in the spinal cord (Alter 2004). This reflex is also called Sherrington's law II, from the founder Sir Charles Scott Sherrington's previous research. If one muscle is stretched, its antagonist will also temporarily relax.

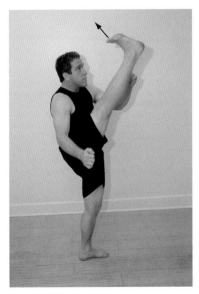

Figure 6.4 • Ballistic flexibility

shown to decrease passive resistive torque during isokinetic passive motion of the ankle joint. It is suggested that regular static stretching exercises by themselves can improve specific exercise performances after 10 weeks (Kokkonen et al. 2007). It has also been presented that a significant increase in hamstring length can be sustained for up to 24 h when using static stretching (de Weijer et al. 2003). A study on prepubertal school children additionally suggests that the build-up of stretching frequency is effective for increasing ROM. Subjects utilizing static stretching four days/week had bigger flexibility gains compared to those that only stretched two times/week (Santonja Medina et al. 2007).

A static stretch involves slowly stretching a muscle/muscle group to the end point, which is where a good stretch is felt, and the stretched target muscle begins to contract as the stretch/myotatic reflex is triggered (Box 6.2). The muscle stretch is held in this position while slow and relaxed breathing is continued (see Fig. 6.5). As the stretch reflex reduces and the muscle relaxes, the stretch is gently taken further until the new end point is reached. This cycle generally continues for 30 s up to 2 min, but can be prolonged in some situations.

Box 6.2

Muscle contraction types

1. **Isometric muscle contraction.** A contraction where the muscle keeps the same length despite increasing tension. There is also no movement in the joint during this contraction.
2. **Isotonic muscle contraction.** A contraction where the tension in the muscle remains unchanged despite a change in muscle length. This takes place when a muscle's maximal contractile force exceeds the total load placed on the muscle. Isotonic contraction is subdivided into concentric and eccentric muscle contraction.
   a. **Concentric muscle contraction.** The force generated by the contraction is sufficient to overcome the added resistance. This makes the muscle shorten as it contracts.
   b. **Eccentric muscle contraction.** The force generated by the contraction is insufficient to overcome the generated resistance. This makes the muscle lengthen as it contracts.
3. **Isokinetic muscle contraction.** The muscle contracts and shortens at a constant rate of speed, despite possible changes in external resistance.
4. **Isolytic muscle contraction.** A muscle lengthens involuntarily during its contraction, and the applied external force is substantially greater than the contractile force from the muscle. This contraction form can be used therapeutically to break down fibrotic tissue in a muscle (see Isolytic MET).

Passive stretching

Passive stretching is when a therapist or an outside force, like a stretch machine or external weight, performs the actual stretch phase. Passive stretching has many benefits for an athlete, especially if the source is a well-educated and experienced sports therapist. It is easier for the athlete to relax into the stretch and a good therapist knows just how far to stretch the muscle to achieve maximal effect. If a therapist is performing static stretching on an athlete, it is called passive static stretching.

The therapist stretches the muscle to the end point where the stretched target muscle mildly begins to contract as the stretch/myotatic reflex is triggered. The muscle stretch is held in this position while slow and relaxed breathing is continued (Fig. 6.6). As the stretch reflex reduces and the muscle relaxes, the stretch is gently taken further until the new end point is reached. This cycle generally continues for 30 s up to 2 min, but can be prolonged in some situations.

Dynamic stretching

Dynamic stretching can generally be defined as stretching during motion. It has been suggested that dynamic stretching can enhance muscular performance, whereas the same study found that static stretching for 30 s neither improved nor reduced the level of muscular performance (Yamaguchi & Ishii 2005).

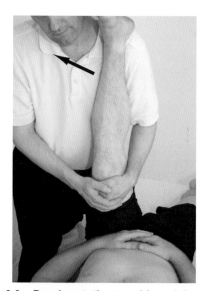

Figure 6.6 • Passive static stretching of the hamstring muscle group

Neural mechanisms play a significant role in increased ROM about a joint from stretching exercises (Guissard & Duchateau 2006), and perhaps a "priming" of the nervous system from increased proprioceptive feedback, stimulated by the movement during dynamic stretching, forms a contributing factor to enhancements in muscular performance (Fletcher & Anness 2007). Due to the beneficial effects of dynamic stretching exercises, it can be recommended to include this form of stretching during warm-up routines prior to athletic performance (MacMillan et al. 2006).

Dynamic stretching is executed by repeatedly and gradually stretching the muscles to the end point by gently using the weight and momentum of the body part (Fig. 6.7).

To safely use this stretching application, it is recommended to start gently and "lead" the body part by simultaneously contracting the antagonistic muscles, e.g. when the ischiocrural/hamstring muscle group is stretched, hip flexors like the rectus femoris and iliopsoas muscles can actively guide the leg upward. The use of antagonistic muscles will activate additional muscle relaxation in the target muscle through the reciprocal inhibition reflex. The ROM is progressively increased as the soft tissue stretches and loosens with each repetition. Dynamic stretching is not forceful, but rather allows the body to gradually increase ROM through each repetition.

Ballistic stretching

Ballistic stretching, a more forceful form of stretching during movement, is when a relaxed muscle is stretched more forcefully beyond its normal ROM. It is usually avoided during regular therapeutic stretching, due to the fear of an increased injury risk and the likelihood of activating the myotatic reflex, which elicits increased muscle contractions during the stretch. In athletic circumstances the conditioning and demands are a bit different, and ballistic stretching has a few important functions. Most involved movements during sports activity are ballistic in nature, and it may be important to prime the nervous system for this type of upcoming movement intensity. It is suggested that ballistic stretching can increase tendon elasticity significantly, something that can have major clinical importance for the treatment and prevention of tendon injuries (Mahieu et al. 2007; Rees et al. 2007; Witvouv et al. 2007). Ballistic stretching has also been shown to increase jump height for basketball players. Test subjects used either static stretching, static stretching with warm-up, warm-up alone, or ballistic stretching. Only the ballistic stretching group showed an acute increase in vertical jump height 20 min after playing basketball (Woolstenhulme et al. 2006).

The leg is rapidly and fairly forcefully lifted in a series of repetitions (Fig. 6.8). It is important

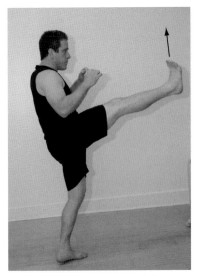

Figure 6.7 • Dynamic stretching of the hamstring muscles

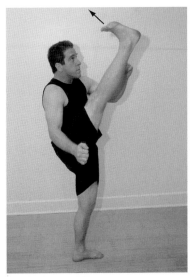

Figure 6.8 • Ballistic stretching of the hamstring muscles

to note that ballistic stretching, whilst performed more explosively, should still contain an element of control.

Active stretching

Active stretching, also named static active stretching, should perhaps be viewed as more as a strength training and neuromuscular reeducation/coordination exercise than a pure soft tissue stretch. It can however serve as an important part of flexibility training since strengthened, conditioned muscles around a joint may make it more balanced, which ideally renders more protection against injuries.

Static active stretching (Alter 1996, Kurtz 1991) is where an antagonistic target muscle is stretched by activation of agonistic and synergistic muscles. For example, the hip flexors, foremost the iliopsoas and rectus femoris muscles, are activated to move the leg into flexion (Fig. 6.9). Once the maximal position is reached, the body part is temporarily held in a static position for 10–15 seconds.

Dynamic active stretching is a variation where an antagonistic target muscle is stretched, in a series of repetitions, by activation of agonistic and synergistic muscles. This modification can also be performed with ballistic movements (Alter 1996). If an external weight or resistance is applied, the term "resistive" may be used. If only the weight of the body part is utilized, the term "free" applies (Alter 1996). Thus a

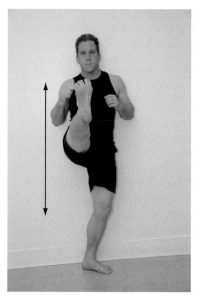

Figure 6.10 • Dynamic active stretching of the hamstring muscles

repetitive active stretch with additional external force would be named resistive dynamic/ballistic active stretching. For example, in dynamic active stretching of the hamstring muscles, the hip flexors, foremost the iliopsoas and rectus femoris muscles, are activated to repetitively move the leg into flexion (Fig. 6.10). Once the maximal position is reached, the leg is slowly lowered toward the start position. The number of repetitions will vary depending on the muscles' condition, the amount of weight/resistance used, and target goal of the exercise.

Proprioceptive neuromuscular facilitation (PNF)

PNF was originally developed by Dr. Herman Kabat as a method for stroke rehabilitation, often combining movement patterns through three planes of movement, e.g. flexion, abduction, rotation. Kabat based part of the PNF theories on three rules generated from previous research by Charles Sherrington (McAtee 1993).

Successive induction

This method involves isotonic or isometric contraction of one muscle, immediately followed by contraction of its antagonist. Sherrington was of the opinion

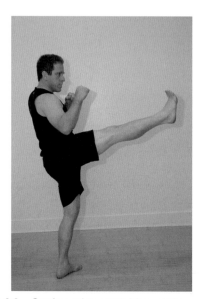

Figure 6.9 • Static active stretching of the hamstring muscles

that this enhances flexibility, i.e. flexion will enhance extension ability, etc. (McAtee 1993).

Reciprocal inhibition

Contraction of one muscle temporarily inhibits the contraction ability of its antagonist; e.g. contraction of the quadriceps muscles will inhibit the ischiocrural/hamstring muscle group and thereby render them in a more relaxed state (McAtee 1993) (see Box 6.1).

Irradiation

When maximal muscle contraction is executed against applied resistance, the excitation from the contracting muscle "irradiates" to nearby synergistic muscles, thus activating them to help overcome the resistance (McAtee 1993).

Besides demonstrating improved rehabilitation results, PNF also revealed flexibility benefits, which is one major reason some of these techniques quickly became popular within athletic training and injury rehabilitation regimens. For instance, it is indicated that static and dynamic PNF programs may be appropriate for improving short-term trunk muscle endurance and trunk mobility (Kofotolis & Kellis 2006). Utilizing hold-relax (HR) revealed a substantial improvement in ROM in the hip joint, compared with the baseline measurements. The application of the findings suggests that clinicians could choose any of the hold times and produce the same result in the patient (Bonnar et al. 2004). Another study suggests that PNF stretching is a useful modality for increasing a joint's ROM and strength (Rees et al. 2007).

A series of techniques is incorporated under the collective name PNF, and as modifications later emerged, a distinction was made between the original PNF and newer "modified PNF" stretching techniques. These techniques commonly utilize muscle contractions prior to and during the stretch to minimize the myotatic reflex from the muscle spindles (Box 6.3) and benefit from muscle-relaxing effects from the inverse myotatic reflex/autogenic inhibition (Box 6.4), and reciprocal inhibition reflex.

During all stretches involving muscle contractions, it is advisable not to hold the breath, but instead breathe normally during the contraction phase.

Holding the breath could elevate the blood pressure unnecessarily, and should be avoided during the treatment.

Slow reversal (SR) (Voss et al. 1985; Alter 2004)

This technique involves the patient moving an extremity through the desired range of motion with continuous resistance. No rest periods occur between the isotonic contractions; i.e. the therapist applies graded resistance to the patient's extremity as it moves from a starting position through the desired ROM. The therapist later applies immediate reversed graded resistance as the patient returns the extremity toward the starting position.

Rhythmic stabilization (RS) (Voss et al. 1985; Alter 2004)

RS is the application of an isometric contraction of muscles performing an agonistic movement pattern, immediately followed by an isometric contraction of the muscles creating the antagonistic movement pattern. The power of the contractions is steadily increased as the ROM is gradually decreased during the complete treatment cycle.

RS may contribute to increased blood circulation to the area thanks to the use of isometric muscle contractions, and equally create a build-up of holding power and stabilization of the trunk, hip, and shoulder girdle. In RS, the patient should simply resist movements utilizing isometric muscle contractions against the manual resistance from the therapist. For example, the therapist can apply simultaneous resistance to the anterior left shoulder and posterior right shoulder or hip for 2–3 s before altering the resistance to the posterior left shoulder and the anterior right shoulder or hip. The movements should preferably be smooth and continuous. RS can be performed at any point of available ROM.

Contract–relax (CR)

CR is normally performed at the end point of a muscle. This is where a good stretch is felt without any unpleasant pain. CR consists of isotonic contractions

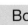

Box 6.3

Muscle spindle

Muscle spindles can be defined as small, spindle-shaped sensory receptors located in skeletal muscle tissue (Fig. 6.11), and they run parallel to the main muscle fibers (extrafusal fibers). A muscle spindle consists of several differentiated muscle fibers (intrafusal fibers) that are enclosed in a spindle-shaped connective tissue sac. The ends of the intrafusal fibers are contractile, but the central portion is noncontractile and innervated by special neurons named gamma motor neurons. Muscle spindles are sensitive to both the phasic stretch (the rate at which a muscle stretches) and the tonic stretch (the extent to which the muscle is stretched). Stimulation of muscle spindles elicits a contraction in the stretched muscle (myotatic reflex, i.e. stretch reflex) and at the same time inhibits action potentials to antagonistic muscles. The muscle spindles also participate in regulating the muscle tone.

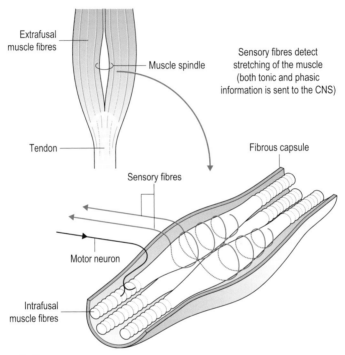

Figure 6.11 • Muscle spindle

of muscles responsible for an antagonistic pattern, followed by passive motion in the agonistic movement pattern. The overall goal of this particular technique is to achieve relaxation of the muscles responsible for agonistic movement pattern where active motion cannot be performed from the stretch range of the same agonistic movement pattern.

1. The hamstring muscles are stretched to the end point.
2. The athlete is asked to perform an isotonic contraction ("push" or "pull") against maximal resistance from the therapist.

3. The athlete is then asked to relax, and the target muscle is stretched in the agonistic movement pattern to the new end point of the muscle (Fig. 6.13). This procedure is repeated many times (Voss et al. 1985). If the athlete is not able to initiate the contraction from the stretched position, they can execute contractions with active motion in the agonistic movement pattern after each contract–relax sequence. This will trigger additional relaxation in the stretched muscle through the reciprocal inhibition reflex.

Box 6.4

Golgi tendon organ (GTO)/neurotendinous spindle

The GTO relays information about force levels in the muscle or tendon to the central nervous system. It consists of small inhibitory mechanoreceptors located near the junction of the muscle and tendon, and monitors the amount of tensile force placed on the tendon structure. Each Golgi tendon organ consists of small bundles of tendon fibers enclosed in a layered capsule with dendrites (fine branches of neurons) coiling between and around the fibers (Fig. 6.12). The organ is activated by muscular contractions or a stretch of the tendons. This results in an inhibition of alpha motor neurons innervating the contractile elements of the same striated skeletal muscle, causing the muscle to relax, and thereby protecting the muscle and connective tissue from excessive loading and potential injury. This reflex is named "inverse myotatic reflex," or "autogenic inhibition." It was once believed that the GTOs were stimulated only by prolonged muscle stretches, but today GTOs are also often considered to be sensitive detectors of tension in specific portions of a muscle (Patrick et al. 1982; Mileusnic & Loeb 2006).

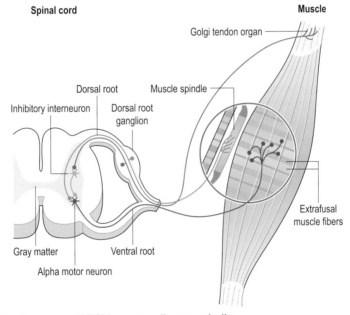

Figure 6.12 • Golgi tendon organ (GTO)/neurotendinous spindle

Hold–relax (HR)

HR can be used at any part of the ROM where a limitation in movement presents itself as muscle spasm as a result of pain. It involves an isometric muscle contraction against maximal resistance. It follows the same pattern as the CR stretch, but the athlete is instructed to "hold" instead of "push" or "pull" (Voss et al. 1985).

Modified CR

1. Here, the target muscle is stretched to its end point, where a good stretch is felt but without any sensation of unpleasant pain.

2. The athlete initiates a moderate isometric muscle contraction of the target muscle against a resistance for 6–10 s.

3. As the athlete is instructed to take a deep breath and exhale during the relaxation phase, the muscle is stretched out to its new end point (Fig. 6.14). The stretch is held for 10–15 s, which completes one cycle. A total of three to five cycles are generally performed for each treated muscle/muscle group.

Reciprocal inhibition

Reciprocal inhibition follows the same pattern as modified contract–relax, with the difference that a moderate isometric muscle contraction of

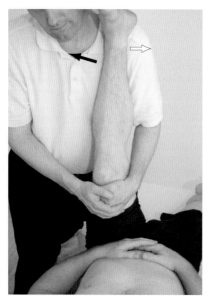

Figure 6.13 • CR of the hamstring muscles

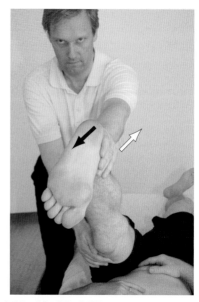

Figure 6.14 • Modified CR

the agonistic muscle(s) instead of the target muscle is executed.

1. Here, the target muscle is also stretched to its end point, where a good stretch is felt but without any sensation of unpleasant pain.
2. The athlete initiates a moderate isometric muscle contraction of the agonistic muscles against applied resistance for 6–10 s.
3. The athlete is then instructed to relax by taking a deep breath followed by an exhale, and the target muscle is stretched to its new end point (Fig. 6.15). The stretch is maintained for 10–15 s, which completes one cycle, and a total of three to five cycles are normally performed for each treated muscle/muscle group.

CRAC (contract–relax antagonist contract) (McAtee 1993)

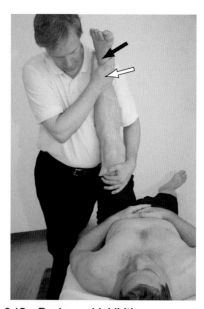

Figure 6.15 • Reciprocal inhibition

CRAC is a combination of both the CR and reciprocal inhibition stretch. It is a beneficial method to use since two reflexes will relax the target muscle. The athlete also participates more actively, which may assist the neuromuscular integration during the stretch. CRAC follows the same pattern as modified contract–relax, with the difference that the athlete actively moves the target muscle to

the new end point after each isometric contraction, by activating the agonistic muscles.

1. The target muscle is stretched to its end point, where a good stretch is felt without any sensation of unpleasant pain.
2. The athlete initiates a moderate isometric muscle contraction against applied resistance for 6–10 s.

3. The athlete is instructed to take a deep breath and exhale and immediately move the muscle out further to its new end point by activating agonist muscles (Fig. 6.16). The stretch is held here for 10–15 s. This completes one cycle, and a total of three to five cycles are normally performed for each treated muscle/muscle group.

MET stretching methods

Muscle energy techniques were developed mainly by practitioners in the osteopathic community, and over the years they have evolved into a wide range of effective soft tissue techniques. MET shares some principles with PNF, but MET stretches often use milder muscle contractions prior to the stretch, and normally have an end position that does not stretch the muscle and connective tissue as far as the end point in PNF, and modified PNF. Instead, the "barrier of resistance" is used, which is the point where resistance to movement is first noted. The milder muscle contractions and slightly gentler stretch phase aim to avoid any tendencies to cramping and/or injury during the stretch. Thanks to the milder stretch intensity, some MET techniques can hold the stretch at the barrier of resistance for a longer period of time, sometimes 45 s or more, to allow an effective but gentle elongation of the soft tissue. Despite a sometimes more gentle approach, the end results are equally impressive.

PIR/post isometric relaxation technique (Karel Lewit's modification)

Post isometric relaxation stretching was originally developed by Mitchell Jr., D.O. He suggested that immediately following an isometric muscle contraction the "neuromuscular apparatus" is in a refractory period, allowing the use of further passive stretching without interference of the myotatic reflex (Ward et al. 2002). PIR was later modified by Karel Lewit, M.D.

1. The hypertonic muscle is taken, without force or bounce, to a length just short of pain, or to the point where resistance to movement is first noted in a stretched position (Chaitow 2001). This is called the "barrier of resistance."

2. The athlete gently executes an isometric contraction of the affected hypertonic muscle for 5–10 s (Fig. 6.17). The contractile force should be only 10–20 % of the available strength. The athlete inhales during this effort (Lewit & Simons 1984).

3. Following the isometric contraction, the patient is asked to exhale and relax completely. The muscle is then stretched to the new barrier. Starting from this new barrier, the procedure is repeated two or three times. To further assist the treatment, the athlete can participate by looking in the direction

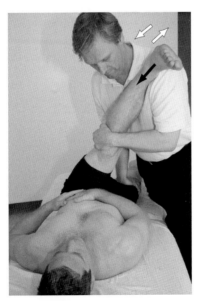

Figure 6.16 • CRAC

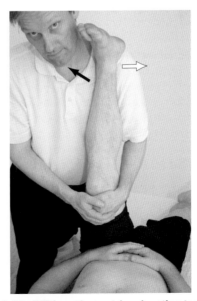

Figure 6.17 • PIR/post isometric relaxation technique

of contraction during the contraction phase, and in the direction of the stretch during the stretching phase of the therapy. Additionally, the breathing is used in the form of an inhalation during the contraction phase and an exhalation during the relaxation and stretch phase.

Reciprocal inhibition (RI)

In RI, the muscle is also moved to the barrier of resistance. The athlete is asked to try to continue the movement by mildly contracting the agonistic muscles against the therapist's resistance. The force of the isometric contraction should be only 10–20 % of available strength. The athlete is then asked to relax and exhale as the muscle is moved through its new barrier of resistance. During this motion the athlete can assist by gently contracting the agonistic muscles. This is valid for chronic problems. For acute problems the stretch is only taken to the barrier of resistance (not through it), and the athlete does not assist during the stretch phase of the treatment (Chaitow 2001).

Pulsed MET/T.J. Ruddy's rapid pulsing duction

This technique (Fig. 6.18) was originally created by T.J. Ruddy, D.O., and later refined by Leon Chaitow, D.O., N.D. By performing rhythmic and gentle isometric muscle contractions of agonistic muscles against applied resistance a gradual increase of ROM is achieved (Chaitow 2001).

1. The tensed soft tissue and/or joint are moved to its "restriction barrier" where the athlete initiates a series of rapid (2/s) small isometric contraction efforts of agonistic muscles toward the resistance barrier created by the practitioner.

2. After the initial 10 s cycles of contractions, the patient relaxes and the tissues or joint are taken to a new barrier of resistance where the process is repeated.

The application of this neural conditioning involves contractions which are short, rapid, and rhythmic with a gradual increase in the amplitude and degree of applied resistance, which is thought to recondition the proprioceptive system involved. The pulsing contractions are also assumed to create improved oxygenation and enhanced venous and lymphatic circulation in the treated area.

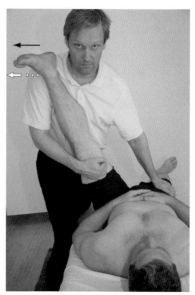

Figure 6.18 • T.J. Ruddy's rapid pulsing duction

Jandas' postfacilitation stretch method (Chaitow 2001)

Vladimir Janda, M.D., D.Sc., made a substantial contribution to the area of manual medicine and soft tissue treatment. Among his many techniques, the post facilitation stretch method (Fig. 6.19) is one example of a stretch method well suited for athletes. The treated muscle is placed in a position about halfway between an entirely stretched and a fully relaxed state. (Figs 6.20–6.22 for the treatment method.)

Isolytic MET (Chaitow 2001)

Isolytic MET is used as a method to stretch and/or break down fibrotic tissue in a muscle. The force applied by the therapist overpowers the patient's attempt to perform an isotonic concentric contraction of the target muscle.

Isolytic MET of the hamstring muscles (Fig. 6.23)

1. The muscle is brought to approximately 50% of its resting length.

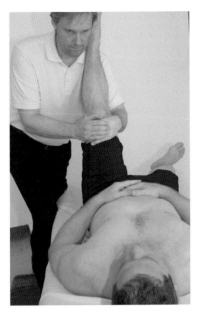

Figure 6.19 • Jandas' postfacilitation stretch method

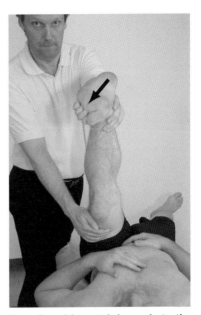

Figure 6.21 • A rapid stretch is made to the new barrier of resistance

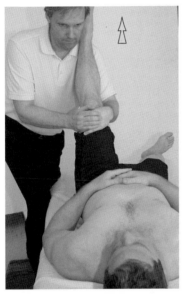

Figure 6.20 • Isometric muscle contraction

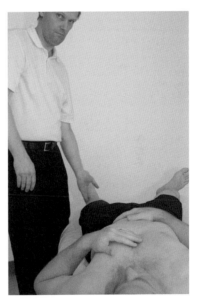

Figure 6.22 • The muscle is then brought to a complete relaxation

2. The athlete is asked to contract the hamstring muscles as the therapist, forcing the leg into extension, overpowers this effort. The succession of contractions and stretches are performed at a rapid pace since the aim of this technique is to break down and/or stretch out fibrotic tissue in the affected muscles.

AIS/Active Isolated Stretching (AIS)

Developed by Aaron L. Mattes, Active Isolated Stretching is a soft tissue stretching technique that recently has gained popularity amongst athletes,

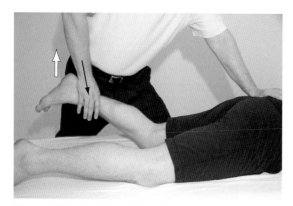

Figure 6.23 • Isolytic MET of the hamstring muscles

sports massage therapists, and others (Mattes 2000). AIS is a method of fascial release that effectively utilizes dynamic facilitated stretches of major muscle groups, and serves as a therapy for superficial and deep muscular and fascial release. To minimize the effects of an onset of the myotatic reflex (stretch reflex), the stretches are generally held in intervals of a maximum of 2 s. According to Mattes, this, combined with active movements in the affected joint(s) and stimulation of the reciprocal inhibition reflex through activation of antagonistic muscles, provides a maximum stretch benefit that can be achieved without conflicting tension or causing trauma.

The basic principles of AIS are as follows (Mattes 2000):

1. Initial identification of which muscle and/or supporting connective tissue structures need treatment.
2. Isolate the muscle in its most relaxed position.
3. Carry on a gradual and gentle stretch, with less than 1 lb of pressure. Stretch to the end point of the soft tissue range, which is slightly beyond the current ROM, and grant a controlled return of the body part back to the original start position.
4. The complete stretch sequence should be no longer than 2 s.
5. Repeat the same stretch sequence up to ten times, with each specific stretch repetition increasing the ROM a few degrees compared with the previous round. This is done without activating the myotatic reflex. To ensure maximal blood circulation and neuromuscular feedback in the treated area, it is important to return the moved body part fully to the original start position between each repetition. This will also reduce the pressure on local blood and lymph vessels.

6. The breathing pattern plays another important role in AIS. The athlete should exhale during the stretch phase and inhale during the recovery phase when moving toward the start position.
7. Evidence of any presence of the myotatic reflex is carefully monitored at the end point and beyond, i.e what Mattes calls the "point of light irritation." The stretch is released at this stage, and the treated body part is returned to the original start position.

To further facilitate the stretching procedure, especially during stretches of the lower extremities, an 8 ft/244 cm rope or strap may be used (Fig. 6.24) This modality is utilized during both self-stretches and therapeutically assisted stretches.

AIS of the semitendinosus and semimembranosus muscles (Mattes 2000) (Fig. 6.25)

1. **Start position.** The athlete lies on their back with one leg in 90 degrees flexion at both the hip joint and knee joint.
2. **Execution.** To isolate the distal part of the semitendinosus and semimembranosus muscles, the leg is rotated laterally. The rope is wrapped around the foot and lower leg to facilitate this lateral rotation, which is held as the knee is kept in an extended position. The stretch is accomplished by increasing the flexion in the hip joint until the end point of the muscles is reached. The stretch is released after 2 s and the leg moved back to the start position, i.e. 90-degree flexion in the hip and knee joint. This stretch sequence is repeated for one or two sets of ten repetitions.

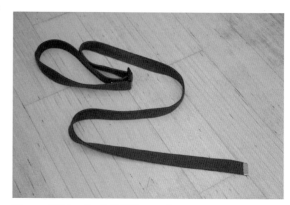

Figure 6.24 • An 8 ft/244 cm strap

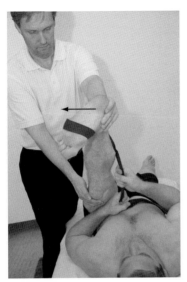

Figure 6.25 • AIS of ischiocrural/semitendinosus and membranosus muscles

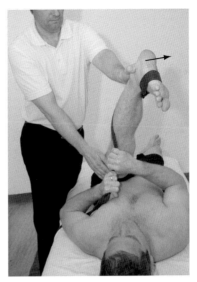

Figure 6.26 • AIS of ischiocrural/biceps femoris muscles

AIS of the biceps femoris muscle (Mattes 2000) (Fig. 6.26)

1. **Start position.** The athlete lies on their back with one leg in 90 degrees flexion at both the hip joint and knee joint.
2. **Execution.** To isolate the distal part of the biceps femoris muscle, the leg is rotated medially.
   The rope is wrapped around the foot and lower leg to facilitate this medial rotation, which is held as the knee is kept in an extended position.
   The stretch is accomplished by increasing the flexion in the hip joint until the end point is reached. The stretch is released after 2 s and the leg moved back to the start position, i.e. 90-degree flexion in the hip and knee joint. This stretch sequence is repeated for one or two sets of ten repetitions.

Traditional Thai massage-influenced stretching techniques (Brust 1990)

The exact origin of traditional Thai massage, or nuad phaen boran, is somewhat unclear. This originally energetic healing art is considered by some to have its roots in India more than 2500 years ago. A medical doctor from northern India by the name of Jivaka Kumar Bhaccha is said to have been a close friend of Buddha, and physician for the community of ordained Buddhist monks and nuns. He may also have served as a personal physician to the Magadha King Bimbisara. Dr. Jivaka Kumar Bhaccha is believed to have introduced not only the art of therapeutic massage to Thailand, but also knowledge about the healing properties of herbs and minerals during his trips to Thailand and Cambodia in the third or second century BC. Many Thai people consider Jivaka Kumar Bhaccha to be the "father of medicine" in Thailand.

Due to the lack of written records, partly owing to an ancient cultural praxis of transferring medical knowledge verbally, but perhaps mainly as a result of the destruction of the majority of recorded scriptures about this medical art form during the Burmese invasion of Thailand in AD 1767, it is unclear if there were any native traditions of massage in Thailand (formerly named Siam) prior to Dr. Jivaka Kumar Bhacchas's arrival, or what extent Chinese medical influence had upon the region. There are currently only a few remaining documented medical texts and images, created in AD 1832 by His Majesty King Rama III, stored at the Wat Phra Chetuphon temple/Wat Pho in Bangkok, Thailand (Brust 1990).

Originally more or less exclusively an energetic healing art, traditional Thai massage focused the treatments along ten main energetic channels called "Sen lines" or "Sen Sib" (Fig. 6.27) with pressure treatment on selected energy points along the Sen lines. Manual stimulation of these points would often alleviate or completely heal a wide range of diseases

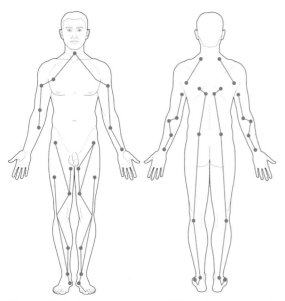

Figure 6.27 • Examples of Sen Sib on the front and back of the human body

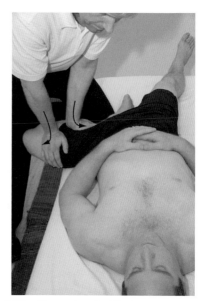

Figure 6.28 • Example of a Thai massage stretch of the right hip joint performed on a massage table

and ailments. Yoga-influenced stretching techniques coupled with specific locking, pushing, and/or pulling massage techniques were later added to form what is known today as traditional Thai massage.

Thai massage does not really use a fixed pattern of movements but can be regarded more as a collection of multiple therapeutic massage and stretching techniques that are applied as needed. The treatments can therefore easily be adapted to many different situations or conditions. In general, there is much focus on the lower extremities during a regular traditional Thai massage, which makes it well suited to the sports massage therapist. Selected traditional Thai massage techniques can be of great value in sports massage since they often combine massage and stretching techniques simultaneously. This can be very useful, particularly in pre-, post-, and interevent sports massage where effect vs. time is important.

Traditional Thai massage is generally performed on a soft mat on the floor, but many of these effective treatment techniques can easily be transferred to most sports massage settings, whether carried out on a regular massage table (Fig. 6.28) or on the ground.

The stretching part of this healing art is usually achieved by either rhythmically compressing the tissue with the either hands, knees, and feet, or by first locking the soft tissue with the heel of the palm, foot, elbow, forearm, or knees, whilst the treated body part is moved sequentially through its range of motion. This creates a very effective stretch that can be accentuated where it is needed thanks to the initial localized fixation.

More recently developed techniques like Aaron Mattes' Active Isolated Stretching (AIS), Michael Leahy's Active Release Technique (ART), and others share some similar traits with this and other ancient treatment methods, albeit the modern techniques encompass further recent advances and are commonly more structurally exact in their approach.

The physical power of the traditional Thai massage system is generated through a refined use of momentum from correct technique and body mechanics. In this way, even a relatively small person can easily create a surprising amount of power. This can of course be very useful when working with strong athletes. It is important, however, to gradually increase the strength of the stretches since the treatment effect is intensified through the frequent addition of simultaneous joint movement. Recognizing the end point of the treated muscles helps to avoid possible overstretch and pain during the treatment. In a typical "on the field" sports massage scenario, Thai massage techniques can be blended into the regular massage routine. The stretches are beneficially applied toward the end of the treatment of each body part, sometimes replacing some of the regular therapeutic stretches normally performed at the end of a pre-, post-, or interevent sports massage.

Example of a hip-opening Thai massage-based treatment sequence

Adductor massage and hip stretch
(Fig. 6.29)

1. The athlete lies supine on a massage table. The treated leg is flexed at the hip and knee joint and placed in a "figure 4" position.
2. The therapist places the palms on each side of the inner thigh, starting close to the groin.
3. The therapist compresses the leg by leaning downward and forward over the hands with straight arms. This creates an additional traction in the hip joint and will eliminate a possible pinching sensation. This compression with traction is worked down the thigh toward the knee. The closer to the knee the pressure is applied, the stronger the stretch effect will be.
4. The thigh is massaged down and up a couple of times until increased softness and flexibility are sensed.

Rectus femoris massage with hip stretch
(Fig. 6.30)

1. The athlete lies supine with the hip and knee joint flexed and the foot on the table.

2. The therapist locks the athlete's foot with the hip, and places the fingertips on each side of the rectus femoris muscle.
3. The muscle is stretched by alternately pulling it medially and laterally from the midline, starting by the knee, superior to the patella, and working up toward the groin.

Palm compression with hip stretch

1. The therapist clasps the hands around the quadriceps muscle, just superior to the knee, by interlocking the fingers and squeezing the thigh with the palms of the hands.
2. The hip joint is stretched as the therapist leans backward with straight arms. The amount of pulling force should slightly lift the hip on the same side off the table (Fig. 6.31).

Gluteus medius and minimus muscles, and lateral thigh stretch

1. The athlete lies supine in the same position as in the previous stretch. In this stretch, the knee is pushed medially to increase the amount of adduction in the hip joint and thereby stretch the gluteal muscles and lateral part of the thigh.
2. The therapist uses one hand to control the amount of adduction in the hip joint, and the palm heel, or

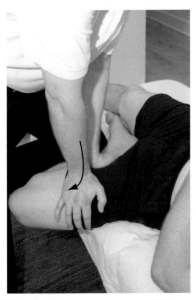

Figure 6.29 • Adductor massage and hip stretch

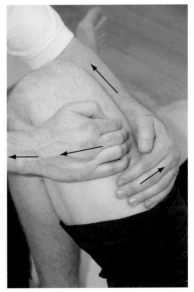

Figure 6.30 • Rectus femoris massage with hip stretch

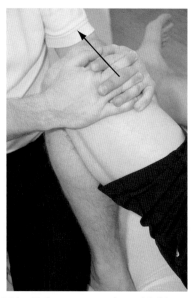

Figure 6.31 • Palm compression with hip stretch

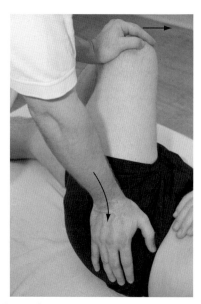

Figure 6.32 • Gluteus medius and minimus muscles, and lateral thigh stretch

forearm of the other arm will perform a slight "rolling" massage during the stretch. To best achieve a good effect in this movement, the treated muscle is first fixated with the palm heel, or forearm whilst the leg is in a more relaxed starting position, and the stretch momentum is added immediately after this. Besides making the stretch more effective, it also negates the need to move the hip joint into a strong adduction and medial rotation, which can easily cause pain or discomfort for the athlete.

3. As the muscle is stretched, the palm heel gradually pushes downward, or the forearm can execute a light rolling motion toward the hip joint. This tends to reduce any potential discomfort this intense movement may create (Fig. 6.32).

4. The stretch/massage is repeated as the palm heel, or forearm works multiple sections of the lateral thigh and gluteal area.

Hip extensor stretch

1. The athlete lies supine with the hip and knee joint flexed, and foot resting on the therapist's forearm, or elbow crease.

2. The adductor muscle group and hip extensors are stretched as the therapist increases the hip flexion by gently lunging forward (Fig. 6.33).

3. It is crucial that the stretch is executed at a smooth and rhythmic pace until flexibility in the hip joint increases.

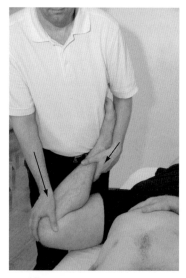

Figure 6.33 • Hip extensor stretch

Enhanced hip adductor stretch

1. The athlete lies supine with the hip and knee joint flexed, and foot resting in the therapist's hip, elbow crease, or shoulder.

2. The adductor muscle group is stretched as the therapist leans forward and pushes the athlete's leg into increased adduction and flexion. One

hand is pushing and/or fixating the muscle as it is stretched (Fig. 6.34).

3. The muscle is systematically pushed along its length as the stretch is repeated.

Stretch of the medial aspect of the thigh, including gracilis muscle

1. The athlete lies supine with the hip joint flexed, knee joint extended, and the leg placed in an abducted position.

2. The gracilis muscle is stretched as the straight leg, with toes pointing toward the head, is gradually pushed into further abduction (Fig. 6.35).

3. The therapist uses one hand or forearm to push, and/or fixate the gracilis muscle during the stretch. This stretch should be done with caution since the straightened leg causes a long and effective lever, and the muscle is long and relatively thin.

Stretch of the ischiocrural muscle group/ hamstring muscles

1. The athlete lies supine with the hip joint flexed and knee joint semiextended. The therapist holds the athlete's ankle with one hand.

2. With the other hand, or elbow, the therapist pushes on and fixates the muscle during the stretch (Fig. 6.36).

3. The muscle is first compressed, as the leg is gently pushed into further flexion at the hip joint. The end point of the stretch is achieved when the knee is also extended slightly further and resistance in the tissue is felt. There should be no major pain or discomfort produced during the stretch.

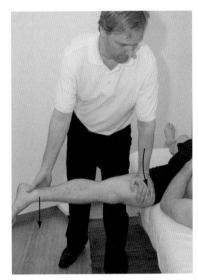

Figure 6.35 • Stretch of the medial aspect of the thigh, including gracilis muscle

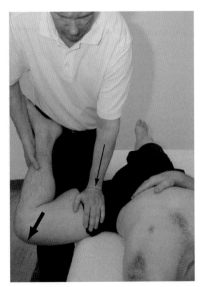

Figure 6.34 • Enhanced hip adductor stretch

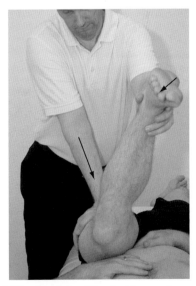

Figure 6.36 • Stretch of the ischiocrural muscle group/hamstring muscles

References

Alter, M., 1996. Science of flexibility, second ed. Human Kinetics, Champaign, IL.

Alter, M., 2004. Science of flexibility, third ed. Human Kinetics, Champaign, IL.

Askling, C.M., et al., 2007. Acute first-time hamstring strains during slow-speed stretching: clinical, magnetic resonance imaging, and recovery characteristics. Am. J. Sports Med. 35 (10), 1716–1724 Epub 2007 Jun 13.

Bonnar, B.P., et al., 2004. The relationship between isometric contraction durations during hold-relax stretching and improvement of hamstring flexibility. J. Sports Med. Phys. Fitness 44 (3), 258–261.

Brandenburg, J.P., 2006. Duration of stretch does not influence the degree of force loss following static stretching. J. Sports Med. Phys. Fitness 46 (4), 526–534.

Brust, H., 1990. The art of Traditional Thai Massage. DK Book House, Bangkok.

Chaitow, L., 2001. Muscle energy techniques. second ed. Churchill Livingstone, Edinburgh, pp. 69–78.

Chaouachi, A., et al., 2010. Effect of warm-ups involving static or dynamic stretching on agility, sprinting, and jumping performance in trained individuals. J. Strength Cond. Res. 24 (8), 2001–2011.

Cramer, J.T., et al., 2007. An acute bout of static stretching does not affect maximal eccentric isokinetic peak torque, the joint angle at peak torque, mean power, electromyography, or mechanomyography. J. Orthop. Sports Phys. Ther. 37 (3), 130–139.

de Weijer, V.C., et al., 2003. The effect of static stretch and warm-up exercise on hamstring length over the course of 24 hours. J. Orthop. Sports Phys. Ther. 33 (12), 727–733.

Egan, A.D., et al., 2006. Acute effects of static stretching on peak torque and mean power output in National Collegiate Athletic Association Division I women's basketball players. J. Strength Cond. Res. 20 (4), 778–782.

Ferreira, G.N., et al., 2007. Gains in flexibility related to measures of muscular performance: impact of flexibility on muscular performance. Clin. J. Sport Med. 17 (4), 276–278.

Fletcher, I.M., Anness, R., 2007. The acute effects of combined static and dynamic stretch protocols on fifty-meter sprint performance in track-and-field athletes. J. Strength Cond. Res. 21 (3), 784–787.

Fletcher, I.M., Monte-Colombo, M.M., 2010. An investigation into the effects of different warm-up modalities on specific motor skills related to soccer performance. J. Strength Cond. Res. 24 (8), 2096–2101.

Ford, P., McChesney, J., 2007. Duration of maintained hamstring ROM following termination of three stretching protocols. J. Sport Rehabil. 16 (1), 18–27.

Guissard, N., Duchateau, J., 2006. Neural aspects of muscle stretching. Exerc. Sport Sci. Rev. 34 (4), 154–158.

Kofotolis, N., Kellis, E., 2006. Effects of two 4-week proprioceptive neuromuscular facilitation programs on muscle endurance, flexibility, and functional performance in women with chronic low back pain. Phys. Ther. 86 (7), 1001–1012.

Kokkonen, J., et al., 2007. Chronic static stretching improves exercise performance. Med. Sci. Sports Exerc. 39 (10), 1825–1831.

Kurz, T., 1991. Science of sports training, How to plan and control training for peak performance. Stadion Publishing, Island Pond, VT.

Lewit, K., Simons, D.G., 1984. Myofascial pain: relief by post-isometric relaxation. Arch. Phys. Med. Rehabil. 65 (8), 452–456.

McAtee, R., 1993. Facilitated stretching. Human Kinetics, Champaign, IL.

McKean, E. (Ed.), 2005. New Oxford American Dictionary. second ed. Oxford University Press, Oxford.

MacMillan, D.J., et al., 2006. Dynamic vs. static-stretching warm up: the effect on power and agility performance. J. Strength Cond. Res. 20 (3), 492–499.

Mahieu, N.N., et al., 2007. Effect of static and ballistic stretching on the muscle-tendon tissue properties. Med. Sci. Sports Exerc. 39 (3), 494–501.

Marek, S.M., et al., 2005. Acute effects of static and proprioceptive neuromuscular facilitation stretching on muscle strength and power output. J. Athl. Train. 40 (2), 94–103.

Mattes, A., 2000. Active Isolated Stretching: The Mattes Method. Aaron Mattes Therapy, Sarasota, FL.

Mileusnic, M., Loeb, G., 2006. Mathematical models of proprioceptors. II. Structure and function of the Golgi tendon organ. J. Neurophysiol. 96 (4), 1789–1802.

Needham, R.A., et al., 2009. The acute effect of different warm-up protocols on anaerobic performance in elite youth soccer players. J Strength Cond. Res. 23 (9), 2614–2620.

Patrick, E., et al., 1982. Sampling of total muscle force by tendon organs. J. Neurophysiol. 47 (6), 1069–1083.

Rees, S.S., et al., 2007. Effects of proprioceptive neuromuscular facilitation stretching on stiffness and force-producing characteristics of the ankle in active women. J. Strength Cond. Res. 21 (2), 572–577.

Ryan, E.E., et al., 2010. The effects of the contract-relax-antagonist-contract form of proprioceptive neuromuscular facilitation stretching on postural stability. J. Strength Cond. Res. 24 (7), 1888–1894.

Santonja Medina, F.M., et al., 2007. Effects of frequency of static stretching on straight-leg raise in elementary school children. J. Sports Med. Phys. Fitness 47 (3), 304–308.

Sekir, U., et al., 2010. Acute effects of static and dynamic stretching on leg flexor and extensor isokinetic strength in elite women athletes. Scand. J. Med. Sci. Sports 20 (2), 268–281. Epub 2009 Apr 15.

Voss, D., et al., 1985. Proprioceptive neuromuscular facilitation, third ed. Harper & Row, Philadelphia, PA.

Ward, R., et al., 2002. Foundations for osteopathic medicine. Lippincott Williams & Wilkins, Philadelphia, PA.

Winke, M.R., et al., 2010. Moderate static stretching and torque production of the knee flexors. J. Strength Cond. Res. 24 (3), 706–710.

Witvouv, E., et al., 2007. The role of stretching in tendon injuries. Br. J. Sports Med. 41 (4), 224–226.

Woods, K., et al., 2007. Warm-up and stretching in the prevention of muscular injury. Sports Med. 37 (12), 1089–1099.

Woolstenhulme, M.T., et al., 2006. Ballistic stretching increases flexibility and acute vertical jump height when combined with basketball activity. J. Strength Cond. Res. 20 (4), 799–803.

Yamaguchi, T., Ishii, K., 2005. Effects of static stretching for 30 seconds and dynamic stretching on leg extension power. J. Strength Cond. Res. 19 (3), 677–683.

Yamaguchi, T., et al., 2006. Acute effect of static stretching on power output during concentric dynamic constant external resistance leg extension. J. Strength Cond. Res. 20 (4), 804–810.

Applied stretches to common muscle groups

7

Soft tissue stretching is an intricate part of sports activity, and is generally a necessity to achieve the desired ROM and musculofascial health each sport requires. Since there are many methods of stretching (see Chapter 6) it is also important to utilize the techniques correctly when applying them to different sports scenarios. Research has demonstrated that static stretching can reduce muscular power output and speed when used immediately prior to athletic activity (Bazett-Jones et al. 2008; Cè et al. 2008; Chaouachi et al. 2008; Herda et al. 2008; Herman & Smith 2008; Holt & Lambourne 2008; McHugh & Nesse 2008; Mirca et al. 2008; Samuel et al. 2008; Torres et al. 2008; La Torre et al. 2010), especially when the muscle is in a shortened position and if performed after active warm-up (Cè et al. 2008; McHugh & Nesse 2008). Static stretching of the upper body seems to generate fewer negative effects in regard to strength (Torres et al. 2008), and it has been suggested that athletes may perform upper-body static stretching without power reduction, provided sufficient time is allowed before the event (Torres et al. 2008). Some studies on static stretching indicate negative effects on speed, endurance, and power performance in muscles of the lower body when carried out close to athletic activity (Samuel et al. 2008; Wilson et al. 2010), while it is also suggested that acute static stretching does not negatively affect high-intensity aerobic exercise performance (Samogin Lopes et al. 2010). On the other hand, dynamic stretching techniques have been demonstrated to produce beneficial effects like increased jump power and sprint performance, especially when combined with elements of resistance (Jaggers et al. 2008; Needham et al. 2009). Dynamic warm-ups have been shown to produce increased strength, sustained power, muscular endurance, anaerobic capacity, and agility among wrestlers (Herman & Smith 2008), and consequently today it is generally recommended to utilize dynamic warm-up routines, including dynamic stretches, prior to imminent athletic performance (Herman & Smith 2008; Torres et al. 2008; Needham et al. 2009; Sekir et al. 2010; Fletcher & Monte-Colombo 2010). It is even suggested that static stretching should be utilized only during post-practice or competition (Bazett-Jones et al. 2008), but also indicated that static stretching utilized in combination with active movements like sprint training reduces some of the negative effects commonly associated with static stretching and sports performance (Chaouachi et al. 2008). Additionally, there is also the opinion that musculotendinous stiffness may contribute to optimizing power output in explosive movements, and furthermore potentially guard an athlete against sports injuries (Wilson & Flanagan 2008).

Focal stretching

To ensure both full control and effect in treated tissues during the stretch, the lever (often an arm, leg, or neck) to which the muscles are attached is moved in specific angles. For example, to focus the stretch on the lateral aspect of a muscle or body part, the lever is moved medially before the stretch commences. An imaginary line can be drawn through the lever to the muscle (or conversely, from the intended section of the muscle out through the lever), taking the general stretch direction into

DOI: 10.1016/B978-0-443-10126-7.00007-1

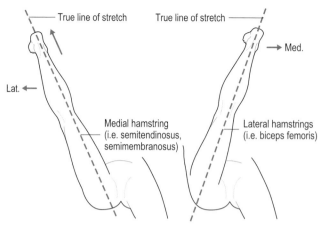

Figure 7.1 • True line of stretch

consideration (Fig. 7.1), to see exactly where the stretch effect will end up. In this way, specific fiber sections of a muscle can be selected for a very precise and effective stretch. This method works well for flexion, extension, abduction, adduction, etc., but not as well for rotational movements, where the lever is better viewed as a "spool" around which the tendon is "rolled up."

Therapeutic stretching is always three-dimensional, and it is important the sports therapist thinks in a functional manner. Therapeutic stretching in sports treatment is commonly performed from many different positions, and it is customary for the therapist to improvise and adapt to the situation at hand. By thinking three-dimensionally, it is easier to assess the "true lines of stretch." The stretch movements are commonly the opposite of the treated muscle's actions, where each movement is performed in sections toward its respective end point. This enables complete control of the stretch, and presents the possibility of focusing on specific restricted movements in a general movement pattern. The therapist must, however, be aware that the actions of a muscle can change depending on the position of the lever. One example of this is the piriformis muscle, which changes action from lateral rotation to medial rotation when the hip joint is flexed more than approximately 60–90 degrees. Another example is the supraspinatus muscle, which performs medial rotation instead of the normal lateral rotation when the glenohumeral joint is positioned in strong adduction. This again stresses the importance of thinking functionally and "three-dimensionally" during therapeutic muscle stretching.

Another important aspect of therapeutic stretching is the concept of an initial manual fixation of origin, insertion, muscle belly, and/or fascia. By fixating the tissue prior to the stretch, the effect is focalized, and joint movement reduced. Fixating can also minimize the stress on an inflamed tendon while the rest of the muscle can still be stretched effectively. The tissue is often fixated obliquely into the muscle and away from the direction of stretch. The muscle can also be pushed into a "C-shape" during the stretch to focalize the effect. A pressure applied after the stretch is initiated tends to have an effect in more superficial layers, whereas if it is applied just prior to the stretch, more deeply situated fibers are affected. Specific massage strokes and soft tissue techniques may also be applied to a stretch to increase its effectiveness. This is described in more detail in Chapter 14.

A tensed muscle will activate the reciprocal inhibition reflex (see Chapter 6) and thereby "weaken" its antagonists. It may therefore be advantageous to precede the stretch with one or more isometric contractions of the antagonist to reactivate the weakened muscle. This may also cause some relaxation in the treated target muscle even before the actual stretch commences. This procedure may generate a more "balanced" joint after the stretch is completed.

The use of accessories

Even though it is desirable for the sports therapist to develop adequate skill to stretch athletes without additional equipment in order to minimize equipment dependency, certain situations may require the use of props. Stretching straps (Fig. 7.2) enable areas

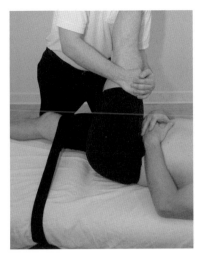

Figure 7.2 • Stretch strap

of the body to be fixated to facilitate specific and effective stretching. Blocks and wedges may be used to help keep heavier body parts elevated during a stretch, and/or assist a smaller therapist to work more effectively on large and strong athletes.

Methods

All stretch methods previously mentioned in Chapter 6 can be used on any stretched muscle or muscle group (Figs 7.3; 7.4). The decision of which method to employ depends on personal preference, desired effect, and the specific need in the athletic scenario.

Common stretches for the lower body

Therapeutic stretch of tibialis anterior muscle

The athlete lies supine. The therapist dorsal flexes the athlete's foot to relax the muscle, and uses the palm heel to fixate the muscle by pushing into the muscle with an additional cranial direction of 45 degrees (Fig. 7.5). The muscle is stretched as the athlete's foot is pushed into plantar flexion and eversion with simultaneous increased fixation force.

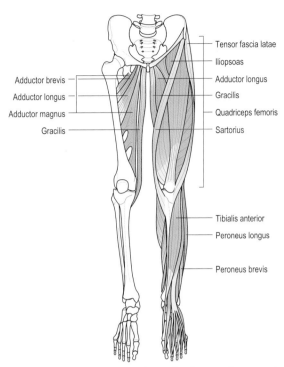

Figure 7.3 • Muscles of the lower body, anterior aspect

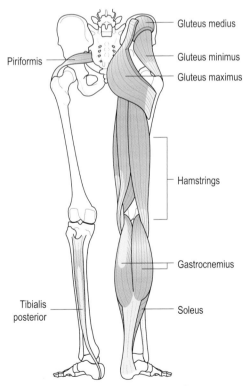

Figure 7.4 • Muscles of the lower body, posterior aspect

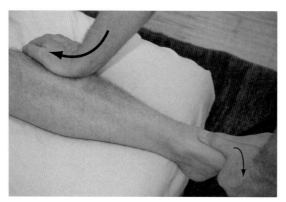

Figure 7.5 • Therapeutic stretch of the tibialis anterior muscle

Therapeutic stretch of tibialis posterior muscle

1. The athlete lies prone with the treated leg in 90-degree flexion at the knee joint.
2. The therapist gently grasps the athlete's heel, and presses the foot into dorsal flexion with the forearm (Fig. 7.6). The pressure is more on the lateral aspect of the ball of the foot, which generates a needed eversion.

Therapeutic stretch of peroneal muscle group

1. The athlete lies prone with the stretched leg in 90-degree flexion at the knee joint.
2. The therapist fixates the muscle proximally with one hands thumb, grasps the ball of the foot with the other hand, and presses the foot into dorsal flexion (Fig. 7.7). The pressure is on the medial aspect of the ball of the foot to generate an additional inversion of the foot.

Therapeutic stretch of triceps surae muscle group

1. The athlete lies supine. The therapist grasps the heel and presses the foot into dorsal flexion with the forearm. The pressure is on the ball of the sole of the foot.
2. To further focus the stretch on either belly of the gastrocnemius muscle, the foot is rotated laterally for medial belly (Fig. 7.8), or medially for lateral belly. The soleus muscle is stretched in the same manner as the tibialis posterior muscle (see Fig. 7.6) but without eversion of the foot.

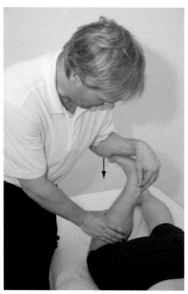

Figure 7.6 • Therapeutic stretch of the tibialis posterior muscle

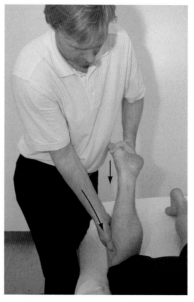

Figure 7.7 • Stretch of the peroneal muscle group

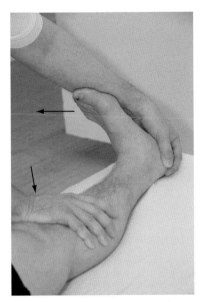

Figure 7.8 • Stretch of the gastrocnemius muscle, with a focalized stretch effect on the medial head.

General stretch of the hamstring muscle group (Fig. 7.9)

Previous injuries should be noted prior to stretching the hamstrings to possibly include potential cautionary measurements, and/or prestretch fibrotic treatment techniques.

1. The athlete lies supine. The therapist places the athlete's leg on one shoulder. The athlete's hip joint is pushed into further flexion while the two hands, placed immediately superior to the knee joint, pull to simultaneously extend the knee joint. The therapist pushes the leg anterior with an additional 45-degree superior angle to keep a certain level of traction, which also prevents the knee from bending during the stretch (see Fig. 7.9A).

2. To stretch the medial hamstrings more specifically, the leg is either abducted until the true line of stretch overlaps the muscles, or laterally rotated, which also will distance origin and insertion (see Fig. 7.9B).

3. The biceps femoris is stretched by adducting the leg, or medially rotating the straightened leg as the hip joint is moved into increased flexion (see Fig. 7.9C).

4. For more flexible athletes, the therapist may place the athlete's heel in the web between the

thumb and index finger. With the therapist's body lined up (see Fig. 7.9D) the athlete's leg is pushed into further hip flexion, traction, and knee extension.

Stretch of quadriceps femoris (Fig. 7.10)

1. The athlete lies prone. The therapist flexes the athlete's knee joint, and the hip and pelvis are fixated to the table by the therapist's forearm or hand (see Fig. 7.10A). The fixation is on the inferior aspect of the sacral area. The athlete's foot is pushed toward the gluteus maximus muscle.

2. To focalize the stretch to the vastus lateralis muscle, the athlete's foot is pushed toward the opposite gluteal area (see Fig. 7.10B). The stretch can also be accentuated if the therapist simultaneously fixates the vastus lateralis muscle by pushing it into a "C-shape."

3. The athlete's foot is pushed laterally to the hip joint to focalize the stretch to vastus medialis. One hand stabilizes the pelvis (see Fig. 7.10C), or can also push the muscle into a "C-shape" prior to the stretch phase.

Note that stretches 2 and 3 are applied only on healthy knee joints. The initial fixation is most important here to minimize the lateral and medial movement.

4. The therapist places one knee under the athlete's thigh, just superior to the patella, to generate extension in the athlete's hip joint. The hip and pelvis are fixated and leveled to the table by the therapist's forearm, and in addition the hand of the same arm pulls the opposite hip toward the therapist (see Fig. 7.10D). The fixation is on the inferior aspect of the sacral area to avoid further extension of the lumbar spine. The therapist slowly generates flexion in the athlete's knee joint to stretch the muscle to the end point.

5. The athlete lies prone on the table with one foot on the floor. The therapist fixates the athlete's heel with one foot (see Fig. 7.10E). One hand stabilizes the athlete's pelvis. The stretched leg is aligned straight to focalize the stretch to the rectus femoris muscle, and the knee is flexed until the end point of the muscle is reached.

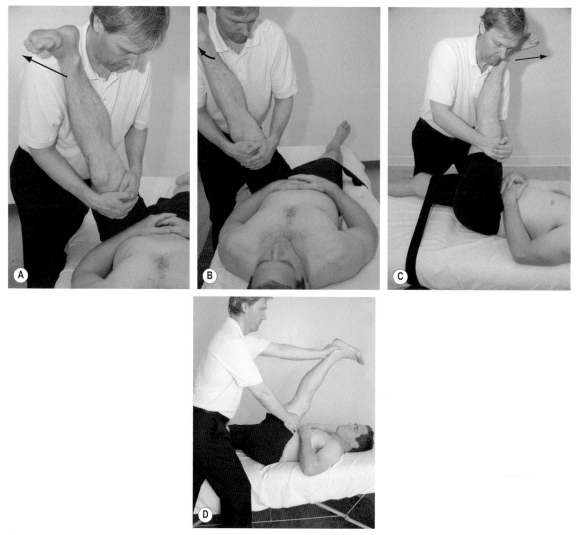

Figure 7.9 • Stretch of the hamstring muscle group • A General stretch of the hamstring muscle group B Semitendinosus/semimembranosus C Biceps femoris D Modified hamstring stretch

Stretch of the adductor group

1. The athlete lies supine with one leg slightly abducted and the lower leg hanging off the treatment table. The therapist locks the athlete's leg with one thigh (Fig. 7.11) and leans gently away from the table to create traction in the hip joint. The muscles are stretched as the leg is pushed into further abduction.

2. Adductor magnus stretch. The posterior aspect of the adductor magnus muscle is stretched by adding a slight flexion in the hip joint.

Stretch of the gracilis muscle

The athlete lies supine with the treated leg straight and slightly abducted. The therapist locks the athlete's leg with one thigh (Fig. 7.12) and leans gently

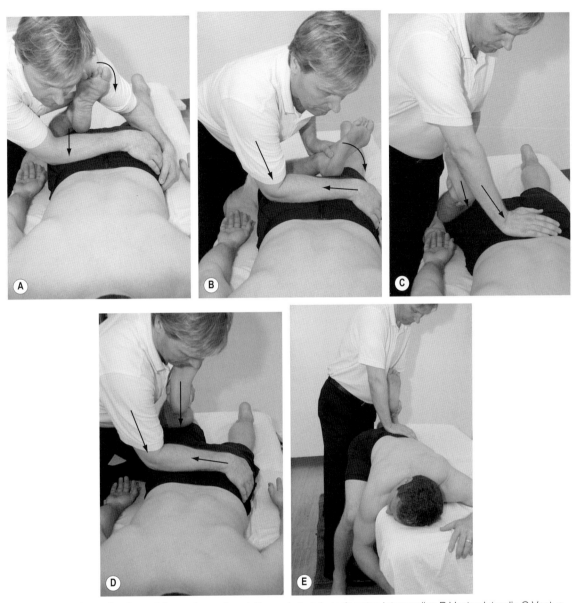

Figure 7.10 • Stretch of quadriceps femoris • A General stretch and vastus intermedius B Vastus lateralis C Vastus medialis D Rectus femoris E Rectus femoris, variation

away from the table to create traction in the hip joint. The toes should point straight up to affect the target muscle and minimize hamstring involvement. The muscle is stretched as the leg is pushed into further abduction.

Stretch of the sartorius muscle

The athlete lies supine with one leg slightly abducted and hanging off the treatment table. The nontreated leg is either hanging over the opposite side of the

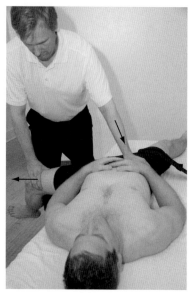

Figure 7.11 • Stretch of the adductor group, i.e. pectineus, adductor magnus, adductor longus, adductor brevis muscles, except gracilis

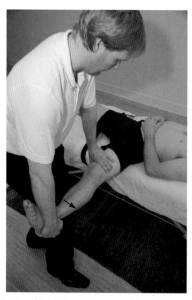

Figure 7.12 • Stretch of the gracilis muscle

table, or is fixated with a stretch strap. The therapist locks the athlete's treated leg by grasping around the thigh and pressing against the shoulder, and leans gently away from the table to create traction in the hip joint. The therapist additionally performs an abduction, extension, and medial rotation of the hip joint to stretch the muscle (Fig. 7.13).

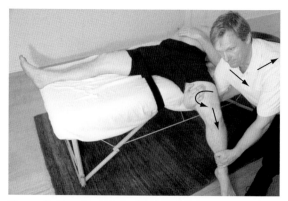

Figure 7.13 • Stretch of the sartorius muscle

Common stretches for the gluteal area and hips

Stretch of the iliopsoas muscle (Fig. 7.14)

1. The athlete lies supine with the nontreated leg flexed toward the chest, and the treated leg hanging off the treatment table (see Fig. 7.14A). The therapist stands with the side of the body fixating the foot of the nontreated leg. The therapist steps in and uses one thigh to push the athlete's leg into slight abduction. This is to move the stretch into the iliopsoas and away from the rectus femoris muscle. The stretch is initiated by pushing the hip joint into further extension. The athlete's shin can additionally be pushed laterally to generate a mild medial rotation in the hip joint.
2. The same stretch can be applied when the athlete is positioned on the side (see Fig. 7.14B).

Stretch of the tensor fasciae latae muscle

The athlete lies obliquely on the side on the treatment table, with the nontreated leg flexed in both the knee joint and the hip joint, and the treated leg straight. The therapist supports the athlete's sacral area with the hip to prevent the athlete from rolling over. The stretch is applied by generating extension and adduction in the hip joint (Fig. 7.15). The stretch is further reinforced by applying a transverse force to the muscle with the flat aspect of an elbow.

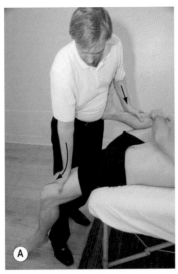
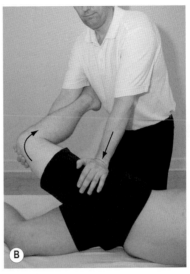

Figure 7.14 • Stretch of the iliopsoas muscle • A Supine B Side

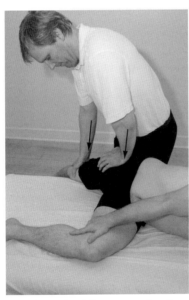

Figure 7.15 • Stretch of the tensor fasciae latae muscle

Stretch of the gluteus maximus

The athlete lies supine. The therapist flexes the athlete's knee and brings the leg toward the opposite shoulder (Fig. 7.16A). The pressure is on the shin close to the foot to minimize compression of the hip joint. If pain is experienced in the hip joint despite this caution, additional traction needs to be administered in conjunction to the stretch. This is done by standing on the opposite side of the table and grasping around the leg at the knee, lifting the athlete's leg over toward the opposite shoulder (Fig. 7.16B).

Stretch of the gluteus medius and minimus muscles

The athlete lies supine. The therapist stands on the opposite side of the table with one hand fixating the athlete's pelvis at the ASIS and the forearm of the other arm resting on the lateral aspect of the athlete's thigh. The therapist further flexes the athlete's knee and brings the leg across the table. The therapist's palm starts face down and as the leg is brought across the table, the palm supinates, generating traction in the hip joint through the forearm. The therapist stretches the muscle by leaning over, moving the athletes leg into further adduction through pressure from the forearm and medial side of the elbow (Fig. 7.17).

Stretch of the piriformis muscle

1. The athlete lies supine. The therapist sits on the opposite side of the table, locking the athlete's nontreated leg, at the hip or thigh, with the hip.

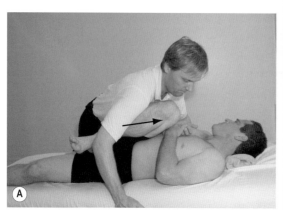
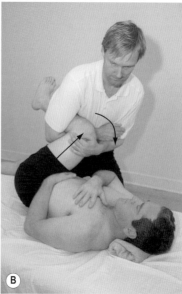

Figure 7.16 • **Stretch of gluteus maximus** • A Regular B With additional traction

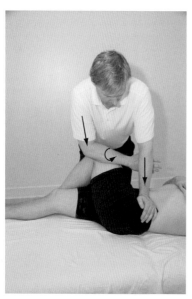

Figure 7.17 • **Stretch of the gluteus medius and minimus muscles**

adduction (commonly by aiming the knee just lateral to the athlete's opposite shoulder), and lateral rotation of the hip joint. The athlete's knee joint is flexed 90 degrees to achieve a good lever. Note that the piriformis muscle here is stretched with lateral rotation in the hip joint, since from this position it has changed function from being a lateral rotator to instead becoming a medial rotator, due to the amount of initial flexion in the athlete's hip joint.

2. The athlete lies prone, with the knee joint in 90 degree flexion. The piriformis muscle is initially slacked as the therapist generates lateral rotation in the athlete's hip joint by pushing the foot toward the opposite leg. The muscle is fixated with the therapist's elbow, and gently stretched as the therapist pulls the athlete's foot, thus generating a medial rotation in the hip joint (Fig. 7.18B). The fixation is released between each stretch to promote the blood circulation in the area.

This prevents the athlete's hip from rolling over during the stretch. The treated leg is brought over and placed at the therapist's chest or shoulder (Fig. 7.18A). The muscle is stretched as the therapist generates additional flexion,

Common stretches for the upper body (Figs 7.19; 7.20)

- Back.
- Erector spinae muscle group (Torres et al. 2008).

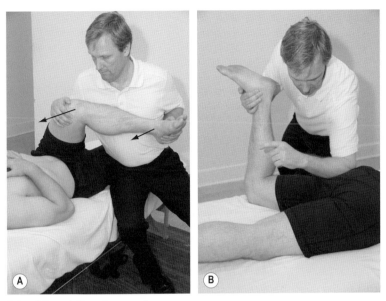

Figure 7.18 • Stretch of the piriformis muscle

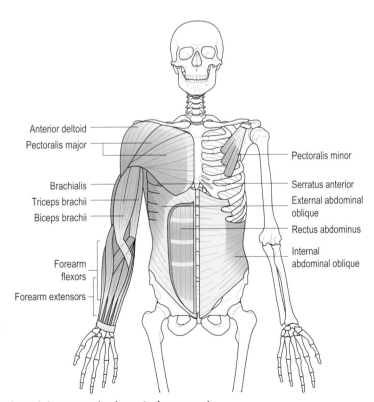

Figure 7.19 • Muscles of the upper body, anterior aspect

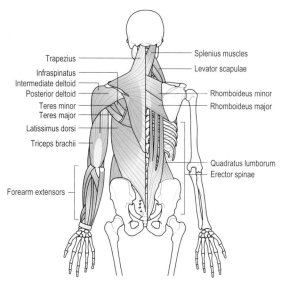

Figure 7.20 • **Muscles of the upper body, posterior aspect**

Erector spinae muscle group

The erector spinae muscle group consists of a number of different muscles, i.e:

- iliocostalis: lumborum, thoracis, cervicis
- longissimus: thoracis, cervicis, capitis
- spinalis: thoracis, cervicis, capitis
- semispinalis: thoracis, cervicis, capitis

- multifidi
- rotatores: thoracis longus, thoracis brevis
- interspinales
- intertransversarii.

The erector spinae group runs from the sacral area and pelvis, all the way up to the occipital bone (Kendall et al. 1971). This creates a very long muscle group and is consequently beneficially stretched in separate segments of the lumbar, thoracic, and cervical areas.

Stretch of the erector spinae muscle group (Fig. 7.21)

1. The athlete is treated in sitting position. A wedge, rolled towel, or firm pillow is positioned unilaterally under the gluteal area on the side that is not to be treated (see Fig. 7.21A). This will drop the pelvis on the treated side and take up the slack in the muscles. The athlete is instructed to grasp the heel of the opposite leg, and the muscle is stretched as the leg on the nontreated side is gradually extended. The therapist accentuates the stretch by applying manual longitudinal or transverse pressure on the muscle belly.

2. The same treatment position pertains, but the therapist applies manual reinforcement with a palm heel or elbow in the thoracic area of the muscle group (see Fig. 7.21B).

3. The athlete lies supine. The therapist lifts the athlete's head into a slight lateral flexion (to

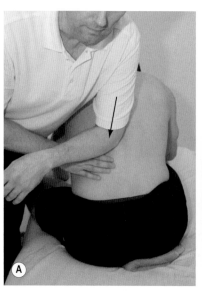
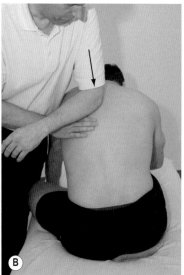
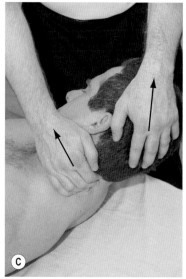

Figure 7.21 • **Stretch of the erector spinae muscle group** • A Lumbar B Thoracic C Cervical region

reduce stress on the nuchal ligament, and to achieve the true line of stretch), conducting flexion and contralateral rotation with one hand. The treated muscle group is grasped with the fingertips of the other hand until the end point is reached. The muscle can be held in this position or the fingertips can slowly glide transversely over the muscle to facilitate a myofascial release effect (see Fig. 7.21C).

Lower back

Stretch of the quadratus lumborum muscle

The athlete lies prone with the legs moved to one side of the table. The upper body is positioned in lateral flexion to the same side. This position generates a gentle basic stretch of the muscle. To improve the stretch, the therapist uses the hypothenar edge of the hand whilst standing on the opposite side of the table, or the flat part of one elbow whilst standing on the same side as the treated muscle (Fig. 7.22). It is important to palpate the 12th rib prior to the stretch to ensure it is not compressed during the stretch.

Abdomen

The athlete rests in a supine position with support under the back, generating extension of the back. The therapist focally stretches the muscle by applying a medial and/or lateral horizontal pressure on the treated area. If the whole muscle is stretched,

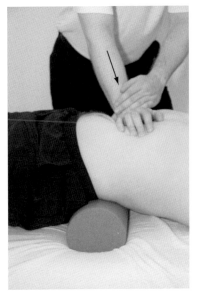

Figure 7.23 • Stretch of the rectus abdominis muscle

the therapist applies sectional pressure for each quadrant (Fig. 7.23). The stretch can also be executed in a side-lying position.

Stretch of the external and internal abdominal oblique (Fig. 7.24)

The athlete lies on the side with the back close to one edge of the treatment table. The therapist supports the athlete's sacral region with one hip, and gently stretches the muscle by pressing the shoulder down toward the table (see Fig. 7.24A). It is important not to push the athlete's pelvis in an anterior direction since this would generate stress on the lumbar area. The stretch is intensified if the therapist gently presses on the muscle belly with the palm heel. The internal abdominal oblique on the opposite side is stretched simultaneously. The stretch is intensified if the therapist gently pulls on the muscle with the fingertips (see Fig. 7.24B).

Upper back

Stretch of the latissimus dorsi muscle

The athlete lies supine. The therapist generates a lateral flexion of the athlete's upper body and abduction of the arm. The therapist locks the athlete's forearm on the hip and leans backward and moves sideways to increase traction and abduction in the glenohumeral joint (Fig. 7.25).

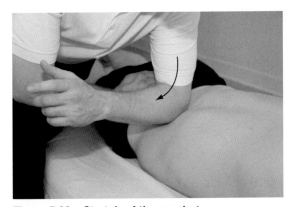

Figure 7.22 • Stretch of the quadratus lumborum muscle

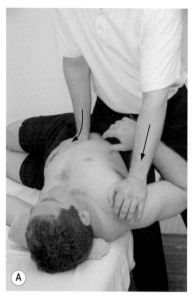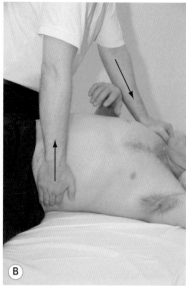

Figure 7.24 • Stretch of the external and internal abdominal oblique

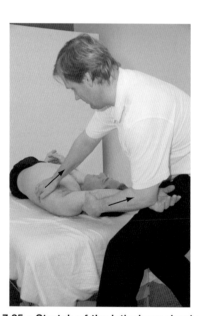

Figure 7.25 • Stretch of the latissimus dorsi muscle

Stretch of rhomboid major and minor muscles

The athlete lies prone with the arm of the treated side abducted. The therapist grasps the athlete's elbow with one hand and places the palm heel of the other hand at the inferior medial border of the scapula. The muscles are stretched by manually pushing the

inferior aspect of the scapula laterally, generating an abduction/protraction with a superior rotation of the scapula. The stretch is fine-tuned by increasing the abduction of the arm by gently pulling the elbow (Fig. 7.26). It is very important not to generate more flexion in the shoulder since this only tends to stress and cause pain in the glenohumeral joint.

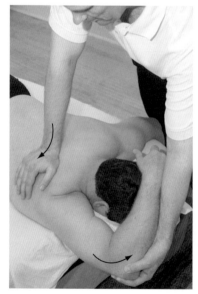

Figure 7.26 • Stretch of rhomboid major and minor muscles

Stretch of the trapezius muscle (Fig. 7.27)

1. The athlete is positioned on the side with both legs bent and the arm of the treated side in full abduction. The therapist stretches the muscle by pushing the inferior angle of the scapula cranially (see Fig. 7.27A). The athlete can assist upon the therapist's command by reaching with the arm above the head.

2. The athlete lies prone with the hand of the treated side on the back. If this generates pain in the anterior aspect of the athlete's shoulder, or if the ROM is too limited, a wedge or rolled towel is placed under the front of the shoulder. The therapist stretches the muscle by horizontally pressing the medial border of the scapulae laterally (see Fig. 7.27B).

3. The athlete is sitting, grasping the back of the table or chair to depress the shoulder. The therapist stretches the muscle by initially fixating the muscle belly close to the shoulder with the flat aspect of one elbow, and additionally generating lateral flexion toward the opposite side, flexion, and lastly an ipsilateral rotation of the head and neck. A good fixation of the shoulder is imperative to minimize the movement and stress on the neck (see Fig. 7.27C).

Stretch of the levator scapula muscle

The athlete is sitting, grasping the back of the table or chair to depress the shoulder. The therapist stretches the muscle by initially fixating the muscle belly at the superior angle of the scapula with the flat aspect of

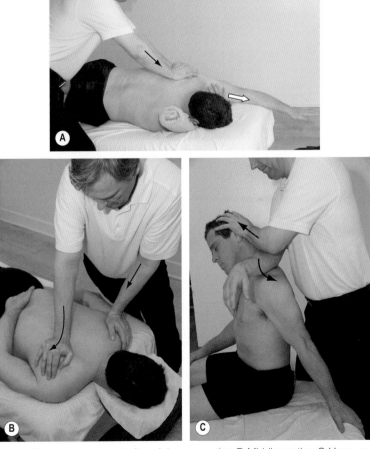

Figure 7.27 • Stretch of the trapezius muscle • A Lower portion B Middle portion C Upper portion

one elbow, and additionally generating lateral flexion toward the opposite side, strong flexion, and lastly contralateral rotation of the head and neck, all made in one movement (Fig. 7.28). A good fixation of the insertion is imperative to minimize the movement and stress on the neck.

Shoulders

Stretch of the infraspinatus and teres minor muscles

The athlete lies supine with the treated arm horizontally adducted. The therapist grasps the athlete's arm in medial rotation where the hand is pointing toward the feet (Fig. 7.29). The athlete's arm is firstly tractioned, followed by a slow and controlled medial rotation. To more specifically stretch the teres minor muscle, the glenohumeral joint is slightly moved into flexion until the line of stretch overlaps the muscle.

Stretch of the supraspinatus muscle (Fig. 7.30)

1. The athlete lies supine with the arm in horizontal adduction and lateral rotation in the glenohumeral joint. The therapist grasps the arm and stretches the muscle by firstly increasing the adduction followed by fine-tuning the stretch through slowly increasing the lateral rotation (see Fig. 7.30A). The initial adduction in the glenohumeral joint is crucial for a successful stretch.

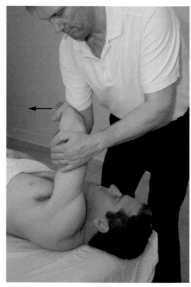

Figure 7.29 • Stretch of the infraspinatus and teres minor muscles

2. The muscle can additionally be fixated prior to the stretch with one hand (see Fig. 7.30B).

Stretch of the subscapularis muscle

The athlete lies supine with the treated arm along the side of the body. The therapist lifts the arm and places the soft pad of one thumb on the anterior aspect of the scapula. The thumb will fixate the muscle during the stretch. With the muscle fixated, the therapist commences a flexion in the athlete's glenohumeral joint until the end point is reached (Fig. 7.31). The procedure is repeated a number of times until the increase of muscle relaxation phases out, or it becomes too painful for the athlete. The thumb is moved between each repetition to fixate a new area of the muscle. Caution should be taken since there are numerous lymph nodes in the area, particularly in the upper aspect of the armpit.

Neck

Stretch of splenius capitis and cervicis muscles

The athlete lies supine. The therapist stretches the muscle by firstly generating lateral flexion in the athlete's neck with one hand, just enough to reduce stress on the nuchal ligament, followed by slowly but firmly flexing the neck with the head toward the chest (Fig. 7.32). Normal ROM is to be able to touch the chin to the chest.

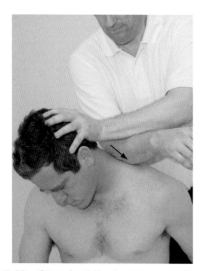

Figure 7.28 • Stretch of the levator scapula muscle

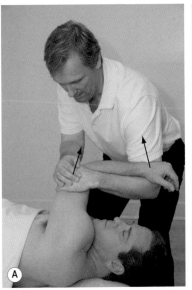
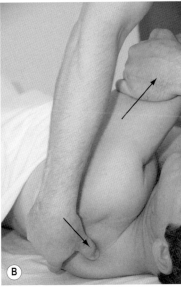

Figure 7.30 • Stretch of the supraspinatus muscle • A Stretch B Fixation

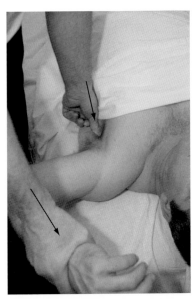

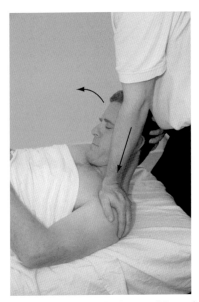

Figure 7.32 • Stretch of splenius capitis and cervicis muscles

Figure 7.31 • Stretch of the subscapularis muscle

Stretch of the deltoid muscle (Fig. 7.33)

1. The athlete lies prone. The therapist uses one arm to hook the athlete's treated arm, and uses the other hand to fixate the shoulder. The muscle is stretched as the therapist increases the extension in the glenohumeral joint. It is important that the athlete's hand points towards the feet during this movement, to avoid any rotation in the glenohumeral joint (see Fig. 7.33A).

2. The athlete lies on the side with the treated arm on the back. The therapist stretches the muscle by firstly tractioning the arm, followed by increasing the adduction in the glenohumeral joint. It is important that the athlete's hand points towards the feet during this movement, to avoid any

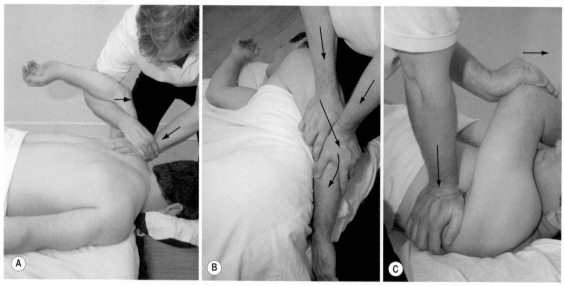

Figure 7.33 • Stretch of the deltoid muscle • A Anterior B Intermedius C Posterior

rotation in the glenohumeral joint (see Fig. 7.33B). The stretch is intensified if the therapist additionally pushes on the muscle with the flat part of an elbow.

3. The athlete lies supine with the treated arm in 90-degree abduction in the glenohumeral joint, and flexion of the elbow joint. The therapist stretches the muscle by firstly fixating the lateral border of the athlete's scapula with the palm heel, and secondly horizontally adducting the arm to the muscle's end point (see Fig. 7.33C).

Stretch of the pectoralis major muscle

The athlete lies supine with the arm abducted, laterally rotated, and with the elbow flexed 90 degrees. The therapist stretches the muscle by grasping the athlete's arm, generating traction, horizontal abduction, followed by a fine-tuning with lateral rotation in the glenohumeral joint (Fig. 7.34). By adjusting the true line of stretch by either increasing or decreasing the abduction/adduction of the athlete's arm, the therapist can stretch all three portions of the muscle, namely the clavicular portion, sternocostal portion, and the abdominal portion.

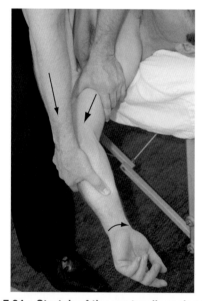

Figure 7.34 • Stretch of the pectoralis major muscle

Stretch of the pectoralis minor muscle

The athlete lies supine. The therapist stands by the athlete's head and grasps the wrist with one hand. The other hand fixates the muscle through the pectoralis major muscle, inferior to the coracoid process.

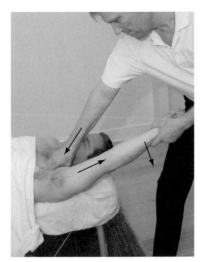

Figure 7.35 • Stretch of the pectoralis minor muscle

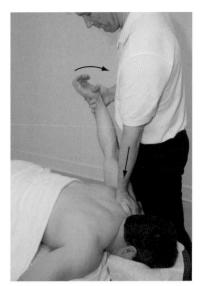

Figure 7.36 • Stretch of the biceps brachii muscle

The muscle is stretched by moving the athlete's arm into traction and strong flexion (Fig. 7.35).

Arms

Stretch of the biceps brachii muscle

The athlete lies prone. The therapist grasps the wrist of the treated arm and performs a mild traction, extension in the glenohumeral joint, extension in the cubital/elbow joint, and pronation in the radioulnar joints until the end point for each movement is reached. The athlete's shoulder is fixated to the treatment table by the therapist's other hand (Fig. 7.36).

Stretch of the triceps brachii muscle

The athlete lies supine with one palm touching the spinous process of the 7th cervical vertebra. This prevents stress on the athlete's wrist during the stretch. The therapist moves the athlete's arm into traction, extension of the glenohumeral joint, and flexion in the cubital/elbow joint (Fig. 7.37). The muscle can additionally be focally reinforced by simultaneously pressing on the muscle with the fist, palm heel and/or pulling with the fingertips.

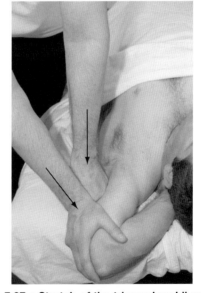

Figure 7.37 • Stretch of the triceps brachii muscle

Stretch of the superficial extensor muscles of the forearm (Fig. 7.38)

1. The athlete lies supine with a straight arm and lightly closed fist. The therapist grasps the athlete's hand and generates flexion in the wrist and rotation towards the ulna (see Fig. 7.38A).
2. The deeply situated extensor muscles are stretched in a similar way with the exception that the cubital/elbow joint is flexed to relax the superficial layer (see Fig. 7.38B).

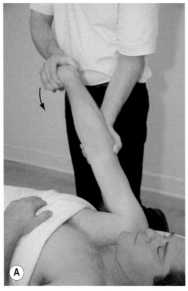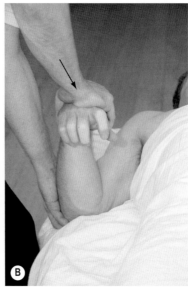

Figure 7.38 • Stretch of the extensor muscles of the forearm • A Stretch of the superficial extensor muscles B Stretch of the deep extensor muscles

Stretch of the superficial flexor muscles of the forearm (Fig. 7.39)

1. The athlete lies supine with a straight arm and an open hand. The therapist grasps the athlete's hand and generates extension in the wrist and rotation towards the ulna (see Fig. 7.39A).

2. The deeply situated extensor muscles are stretched in a similar way with the exception that the cubital/elbow joint is flexed to relax the more superficial layer (see Fig. 7.39B).

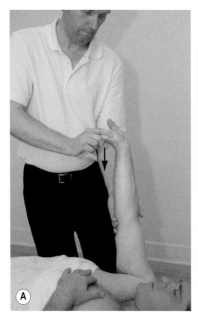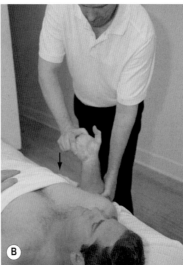

Figure 7.39 • Stretch of the flexor muscles of the forearm • A Stretch of the superficial flexor muscles B Stretch of the deep flexor muscles

References

Bazett-Jones, D.M., et al., 2008. Sprint and vertical jump performances are not affected by six weeks of static hamstring stretching. J. Strength Cond. Res. 22 (1), 25–31.

Cè, E., et al., 2008. Effects of stretching on maximal anaerobic power: the roles of active and passive warm-ups. J. Strength Cond. Res. 22 (3), 794–800.

Chaouachi, A., et al., 2008. Stretch and sprint training reduces stretch-induced sprint performance deficits in 13- to 15-year-old youth. Eur. J. Appl. Physiol. Jun 27. [Epub ahead of print].

Fletcher, I.M., Monte-Colombo, M.M., 2010. An investigation into the effects of different warm-up modalities on specific motor skills related to soccer performance. J. Strength Cond. Res. 24 (8), 2096–2101.

Herda, T.J., et al., 2008. Acute effects of static versus dynamic stretching on isometric peak torque, electromyography, and mechanomyography of the biceps femoris muscle. J. Strength Cond. Res. 22 (3), 809–817.

Herman, S.L., Smith, D.T., 2008. Four-week dynamic stretching warm-up intervention elicits longer-term performance benefits. J. Strength Cond. Res. 22 (4), 1286–1297.

Holt, B.W., Lambourne, K., 2008. The impact of different warm-up protocols on vertical jump performance in male collegiate athletes. J. Strength Cond. Res. 22 (1), 226–229.

Jaggers, J.R., et al., 2008. The acute effects of dynamic and ballistic stretching on vertical jump height, force, and power. J. Strength Cond. Res. 22 (6), 1844–1849.

Kendall, H.O., et al., 1971. Muscles, testing and function, second ed. Williams & Wilkins, Baltimore, MD.

La Torre, A., et al., 2010. Acute effects of static stretching on squat jump performance at different knee starting angles. J. Strength Cond. Res. 24 (3), 687–694.

McHugh, M.P., Nesse, M., 2008. Effect of stretching on strength loss and pain after eccentric exercise. Med. Sci. Sports Exerc. 40 (3), 566–573.

Mirca, M., et al., 2008. Pain syndromes in competitive elite level female artistic gymnasts. Role of specific preventive–compensative activity. Ital. J. Anat. Embryol. 113 (1), 47–54.

Needham, R.A., et al., 2009. The acute effect of different warm-up protocols on anaerobic performance in elite

youth soccer players. J. Strength Cond. Res. 23 (9), 2614–2620.

Samogin Lopes, F.A., et al., 2010. Is acute static stretching able to reduce the time to exhaustion at power output corresponding to maximal oxygen uptake? J. Strength Cond. Res. 24 (6), 1650–1656.

Samuel, M.N., et al., 2008. Acute effects of static and ballistic stretching on measures of strength and power. J. Strength Cond. Res. 22 (5), 1422–1428.

Sekir, U., et al., 2010. Acute effects of static and dynamic stretching on leg flexor and extensor isokinetic strength in elite women athletes. Scand. J. Med. Sci. Sports 20 (2), 268–281. Epub 2009 Apr 15.

Torres, E.M., et al., 2008. Effects of stretching on upper-body muscular performance. J. Strength Cond. Res. 22 (4), 1279–1285.

Wilson, J.M., Flanagan, E.P., 2008. The role of elastic energy in activities with high force and power requirements: a brief review. J. Strength Cond. Res. 22 (5), 1705–1715.

Wilson, J.M., et al., 2010. Effects of static stretching on energy cost and running endurance performance. J. Strength Cond. Res. 24 (9), 2274–2279.

Positional release techniques applied in sports massage

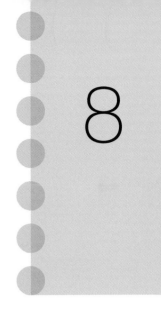

8

Positional release techniques (PRT) are a group of noninvasive effective manual techniques utilizing fine-tuned positions of optimal soft tissue relaxation and pain relief as a treatment for musculoskeletal dysfunctions. PRT techniques produce valuable physiological effects, stemming from both neurological and circulatory changes, when a dysfunctional area is placed in a position of optimal comfort and pain relief (Chaitow 1997). The creation of PRT techniques can be attributed to a number of practitioners, all of whom have contributed significantly to the advancement of manual soft tissue treatment.

The benefits of PRT for the sports massage therapist are many and its practical applications should not be overlooked. Due to the gentle nature of PRT, the techniques can be included in almost any athletic treatment situation. PRT applied in preevent massage can assist relaxation of overly tensed muscles; in postevent massage the techniques may reduce or prevent cramping tendencies; and PRT may assist quick recovery of muscles during interevent sports massage, especially when combined with massage and stretch techniques.

It is believed that during certain conditions, the flow of information between muscles and the central nervous system becomes dysfunctional. A trauma, rapid stretch of a previously approximated and relaxed muscle, or some other stressor may generate a disruption of the normal neural proprioception, causing overstimulation of the muscle spindles and nociceptors (Jones 1995), rendering them hypersensitive and triggering affected muscles into prolonged contraction (Fig. 8.1). Since the affected muscles in this condition commonly are positioned in an extremely shortened and relaxed position at first,

the muscle spindles are quiet. As the affected muscles are stretched rapidly, the spindles commence intense signaling to the central nervous system, triggering a myotatic reflex response with subsequent muscle contractions. The rapid change of state in the muscles concurrently renders the muscle spindles hypersensitive, and the central nervous system continues to interpret the neural proprioceptive inflow as if the affected muscles are truly in a state of stretch, even after the muscles are returned to their normal resting length, which triggers continued contractions. The perpetuated state of contraction concurrently activates spontaneous relaxation of antagonistic muscles (Jones 1995; Chaitow 1997), causing muscular imbalance that places stress on the affected joints and surrounding tissues, leading to persistent pain and dysfunction. If left untreated, the condition may remain for a long time, so that any attempt at increasing stretch or joint movement only generates additional tension and pain.

The sports massage therapist may perceive this as if the treated muscles are incapable of relaxing. Instead of struggling with the tissue by merely attempting to increase the applied stretch force, whether generated from sports massage techniques or therapeutic muscle stretching, the opposite approach is more beneficial. By palpating either the distressed tissue or a "tender point" (see "Strain Counterstrain," below), the dysfunctional part of the athlete's body is gently moved into a position of optimal soft tissue relaxation and pain relief. Subsequently holding this "position of ease" for a predetermined period of time will commonly release the dysfunctional state of spasm and/or tension in the tissue by lessening proprioceptor activity.

DOI: 10.1016/B978-0-443-10126-7.00008-3

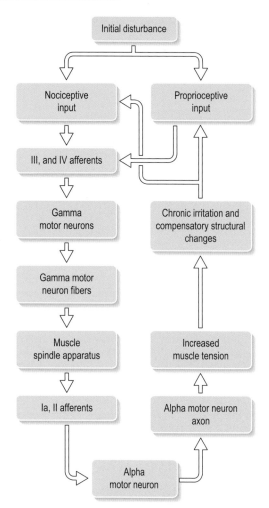

Figure 8.1 • **Proprioceptive dysfunction**

The noninvasive nature of PRT makes it very useful even in more delicate situations. Since it is virtually impossible to injure or traumatize an athlete using PRT, it makes these techniques a very useful tool also for early sports injury rehabilitation treatment. The basic concept behind PRT may be perceived as ingeniously simple and straightforward, but the possible initial therapeutic challenge lies more in the ability to register the subtle tissue reactions the athlete's body generates during the treatment. It often takes a bit of initial training and practice to be able to work efficiently with PRT, but the therapeutic rewards once adequate palpatory skill is acquired are substantial.

Fascial release (Chaitow 1997)

One effective soft tissue technique based on PRT principles is to simply approximate an area, large or small, of tensed soft tissue, and hold it for 3 min, followed by a slow release toward normal length. This tends to lower the tone in the tissue, and is an excellent tool for tensed well-developed muscles in athletes. The soft tissue is either pushed together with the hands (Fig. 8.2), or a part of the athlete's body is moved as a lever to relax the treated tissue. It is easier to utilize massage and stretch techniques after the elevated soft tissue tone is lowered.

Functional technique

Functional technique is based on osteopathic manipulation techniques focusing on function rather than structure alone (Hoover 2001). Osteopathic practitioners at the New England Academy of Applied Osteopathy coined the term "functional technique", during the 1950s (Bowles 1981) (Box 8.1). This early PRT method, with roots tracing back to the origin of osteopathic medicine (Bowles 1981; Chaitow 1997), utilizes movement of the dysfunctional tissue or segment, with simultaneous subjective palpation for the "position of ease" in the treated soft tissue. Functional technique establishes a state of "demand-response" where identified somatic dysfunctions are restored to normal functions (Pedowitz 2005). The method is based on reducing afferent information from mechanoreceptors and nociceptors in the affected tissues (Chaitow 1997).

As the treated area is moved toward "ease," normally involving a certain degree of approximation of the soft tissue, a noticeable palpable sensation of

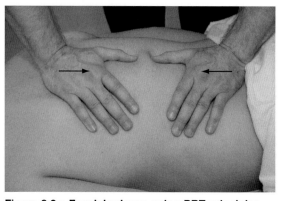

Figure 8.2 • **Fascial release using PRT principles**

Box 8.1

Functional technique terminology (Hoover 2001):

Motive hand – Something generating a motion demand through the treated tissues under the listening hand. It can be hands, fingers, thumbs, or even a verbal command to the athlete to generate motion.

　Motion demand – a desired movement for assessment, i.e. flexion, extension, lateral flexion, abduction, adduction, rotation, circumduction, etc. generated by the motive hand.

　Response – The response from the motion demand in the tissue or segment, reaching the listening hand for assessment.

　Listening hand – Any tactile part of the therapist used to assess the response in the treated tissue or segment.

relaxation occurs as the muscle tone decreases (Chaitow 1997). This natural relaxation was termed "dynamic neutral," and is defined as the state where soft tissues discover balance when the motion of the structure they assist is free and within normal physiological limits (Bowles 1981). Dynamic neutral should not be viewed as a static condition, but instead as a continuous normal state during daily activity (Chaitow 1997). It is the natural state to which all treated dysfunctional areas should be restored (Hoover 2001).

In the basic therapeutic execution of functional technique, one hand will serve as a motive hand (Chaitow 1997; Hoover 2001), creating motion demands by moving a joint or tissue in all directions, whilst the other hand acts as the listening hand (Chaitow 1997; Hoover 2001), registering any change (from the response) of tension in the palpated soft tissue. The listening hand must not move, and should register only compliance or noncompliance, i.e. "ease" or "bind," in the tissue (Bowles 1981; Hoover 2001). The motive hand (Chaitow 1997; Hoover 2001) moves the tissue or body part in all potential directions, whilst the listening hand registers binding tendencies in the soft tissue (Chaitow 1997). If only a sensation of ease is noted from the movements, the tissue function is considered normal. If there is however a sensation of binding, in any direction, a dysfunctional pattern is present in the palpated area (Chaitow 1997; Hoover 2001).

During treatment, the motion that produced the binding response is repeated, and the listening hand monitors the tissue as the movements are subsequently modified until the greatest feeling of ease is restored (Chaitow 1997; Hoover 2001).

There are two main variations of functional technique:

- Balance and hold.
- Dynamic functional.

Balance and hold

The listening hand lightly palpates the treated soft tissue while conforming to its shape. Each motion demand generated by the motive hand is, one by one, assessed for its respective position of ease. The dysfunctional joint is moved through all possible directions, with each separate movement starting at the previously applied movement's position of ease, making one position of ease "stack" on top of another (Chaitow 1997) until all combined positions of ease are accumulated, clearing the previous dysfunctional condition.

Example of balance and hold of the shoulder

1. The listening hand lightly touches the area of pain in the shoulder, simultaneously conforming to its shape (Fig. 8.3).
2. The motive hand grabs the upper part of the arm, generating a motion demand by moving the glenohumeral joint into flexion.
3. The listening hand registers the responses of bind and ease in the tissue, until the position of ease is detected.

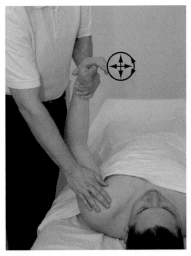

Figure 8.3 • Example of balance and hold of the shoulder

4. From this newly found position of ease, the next movement is initiated by the motive hand. The motive hand generates different motion demands, and the listening hand registers binding and ease, until only positions of ease remain. Dynamic neutral is restored.

Dynamic functional

Dynamic functional utilizes a constant change of tension in the tissue as the motive hand continuously, and in minute increments, moves the dysfunctional tissue or segment toward a position of ease. There is no pause between the motion demands, and the listening hand constantly assesses the tissue response. The end result is identical to the balance and hold method.

Example of dynamic functional of the hip joint

1. The listening hand lightly touches the area of pain or dysfunction at the hip area, simultaneously conforming to its shape (Fig. 8.4).
2. The motive hand moves the athlete's leg in small increments, starting with one of the possible movements.
3. The listening hand continuously registers the response of bind and ease in the tissue during the movements.

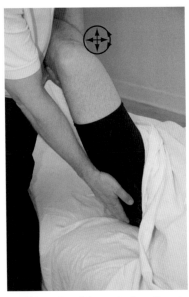

Figure 8.4 • Example of dynamic functional of the hip joint

4. The motive hand continuously adapts to the information the listening hand registers, and fluently guides the athlete's leg with motion demands until only positions of ease remain. Dynamic neutral is restored.

Strain Counterstrain

Strain Counterstrain (SCS) was one of the first major steps in osteopathic medicine to methodically map and treat musculoskeletal dysfunction (Jones 1995). Lawrence Jones, D.O., developed SCS in the 1950s after initially discovering that placing a pain patient, who was unresponsive to treatment, in a comfortable resting position for 20 min, produced unexpected pain relief that also had a lasting effect (Chaitow 1997). It is indicated that symptoms of iliotibial band syndrome are reduced with Strain Counterstrain techniques, allowing for tender point pain relief by moving the affected body part into its position of greatest comfort, which assists in lessening proprioceptor activity (Pedowitz 2005). Osteopathic manipulation techniques like SCS have also demonstrated to significantly reduce soreness, stiffness, and swelling from Achilles tendinitis (Howell et al. 2006). SCS has also shown promise in the treatment of chronic supraspinatus tendinitis and tendinosis, especially when combined with home exercises and modification of work posture (Jacobson et al. 1989).

The mobile point

Dr. Jones discovered that the position of maximal ease is achieved by slowly moving the body toward its original position of strain. This position is often an exaggeration of the presented adaptive distortion pattern at a given time. For example, if one wrist were initially strained in excessive flexion, the position of ease would later normally be somewhere in a more or less flexed position. The position of maximal ease and pain relief Jones named the "mobile point" (Fig. 8.5). During treatment, this position is sustained for 90 s, after which the treated body part or tissue is slowly eased out of the treatment position.

Tender points (TPs)

Dr. Jones noticed the presence of tender spot-like areas on the surface of the skin in fairly close proximity to the musculoskeletal dysfunction. The sensitivity of these points is generally around four times

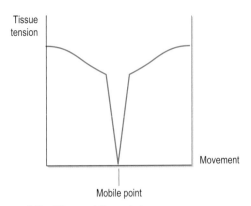

Figure 8.5 • The mobile point

higher than that of normal skin (Jones 1995), and can be described as a sensation similar to that of pressing on a bruise.

The tender points are used in SCS as monitoring and/or diagnostic tools, and should not be fully compared to myofascial trigger points (described in Chapter 11) or fibromyalgic tender points. Jones mapped over 200 TPs, relating to different types of strain, during years of clinical work. The TPs has specific locations and are clinically proven to serve as an important source of monitoring tenderness or tissue changes during SCS treatments. Chaitow has compared Jones TPs to A Shi acupuncture points, which are situated locally, often close to a joint, and tender to pressure (Chaitow 1997).

Besides finding the 'mobile point' through tissue relaxation at either the treated tissue site or via tender points during a treatment, the degree of palpatory pain from the TPs can serve as another monitoring method. Pain should decrease by at least 70%, and there should not be any additional pain created in the symptomatic area or any other area of the client's body (Chaitow 1997). The degree of sensitivity of the TP is verified by asking the client to rate the pain on a scale between zero and ten, where ten is the highest level of pain as the treatment begins. A rate of three or lower is a satisfactory level of ease for achieving respectable treatment results. During the treatment phase, the TP is periodically probed to ensure that the mobile point is maintained.

Examples of a few SCS techniques

SCS of the piriformis muscle (Jones 1995)

1. The athlete lies prone on the treatment table with the treated leg hanging off the table at

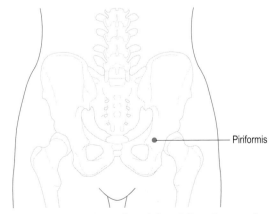

Figure 8.6 • SCS of the piriformis muscle (Jones 1995)

approximately 135-degree flexion in the hip joint, and the shin resting on the therapist's thigh (Fig. 8.6). This enables the therapist to easily adjust the position of the athlete's heavy leg. The femur is strongly abducted and laterally rotated to slacken the muscle.

2. The therapist palpates the tender point (Fig. 8.7) and either feels for tissue relaxation at the TP, or starts with a pain value of ten when lightly pressing on the TP. As the TP is compressed, the leg is fine-tuned by moving it into more (or less) flexion, abduction, and lateral rotation until the pain at the TP is relieved.

3. When the mobile point is reached, the tissue feels soft at the TP or the pain is relieved.

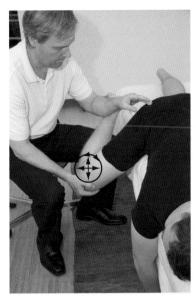

Figure 8.7 • Tender point of the piriformis muscle

123

During TP pain evaluation, a pain sensation with a value of three or less over the TP is considered satisfactory.

4. The position is held for from 90 s up to 3 min (modification), after which the pressure is slowly released.

SCS of the medial meniscus (Jones 1995)

1. The athlete lies supine on the treatment table with the treated lower leg hanging off the table at 60-degree flexion in the knee joint (Fig. 8.8). The tender point is level with the lower border of patella, on the medial aspect of the knee joint (Fig. 8.9).

2. The tibia is gradually medially rotated and slightly adducted with one hand, as the other hand palpates the tissue tension or pain level of the TP. The pain value starts at ten when lightly pressing on the TP. As the TP is compressed, the leg is fine-tuned by moving it into more (or less) flexion, adduction, and medial rotation until the TP tenderness is relieved.

3. When the mobile point is reached, the tissue feels soft at the TP or the pain is relieved. During TP pain evaluation, a pain sensation with a value of three or less over the TP is considered satisfactory.

4. The position is held for from 90 s up to 3 min (modification), after which the pressure is slowly released.

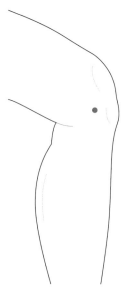

Figure 8.9 • Tender point of the medial meniscus located in the medial joint space of the knee joint, level with the inferior border of patella • Apply pressure laterally on the tender point

SCS of calcaneus (Jones 1995)

1. The athlete lies prone on the treatment table (Fig. 8.10). The tender point is on the anterior or medial part of the inferior side of the calcaneus (Fig. 8.11), and is often painful during plantar faciitis.

2. The therapist pulls the heel toward the ball of the foot with both hands, at the same time as the foot

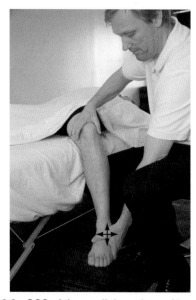

Figure 8.8 • SCS of the medial meniscus (Jones 1995)

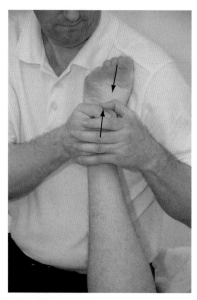

Figure 8.10 • SCS of calcaneus

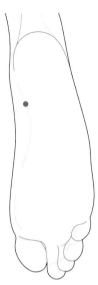

Figure 8.11 • Tender point of calcaneus

is pushed into plantar flexion by pressing toward the therapist's chest or shoulder. The thumb of one hand palpates the tissue tension or pain level of the TP. The pain value starts at ten when lightly pressing on the TP. The calcaneus and foot are fine-tuned until the TP tenderness is relieved.

3. When the mobile point is reached, the tissue feels soft at the TP or the pain is relieved. During TP pain evaluation, a pain sensation with a value of three or less over the TP is considered satisfactory.

4. The position is held for from 90 s up to 3 min (modification), after which the pressure is slowly released.

SCS of long head of biceps brachii muscle (Jones 1995)

The tendon is often involved during impingement syndrome of the shoulder.

1. The athlete lies supine on the treatment table (Fig. 8.12). The tender point is located in the bicipital groove (Fig. 8.13).

2. The therapist holds the athlete's forearm and places the athlete's dorsal side of the wrist on the forehead while palpating the TP with the other hand. The pain value starts at ten when lightly pressing on the TP. The athlete's arm is fine-tuned until the TP tenderness is relieved.

3. When the mobile point is reached, the tissue feels soft at the TP or the pain is relieved. During TP pain evaluation, a pain sensation with a value of three or less over the TP is considered satisfactory.

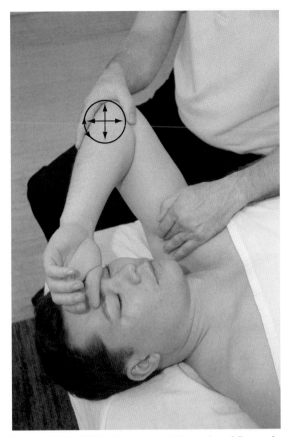

Figure 8.12 • SCS of long head of biceps brachii muscle

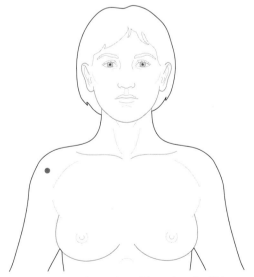

Figure 8.13 • Tender point of long head of biceps brachii muscle located on the tendon in the bicipital groove (intertubercular sulcus) • Apply the pressure on the tender point posteriorly

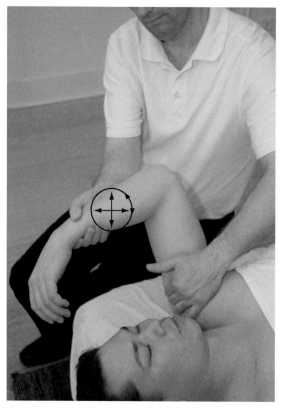

Figure 8.14 • SCS of the subdeltoid bursa

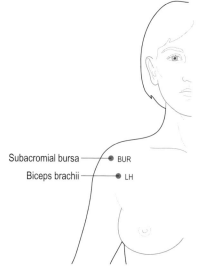

Figure 8.15 • Tender point of the subdeltoid bursa

4. The position is held for from 90 s up to 3 min (modification), after which the pressure is slowly released.

SCS of the subdeltoid bursa (Jones 1995)

A part of this bursa is often involved during impingement syndrome of the shoulder.

1. The athlete lies supine on the treatment table (Fig. 8.14). The tender point is high on the anterolateral part of humerus (Fig. 8.15)

2. The therapist holds the athlete's forearm with 90-degree flexion in the forearm, and flexion in the glenohumeral joint. The therapist's other hand palpates the TP. The pain value starts with 10 when lightly pressing on the tender point. The athlete's arm is fine tuned with flexion until the TP tenderness is relieved.

3. When the mobile point is reached, the tissue feels soft at the TP, or the pain is relieved. During TP pain evaluation, a pain sensation with a value of 3 or less over the tender point is considered satisfactory.

4. The position is held for from 90 s up to 3 min (modification), after which the pressure is slowly released.

References

Bowles, C.H., 1981. Functional technique: a modern perspective. JAOA 80 (5), 326/45–331/50.

Chaitow, L., 1997. Positional release techniques, second ed. Churchill Livingstone, Edinburgh.

Hoover, H.V., 2001. Functional technique in osteopathic manipulative treatment. JAOA 101 (3), 233–237.

Howell, J.N., et al., 2006. Stretch reflex and Hoffmann reflex responses to osteopathic manipulative treatment in subjects with Achilles tendinitis. J. Am. Osteopath. Assoc. 106 (9), 537–545.

Jacobson, E.C., et al., 1989. Shoulder pain and repetition strain injury to the supraspinatus muscle: etiology and manipulative treatment. J. Am.

Osteopath. Assoc. 89 (8), 1037–1040, 1043–1045.

Jones, L.H., 1995. Jones Strain-Counterstrain. Jones Strain-Counterstrain, Carlsbad, CA.

Pedowitz, R.N., 2005. Use of osteopathic manipulative treatment for iliotibial band friction syndrome. J. Am. Osteopath. Assoc. 105 (12), 563–567.

Acupressure and Tui Na in sports massage

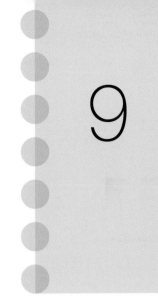

9

According to Asian philosophy, Qi (literally "air, breath") is the circulating life force without which all living things cannot exist. It pervades all living beings, including the human body, and when it is circulating in a natural way, health is the prevalent state. Qi circulates in specific pathways named channels and collaterals, together often referred to as "meridians," which form layers of energy that permeate the body. Major points of access to this energy flow are called "acupuncture points," or "acupoints," and are divided into three basic groups:

1. **Regular acupoints.** These acupoints are located bilaterally on the 12 regular channels, and individually on the "extraordinary channels" Du Mai and Ren Mai, which run on the anterior and posterior midline of the body (Fig. 9.1).
2. **Extraordinary points.** These points have distinct names and locations not always immediately associated with the regular channels. Even though they are situated in many different areas of the body, they are still related to the meridian system, and are commonly used to treat specific conditions.
3. **Ah Shi points.** Local acupoints, tender upon pressure, which are often used during treatment of different pain syndromes.

Acupuncture channels (Fig. 9.1)

The acupoints have distinctly uniform locations, given through a combination of anatomical landmarks and the personally adapted measurement units called "cun." The cun units are measured from the treated athlete's body.

Examples of cun measurements (Fig. 9.2)

Head

- Anterior to posterior hairline: 12 cun.

Chest and abdomen

- Between two nipples: 8 cun.
- Tip of xiphoid process to center of umbilicus: 8 cun.
- Center of umbilicus to superior ramus of the pubic bone: 5 cun.

Back

- Between the two medial borders of the scapulae: 6 cun.
- Medial border of scapulae to center of the spinous process of same-level thoracic vertebrae: 3 cun.

Upper extremities

- End of the axillary fold to the transverse cubital crease: 9 cun.
- Transverse cubital crease to the transverse wrist crease: 12 cun.
- Distance between four fingers (excluding the thumb): 3 cun.
- Width of thumb at the interphalangeal joint: 1 cun.

DOI: 10.1016/B978-0-443-10126-7.00009-5

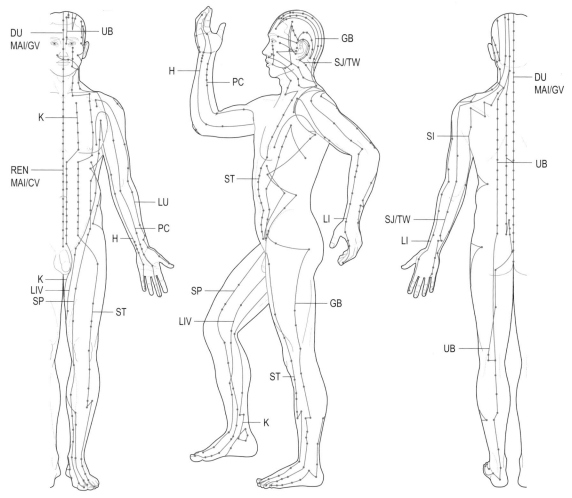

Figure 9.1 • Acupuncture channels

Lower extremities

- Greater trochanter to the middle of patella: 19 cun.
- Center of patella to tip of lateral malleolus: 16 cun.
- Superior ramus of the pubic bone to the superior border of the medial femoral epicondyle ridge: 18 cun.
- Inferior border of the tibial condyle to the tip of medial malleolus: 13 cun.
- Lateral malleolus to lateral edge of the heel: 3 cun.

According to more recent research, the energy channels are commonly found to be located adjacent to larger fascias. A high correlation between fascial formations and the meridian-based channel system was discovered when scanning connective tissue structures in the human body and further combining them with the traditional meridian system and acupoints (Huang et al. 2006). The channels can also be mapped through refined measurement methods of skin impedance (Hu et al. 1993).

Stimulation of the body's energetic system through needles, heat, electricity, and manual pressure has long been part of the Asian medical tradition. Studies have indicated that acupuncture can significantly increase maximum performance capacity and physical performance at the anaerobic threshold (Ehrlich & Haber 1992), and that electrical acupoint stimulation can enhance athletes' rapid strength (Yang et al. 2006). The application of pressure on acupoints using fingers, elbows, or specific tools

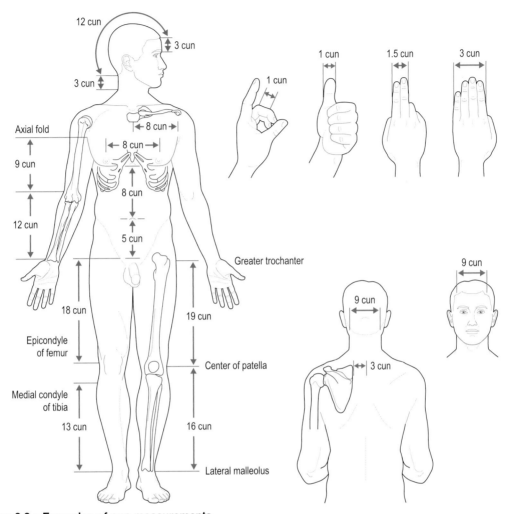

Figure 9.2 • Examples of cun measurements

can be a great supplement to sports massage therapy. Manual stimulation of acupuncture points is often referred to as acupressure, and can be beneficially combined with Chinese manual therapy forms like Tui Na (i.e., push-grasp.) or the Japanese equivalent, Shiatsu.

It has been shown that manual pressure on acupuncture points can substantially influence the cardiovascular system (Felhendler & Lisander 1999). Research has also found that acupressure can be another useful treatment method for reducing low back pain, including when combined with aromatic essential lavender oil treatment (Hsieh et al. 2004; Yip & Tse 2004).

Yin–yang

A well-known concept of balance and change of all material and energetic manifestations is the symbol of yin–yang (Chengnan 1993) (Fig. 9.3). This is the principle of "heaven and earth" that is the guiding force of all existing things: two opposing forces that are mutually dependent. Yet in spite of their opposing nature, yin contains a part of yang within itself, as yang contains a piece of yin, as they constantly transform into one another. Yin–yang can be described as two sides of the same coin, where one is equally vital to the existence of the other. Yin is often described as "the shady side of the hill"

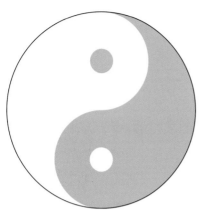

Figure 9.3 • Yin–yang

whereas yang is accordingly depicted as "the sunny side of the hill" (Box 9.1).

The symbol of yin–yang illustrates in an ingenious way the reality of constant change affecting all things in the universe, from the absolutely smallest to the very largest. Health is maintained through keeping a state of balance throughout life rather than striving for a more static or permanent condition. A static condition would only cause stagnation, which according to Asian medicine is a major cause of pathological conditions and should be avoided at all cost. Working with the energy system of the body, releasing blockages through stimulation of the energy channels and acupoints, is therefore an excellent tool to assist balance and the free flow of Qi.

Sports massage treatments are often applied along the concept of yin–yang. For an athlete that is too nervous and mentally overactive before a competitive event (dominant yang), a slower yin-based preevent massage treatment is used to help balance the mental and physical state. For an athlete that is too relaxed (dominant yin) and not yet in the desired mental

peak state, a brisker and faster yang-based massage treatment would be used for stimulation.

Acupressure

Actively stimulating acupoints with either digital or elbow pressure can release energetic blocks in the channels. Acupressure is performed by either pressing or massaging on selected acupoints chosen for their specific effects (regular and extra points), tenderness (Ah Shi points), or where increased tissue tension is noted. According to Asian medicine, pain is created through stagnation of Qi and Blood. A dull, aching pain is considered to be more Qi-based whereas a sharper, more intense pain results from added Blood stagnation. By resolving energetic and circulatory blockages through acupressure, Qi and Blood can flow more freely and tension, pain, or dysfunction is reduced (Hsieh et al. 2004).

Digital pressure

The most common method of applying acupressure is through digital pressure. This is performed with braced thumbs, or long or index fingers, and is applied to selected acupoints during the treatment. The pressure is directed either straight into the point with gradually increased intensity, or as a focalized circular massage. Pressure with longitudinal local massage along the treated channel, crossing acupoints during the stroke, is also an effective technique to reduce stagnation.

Thumb pressure with simultaneous massage along the channels (Fig. 9.4)

The soft tissue is massaged with short strokes, back and forth along the affected energy channels, while simultaneously crossing local acupoints. All the channels in the region of tension or pain are treated to support an unrestricted flow of Qi and Blood.

Tui Na

While acupressure is generally performed by manually stimulating acupoints through direct pressure or focal massage, Tui Na also encompass a wide range of strokes and body movements. Both acupressure and Tui Na can treat a multitude of physical ailments, but for the sports massage therapist, soft tissue

---

Box 9.1

Examples of attributed qualities of yin–yang

Yin	Yang
Cold	Warm
Night	Day
Shadow	Sunshine
Slow	Fast
Wet	Dry
Resting	Active
Large	Small

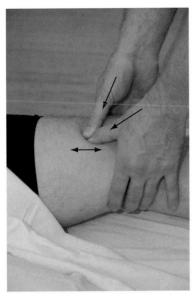

Figure 9.4 • Thumb pressure with simultaneous massage along the channels

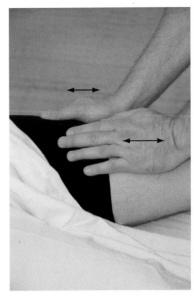

Figure 9.5 • Palm scrubbing

dysfunction is the primary focus here. The treated tissue is pushed, grasped, stretched, compressed, etc., in combination with manual acupoint stimulation, to effectively alleviate the condition. Even though Tui Na often has a strong execution, an emphasis is placed on not overstimulating the body (Xiangcai 2002).

Examples of common Tui Na strokes

Scrubbing

Scrubbing strokes effectively warm the body through friction. Rubbing the skin briskly will increase blood circulation and the heat generated can traverse the treated channels to dispel cold. The pressure is generally light and the stroke is executed at a frequency of 50–100 strokes a minute (Mengzhong 1997). Scrubbing strokes are excellent to use if the athlete feels cold during pre-, post- or interevent sports massage. It is imperative that the therapist keep the arms and shoulders relaxed to avoid early fatigue.

Palm scrubbing (Fig. 9.5)

The flatly positioned palms alternately rub the athlete's skin along the body part and channels until the desired heat is generated. The whole palm serves as the contact surface. On curved areas like the arms and legs, the palms must conform to the rounder

shape for maintained friction. When both hands are used, palm scrubbing is performed alternately with each hand.

Pressing

Pressing of muscles and/or acupoints is executed with the palms, fingers, or elbows. The pressure, directed deep within the muscles, is commonly used to alleviate pain (Mengzhong 1997).

Palm pressing

Palm pressing is executed with the whole palm, heel of the palm, hypothenar, or thenar eminence, depending on the size of the treated area (Fig. 9.6).

Digital pressing

Digital pressing is generally performed with either braced thumbs, the knuckle of the proximal interphalangeal joint of a bent index or long finger, or the interphalangeal joint of a bent thumb (Fig. 9.7).

Elbow pressing

Elbow pressing uses the tip of the olecranon process to push deep into the soft tissue. This stroke is used when working on areas with larger or more deeply situated muscles (Fig. 9.8).

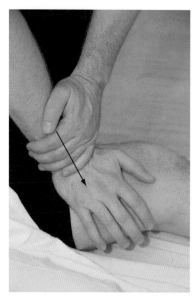

Figure 9.6 • Palm pressing

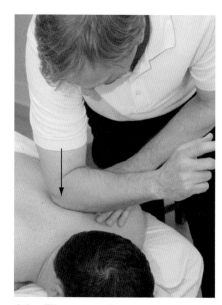

Figure 9.8 • Elbow pressing

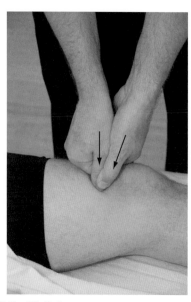

Figure 9.7 • Digital pressure

Rubbing

Rubbing strokes are executed at a rapid pace along a straight line, back and forth, while minimizing gliding on the skin. For the sports massage therapist, the main purpose is to stimulate blood circulation, disperse stagnant Qi to reduce pain, and minimize soft tissue tension. The applied pressure is initially gentle but increases as the tissue softens. Rubbing strokes are also effective on larger areas of Qi stagnation and muscle tension. Due to its rapid execution, it is very important to keep the arms and hands relaxed.

Thumb rubbing

Thumb rubbing is used on specific areas of tension, where the thumb "vibrates" down through the acupoint or tensed soft tissue. While the index finger is bent to brace the thumb, the tip of the thumb is placed on the tensed area. Small shaking movements of the arm make the springing thumb gradually penetrate more deeply into the soft tissue (Fig. 9.9). A correctly executed stroke will give the therapist a feeling of having the thumb "sink" through the tissues.

Thenar rubbing

The proximal base of the thenar eminence of one hand is placed on the area of tensed soft tissue. The wrist is relaxed and the hand is rapidly moved back and forth in a straight line or spiral movement (Mengzhong 1997) (Fig. 9.10). As the tissue relaxes, the stroke moves to an adjacent area.

Hypothenar rubbing

The hypothenar edge of one hand is pressed on the tensed soft tissue. With a relaxed wrist, the hand smoothly but rapidly moves back and forth in a straight line (Fig. 9.11). The hand is also pressed fairly firmly into the soft tissue to achieve greater depth with the stroke.

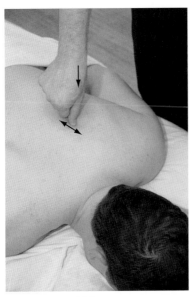

Figure 9.9 • Thumb rubbing

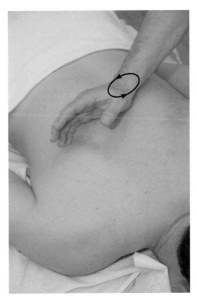

Figure 9.11 • Hypothenar rubbing

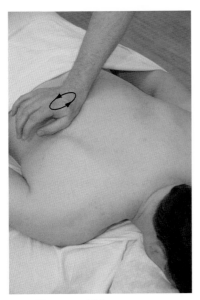

Figure 9.10 • Thenar rubbing

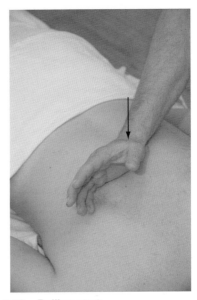

Figure 9.12 • Rolling start

Rolling (Xiangcai 2002) (Figs 9.12–9.14)

The rolling stroke is perhaps one of the more commonly known Tui Na strokes, and takes some practice to master. Described effects are muscle relaxation, promoted blood circulation, warming the channels, relieving muscle spasm, "weakening" adhesions, and "lubricating" joints (Xiangcai 2002). Rolling is applied on larger areas of the body and is executed at a frequency of 140–160 strokes/minute (Xiangcai 2002).

The hypothenar eminence is pressed into the tissue, and as the stroke rolls toward the dorsum of the hand, the wrist, elbow and shoulder bend simultaneously. The rolling stroke moves back and forth, and gradually covers a larger area. The

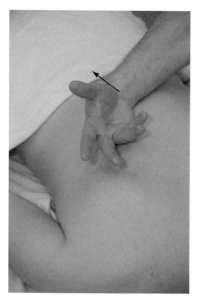

Figure 9.13 • Rolling finish

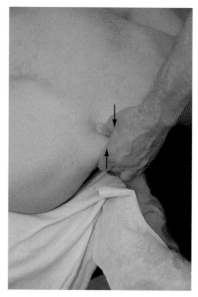

Figure 9.15 • Grasping

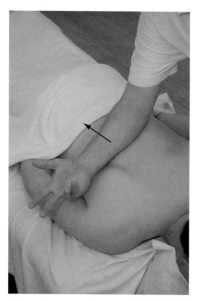

Figure 9.14 • Forearm rolling

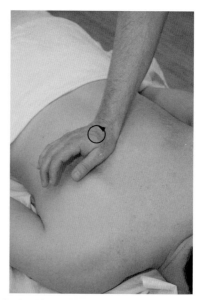

Figure 9.16 • Kneading

forearms are used for rolling in a similar manner. The pressure on the tissue is firm.

Grasping

The tissue or acupoint is grasped between the thumb and remaining four fingers. Grasping is executed by slowly lifting, holding, and simultaneously twisting the treated soft tissue (Fig 9.15). Some of the effects are increased blood circulation, and relieving muscle tension and spasm. Grasping is used on the neck, shoulder, extremities, and lower back.

Kneading

Kneading is executed by moving the palm, palm heel, thenar, or hypothenar eminence in a circular motion as the soft tissue is compressed (Fig. 9.16).

Examples of some basic Tui Na treatments for remedial sports massage

Lumbar strain (Mengzhong 1997)

Treated acupoints (Fig. 9.17)

- **Du 4.** On the posterior midline, inferior to the spinous process of L2.
- **UB 23.** 1.5 cun lateral to the posterior midline, level with the spinous process of L2.
- **Yaoyan.** 3.5 cun lateral to the posterior midline, level with the spinous process of L4.
- **UB 25.** 1.5 cun lateral to the posterior midline, level with the spinous process of L4.
- **GB 30.** At the junction of medial two-thirds and lateral one-third of the distance from the hiatus of sacrum to the greater trochanter of femur.
- **UB 40.** At the midline of the transverse crease of the popliteal fossa between the tendons of the semitendinosus and biceps femoris muscles.
- **Ah Shi points.** Locally tender acupoints.

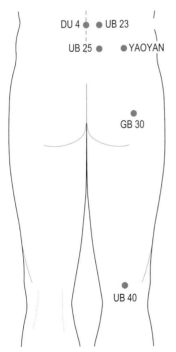

Figure 9.17 • Treated acupoints in lumbar strain

Palm pressing

The therapist applies palm pressing on the acupoints, including local Ah Shi points. As the tissue softens, digital pressing with the thumbs replaces palm pressing. For more massive and well-developed muscles, elbow pressing can substitute for digital pressing.

Grasping and forearm rolling of muscles in the lower back

The therapist employs strong bilateral grasping and forearm rolling of the muscles in the lower back and gluteal region for 10 min, or until the treated muscles feel warm.

Elbow pressing

Strong focal elbow pressing is applied to larger muscles in the area, and bilaterally to UB 25.

Chronic rotator cuff pain (Mengzhong 1997; Xiangcai 2002)

Treated acupoints (Fig. 9.18)

- **St 12.** Midpoint of the supraclavicular fossa, 4 cun lateral to the anterior midline.
- **LI 15.** Inferior to the acromion, at the superior part of the deltoid muscle, and in the depression formed by the anterior border of the acromioclavicular joint as the arm is abducted.
- **GB 21.** Midway between the spinous process of C7 and the acromion process, at the highest point of the superior part of the trapezius muscle.
- **SI 11.** In the infraspinous fossa, at the junction between the superior one-third and mid one-third of a line connecting the lower border of the scapular spine and the inferior angle of the scapulae (Schanke et al. 2001).
- **Ah Shi points.** Locally tender acupoints.

Digital pressing

The athlete rests in a seated position. The therapist performs digital pressing on the selected acupoints, including local Ah Shi points.

Palm pressing and grasping

The therapist uses gentle grasping and pressing of the shoulder and scapular region, focusing on the subacromial and deltoid areas (Fig. 9.19). Pressing and grasping the supraspinatus, subscapularis, infraspinatus, and teres minor muscles facilitates movement of stagnant Qi and Blood.

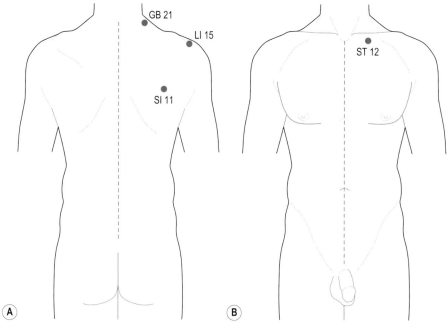

Figure 9.18 • Treated acupoints in chronic rotator cuff pain

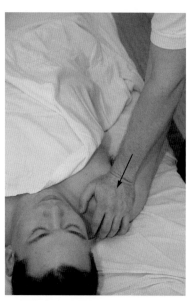

Figure 9.19 • Palm pressing and grasping

Arm movement

The athlete's arm is passively abducted, adducted, and rotated within the pain barrier to ensure stronger stimulation. This can be combined with simultaneous thumb pressing on selected Ah Shi points. To loosen potential adhesions, the shoulder is scrubbed, and finally gently shaken as it is moved through the available ROM.

Lateral knee pain/"runner's knee"

Treated acupoints (Cash 1996; Mengzhong 1997; Schanke et al. 2001) (Fig. 9.20)

- **GB 31.** 7 cun above the transverse popliteal crease on the midline of the lateral side of the thigh.
- **GB 33.** In the depression superior and posterior to the lateral condyle of femur, between the tendon of the biceps femoris muscle and the femur.
- **GB 34.** In the depression anterior and inferior to the head of fibula.
- **St 35.** With the knee flexed, on the lower border of patella in the depression lateral to the patellar ligament.
- **ST 36.** 3 cun below St 35, one finger width from the anterior crest of tibia.
- **UB 37.** On the posterior aspect of the thigh, 6 cun below UB 36, on the line connecting UB 36 and UB 40.
- **UB 39.** At the lateral end of the popliteal transverse crease, on the medial side of the biceps femoris tendon.
- **UB 40.** At the midline of the transverse crease of the popliteal fossa between the tendons of the semitendinosus and biceps femoris muscles.

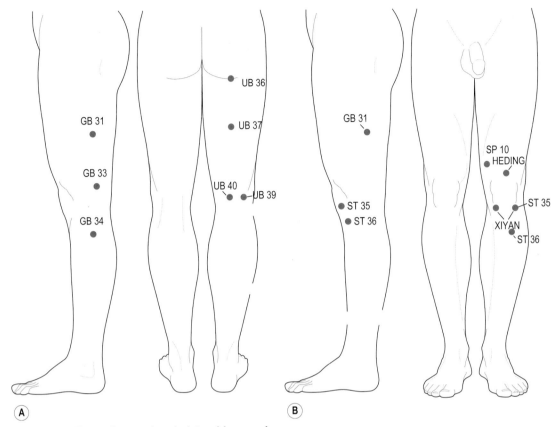

Figure 9.20 • Treated acupoints in lateral knee pain

- **Heding.** Superior to the knee, in the depression at the midpoint of the superior patellar border.
- **Sp 10.** With the knee flexed, on the medial side of the thigh, 2 cun above the superior medial corner of the patella, on the prominence of the vastus medialis muscle.
- **Xiyan.** When the knee is flexed, the point is in the depression medial to the patellar ligament.
- **Ah Shi points.** Locally tender acupoints.

Rolling

The athlete lies on the side as the therapist performs hypothenar and forearm rolling on the lateral aspect of the thigh, especially in the area closer to the knee.

Pressing

To soften the tissue, the therapist applies strong longitudinal and transverse palm pressing on the iliotibial tract, tensor fasciae latae, and vastus lateralis muscle, working the area from the hip to the knee. This is followed by thumb pressing on the acupoints.

Leg movement

The sports massage therapist finally performs circular thumb massage in the painful area of the knee as the leg is simultaneously flexed and extended.

References

Cash, M., 1996. Sports & remedial massage therapy. Ebury Press, London.

Chengnan, S., 1993. Chinese bodywork: a complete manual of Chinese

therapeutic massage. Pacific View Press, Berkeley, CA.

Ehrlich, D., Haber, P., 1992. Influence of acupuncture on physical performance capacity and haemodynamic

parameters. Int. J. Sports Med. 13 (6), 486–491.

Felhendler, D., Lisander, B., 1999. Effects of non-invasive stimulation of acupoints on the cardiovascular system. Complement. Ther. Med. 7 (4), 231–234.

Hsieh, L.L., et al., 2004. A randomized controlled clinical trial for low back pain treated by acupressure and physical therapy. Prev. Med. 39 (1), 168–176.

Hu, X., et al., 1993. Studies on the low skin impedance points and the feature of its distribution along the channels by microcomputer. II. Distribution of LSIPS along the channels. Zhen Ci Yan Jiu 18 (2), 163–167.

Huang, Y., et al., 2006. Study on the meridians and acupoints based on fasciaology: an elicitation of the study on digital human being. Zhongguo Zhen Jiu 26 (11), 785–788.

Mengzhong, X., 1997. Manual treatment for traumatic injuries. Foreign Language Press, Beijing.

Schanke, E., et al., 2001. Qdex: a quick index of acupoints. Qpuncture, Anaheim, CA.

Xiangcai, X., 2002. Chinese Tui Na massage: the essential guide to treating injuries, improving health &

balancing Qi, vol. 13. YMAA Publication Center, Wolfeboro, NH.

Yang, H.Y., et al., 2006. Electrical acupoint stimulation increases athletes' rapid strength. Zhongguo Zhen Jiu 26 (5), 313–315.

Yip, Y.B., Tse, S.H., 2004. The effectiveness of relaxation acupoint stimulation and acupressure with aromatic lavender essential oil for non-specific low back pain in Hong Kong: a randomized controlled trial. Complement. Ther. Med. 12 (1), 28–37.

Myofascial release techniques and connective tissue massage

10

Connective tissue (Fig. 10.1) is one of the most abundant tissue forms in the human body. It serves to connect, support, bind, and separate either organs or other forms of tissue. It is divided into ordinary and specialized connective tissue subgroups.

Ordinary connective tissue provides a mechanical link between muscles and bones, or bones and joints, and binds cells together into tissues, organs, and systems (Watkins 1999). Examples include: tendons, aponeuroses, ligaments, fasciae, Sharpey's fibers, joint capsules, loose irregular connective tissue that serves as a pathway for nerves and blood vessels, and adipose tissue (Watkins 1999; Stanborough 2004).

Specialized connective tissue comprises bone, cartilage, and blood (Watkins 1999; Stanborough 2004).

Examples of ordinary connective tissue structures frequently treated by sports massage therapists are fasciae, tendons, aponeuroses, ligaments, joint capsules, and dysfunctional states like fibrotic tissue and adhesions. The fascial connective tissue in the human body is often described as a three-dimensional web or network, to which many other structures are linked in one way or another as it runs through the body. Ida Rolf, one of the pioneers of myofascial work, called this fascial web "the organ of structure" (Smith 2005).

Connective tissue (Fig. 10.1)

In reality, it may be somewhat difficult to functionally separate muscles, fasciae, nerves, and blood vessels from each other since these structures work in unison during movement (Myers 2002). Additionally, most manual treatment forms will affect all these structures simultaneously, albeit more or less effectively. The realization of the structural importance of fascial connective tissue, and its consequences on function or health if dysfunctional, inspired the development of more specific connective tissue and myofascial treatment techniques.

Exercises strongly affecting the myofascial system can be traced back to at least as far as the roots of Hatha yoga, and several manual treatment forms, including massage, have existed since ancient times. In Sweden, Per Henrik Ling founded in the early 1800s the "Swedish movement cure," where massage, stretching, and exercise were combined to generate health. In the USA, Dr. Andrew Taylor Still founded osteopathy in 1874 (Chikly 2005), which addressed movement restrictions and compression of nerves, blood, and lymph vessels by bone, muscles, or inflammatory swelling (Chikly 2005). These conditions were initially treated by gently manipulating the joints, particularly in the spine. Osteopathy later evolved to include a wide range of specific myofascial and other soft tissue techniques.

Dr. Oakley Smith, one of the first dozen chiropractors in the USA, founded the manual therapy discipline naprapathy in 1905 after realizing the extent to which scar and/or generally shortened connective tissue could interfere with the function of blood vessels, nerves, and other structures, ultimately causing pathology (Smith 1919, 1966, 1932). He stated that not only traumatic injuries could cause debilitating changes in connective tissue, but poor diet, insufficient rest, and poor personal hygiene might as well (Smith 1932). Smith established that through different angles in sequence, repeatedly stretching the connective tissue fibers of contractures with specially developed

DOI: 10.1016/B978-0-443-10126-7.00010-1

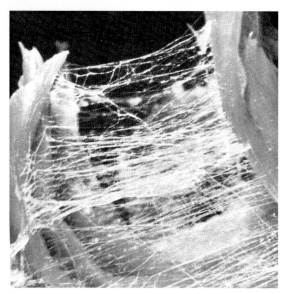

Figure 10.1 • Connective tissue

manipulation techniques could normalize dysfunction and also release nerve interference along the spinal column (Smith 1932). He consequently called the techniques "stretchments" (or "naprapathic directos") instead of "adjustments," to emphasize the treatment intention, and considered this a key to producing more lasting relief for the patient (Smith 1932). Moreover, Smith considered scar tissue to be one of the most stubborn conditions the body must deal with, and that it could account for the chronic nature of many symptoms (Smith 1932).

After many years of extensive research, Dr. Ida Rolf founded "structural integration" in the 1960s (Smith 2005) to address structural and postural dysfunctional patterns in the body. This treatment form is commonly referred to nowadays as Rolfing (Stanborough 2004), and it is practiced by many manual therapists around the world. Rolfing has been demonstrated to produce physiological effects on myofascial structures and the peripheral nervous system (Jones 2004). The method is traditionally performed in a series of ten treatments, each addressing different areas or conditions of the body.

Several other myofascial treatment systems have emerged over the years, each offering different perspectives and additions. Some were created by former students of Ida Rolf, or her institute, such as Joseph Heller—Heller work, Judith Aston—Aston patterning, Tom Myers—anatomy trains, and Erik Dalton—myoskeletal alignment techniques; whilst additional methods were formed by other therapists

like Dr. Leon Chaitow—soft tissue manipulation, John F. Barnes—one of the forces behind myofascial release, Jack Painter—postural integration, William Leigh—Zen bodytherapy, and others (Myers 2002; Smith 2005). Today, myofascial release is a very popular soft tissue treatment method comprising several styles, some gentler whilst others present a more forceful approach.

Myofascial release techniques are valuable in sports massage therapy since they can assist the athlete toward optimal posture, movement ability, and recovery. For instance, it has been shown that myofascial release massage supports recovery back to preexercise levels with regard to heart rate variability and diastolic blood pressure after high-intensity exercise (Arroyo-Morales et al. 2008). It is indicated that patients with carpal tunnel syndrome treated with myofascial release manipulation and self-stretching improved clinically (Sucher 1993). Myofascial release also produces effects on the autonomic nervous system (Henley et al. 2008), and it is suggested that runners who present coexisting sacroiliac joint dysfunction and internal snapping hip syndrome may benefit from myofascial release in combination with proprioceptive neuromuscular facilitation (Konczak & Ames 2005). Fascia is somewhat pliable, and myofascial release uses this tissue plasticity in the treatment to achieve more lasting results. Research suggests that the integration of plasticity from connective tissue with the nervous system may possibly clarify mechanisms of an assortment of treatment methods that may reverse chronic lower back pain by employing mechanical forces to soft tissue (Langevin & Sherman 2007).

Fascial connective tissues have previously been viewed as solely passive structures, capable only of conveying mechanical tension produced by muscle activation or an external force (Schleip et al. 2005). It is now suggested, however, that there is evidence of contractile cells in fascia, possibly enabling a contraction with similar behavior to smooth muscle (Schleip et al. 2005). Successful demonstrations of autonomous contraction of human lumbar fascia, in vitro studies with fascia, and pharmacological stimulation of temporary contractions in ordinary fascia in rats, support this hypothesis (Schleip et al. 2005). If confirmed by additional research, active fascial contractibility could present remarkable benefits for the comprehension of certain musculoskeletal pathologies, and a deeper understanding of the effects of treatments like myofascial release techniques (Schleip et al. 2005).

Effects in the fascial network

Fascia comprises three layers in the human body: the superficial fascia secures the dermis of the skin to underlying structures, deep fascia surrounds individual organs and muscles, and the subserous fascia, situated between the internal layer of the deep fascia and the serous membranes, lines the cavities of the body.

The fascial "network" in the body is formed when several fascial structures are linked to each other in specific patterns. A shortening of the connective tissue in one part will therefore have an effect in another, possibly more distant, area of the body (Fig. 10.2). A recent study demonstrated the presence of myofascial force transmission between antagonistic muscles. Lengthening of the extensor digitorum longus muscle in the lower leg changed forces applied on the tibia and forces exerted by the antagonistic peroneal muscle group, which could be possible only through existing "extramuscular myofascial connections" (Huijing & Baan 2008).

Thomas Myers describes the linked fascial structures as "myofascial meridians" (Myers 2002) that form specific pathways, or individual "anatomy train lines" (Myers 2002), as they run through the body.

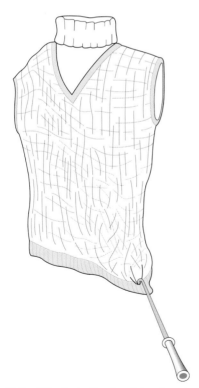

Figure 10.2 • Effects in the fascial network.

These pathways generate structural tensile strength and support in the body, but can create dysfunctions if adaptively shortened or injured. Having an understanding of the principle of the fascial trajectory enables the sports massage therapist to more effectively assess and treat structural connective tissue distortions.

Myers' (2002) principle of "anatomy trains" presents myofascial meridian lines represented in seven groups:

1. Superficial back line.
2. Superficial front line.
3. Lateral line.
4. Spiral line.
5. Arm lines.
6. Deep front line.
7. Functional lines.

Techniques

As a general rule, myofascial release techniques are at first applied to superficial layers and then deeper structures are addressed as the more superficial fascial distortions treated release. Anterior–posterior balance is addressed firstly by working on the posterior and anterior superficial lines (Smith 2005). This is commonly followed by treatment of lateral distortions, followed by rotational issues.

Examples of myofascial release stroke applications

The myofascial release strokes are performed with fingers, loose fists, forearms, or elbows (Fig. 10.3), and are executed slowly to minimize activation of the myotatic/stretch reflex. The stroke is taken to the appropriate depth, and it is important the therapist continuously feels contact with the fascial layer and registers the body's response. By applying body weight, the stroke slowly slides through the tissue (Smith 2005). Should the glide ratio be too high, the "grip" in the fascia is lost, and the stroke must be reapplied. The amount of emollient used is consequently sparse to ensure maximal stretch effect without injuring the skin.

The stroke angle can also be modified during implementation to ensure a continued stretch effect in the fascial structure. Typically, a 45-degree angle into both the tissue and treatment direction will ensure the desired stretch effect, but a supplementary

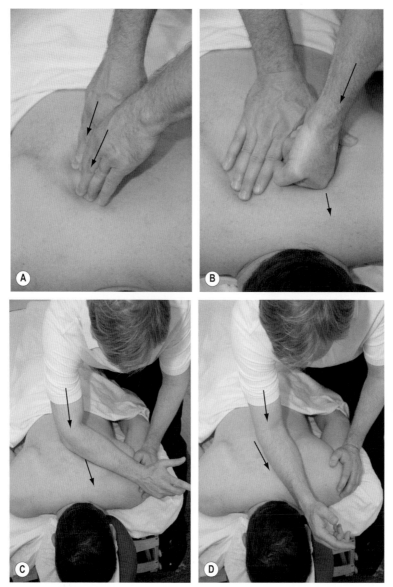

Figure 10.3 • Example of myofascial release stroke applications • A Fingers/"chisel" (Smith 2005) stroke B Fist stroke C Forearm stroke D Elbow stroke

45-degree angle across the fiber direction may also be required. The athlete can also assist upon the therapist's command by actively generating slow movements, thus lengthening the treated tissue into an augmented stretch, and moreover simultaneously assisting in proprioceptive conditioning (Smith 2005).

The following are examples of basic myofascial release techniques of the back, front, and lateral lines. Additional techniques are presented in Chapter 14.

Superficial back line

The superficial back line (SBL) connects the whole posterior aspect of the body (Fig. 10.4). It consists of two lines, parallel to the midline, running from the bottom of the feet to the top of the head. The SBL holds an important postural function, which generally renders fascial structures thicker and stronger.

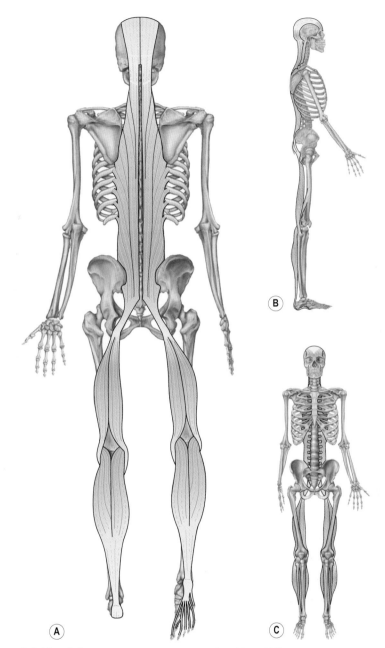

Figure 10.4 • Superficial back line Reproduced with permission from Myers 2002

Important myofascial structures of the SBL (Myers 2002)

- Plantar aponeurosis.
- Calcaneus tendon.
- Ischiocrural/hamstring fasciae including the tendons.
- Sacrotuberous ligament.
- Thoracolumbar fascia.
- Longitudinal fascial aspect of the erector spinae group.
- Structures at the occipital ridge.

Fist glide of the plantar aponeurosis

The therapist uses the fist with major contact on the second and third knuckle area to initiate the stroke just anterior to the calcaneus bone (Fig. 10.5). As the stroke slowly glides toward

143

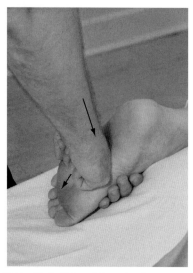

Figure 10.5 • Fist glide of the plantar aponeurosis

the toes, the athlete is simultaneously asked to slowly extend the toes.

Fist glide and thumb glide on triceps surae muscle

The athlete lies prone. The therapist glides with the fist supported by the other hand, or with a reinforced thumb (Fig. 10.6) from just superior to the athlete's heel. The stroke is gradually worked up to the posterior aspect of the knee. The athlete can assist with slow active dorsiflexion of the ankle joint.

The ischiocrural/hamstring muscle group

The athlete remains prone but with the knee resting in flexion (Fig. 10.7). The therapist uses the flat part of the elbow to gradually massage and stretch the

fascial layers up to the ischial tuberosity. The athlete can assist with active extension of the knee joint.

The ischiocrural/hamstring muscles and tendons located at the knee serve to assist the anterior cruciate ligament by supporting the integration between the tibia and femur when forces stress the tibia anteriorly (Di Fabio et al. 1992).

Thoracolumbar fascia

The athlete rests prone in the yoga pose named "child's pose" (Smith 2005) (Fig. 10.8). The therapist uses the forearm or palm heel to slowly glide up toward the 12th rib area. The stroke is performed both in a direction along the spine and at a 45-degree angle away from the spine.

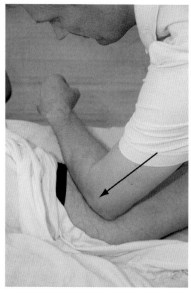

Figure 10.7 • The ischiocrural/hamstring muscle group

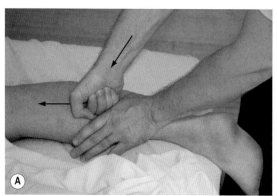

Figure 10.6 • Triceps surae muscle • A Reinforced fist glide B Reinforced thumb glide on the triceps surae muscles

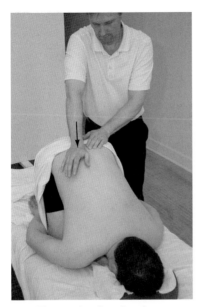

Figure 10.8 • Thoracolumbar fascia

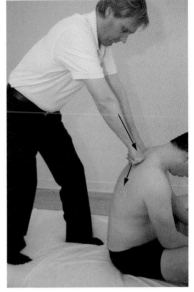

Figure 10.9 • Erector spinae fasciae

Erector spinae fasciae

The athlete rests in a sitting position. The therapist uses the fists of both hands on both sides of the athlete's spine, starting in the lower neck area (Fig. 10.9). The athlete is asked to slowly and gradually bend forward, starting with the head, as the therapist's fists slowly glide downward, stretching the longitudinal fascial layers all the way to the sacrum.

Posterior aspect of the neck

The athlete lies supine. The therapist hooks the fingertips on one side of the neck just lateral to the spine in the T1/C7 area (Fig. 10.10). The therapist slowly lifts the head, with active assistance from the athlete, as the fingers slowly glide laterally. The stroke is segmentally performed up to the occipital bone, and then repeated on the opposite side.

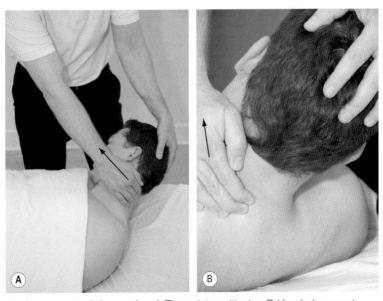

Figure 10.10 • Posterior aspect of the neck • A Therapist positioning B Hand placement

Superficial front line

The superficial front line (SFL) connects the whole anterior aspect of the body, starting from the dorsum of the toes and feet, and running up to the lateral aspects of the skull (Fig. 10.11). The SFL and SBL mutually support and balance each other during postural activity (Myers 2002).

Important myofascial structures of the SFL (Myers 2002)

- Deep and superficial toe extensor muscles.
- Tibialis anterior (including the anterior crural compartment).
- Patellar ligament.
- Quadriceps femoris.

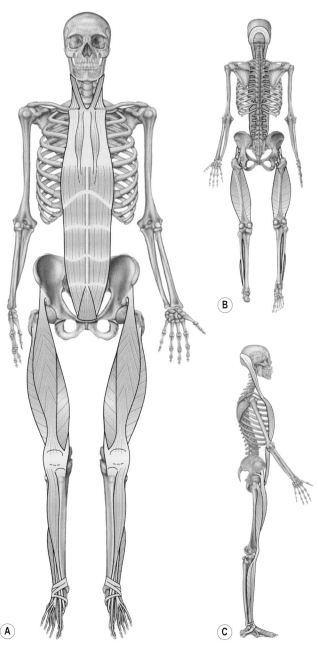

Figure 10.11 • Superficial front line Reproduced with permission from Myers 2002

- Rectus abdominis.
- Sternalis/sternochondral fascia.
- Sternocleidomastoid/SCM muscle.
- Scalp fascia.

Deep and superficial toe extensor muscles and tibialis anterior

The athlete lies supine. The therapist places a flat fist or palm just superior to the ankle joint (Stanborough 2004). The fasciae of the extensor group and tibialis anterior including the anterior compartment are stretched as the fist slowly, in sections of 5–7 in, glides up toward the knee (Fig. 10.12). As the tissue softens, the pressure can increase. The athlete can actively plantarflex the foot on the therapist's command.

Patellar ligament

The athlete lies supine. The therapist places the thumb of one hand just superior and lateral to the tibial tuberosity, whilst the heel of the other hand reinforces from the top. The tissue is slowly stretched in short straight lines, at a 45-degree angle to the fiber direction (Fig. 10.13).

Quadriceps femoris

The athlete lies supine. The therapist places the fingertips of one hand just superior to the patella. The fascial structures are worked as the elbow glides up toward the hip joint in sections of 8–12 in (Fig. 10.14).

Rectus abdominis

The athlete lies supine. The therapist places the fingertips just lateral to the rectus abdominis (Stanborough 2004; Smith 2005). The pressure is directed obliquely "under" the rectus abdominis with a

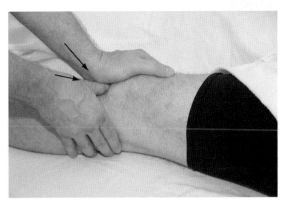

Figure 10.13 • Patellar ligament

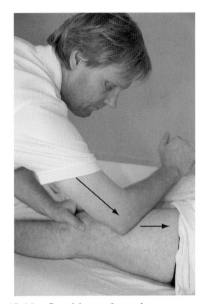

Figure 10.14 • Quadriceps femoris

simultaneous cranial or caudal gliding pressure (Fig. 10.15). The stroke begins or ends at either the costal arch, or 2 in superior to the pubic bone.

Sternalis/sternochondral fascia

The athlete lies supine. The therapist places the fingertips at the inferior tip of the sternum (Fig. 10.16), and slowly glides upward to the sternal notch, bilaterally passing over the sternal origin of the pectoralis major muscle (Smith 2005).

SCM

The athlete lies supine with a rolled towel under the neck, creating a mild extension and a slight contralateral rotation (the neck extension and finger pressure will

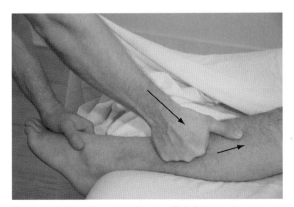

Figure 10.12 • Deep and superficial toe extensor muscles and tibialis anterior

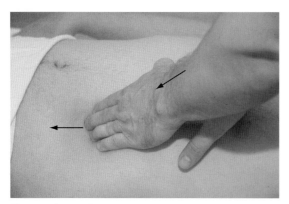

Figure 10.15 • Rectus abdominis

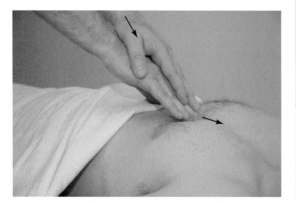

Figure 10.16 • Sternalis/sternochondral fascia

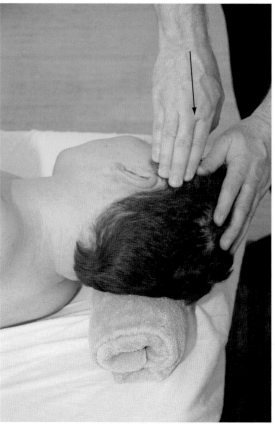

Figure 10.18 • Lateral scalp fascia

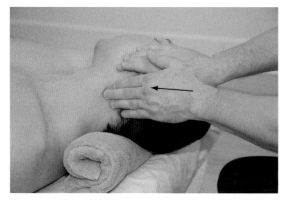

Figure 10.17 • SCM

compensate for rotating in the "wrong" direction). The therapist places the fingertips at the inferior part of the mastoid process, and slowly glides to the sternum to include both the sternal and clavicular insertion (Fig. 10.17). If the muscle is large, each muscle belly is treated separately in its lower portion.

Lateral scalp fascia

The athlete lies on the side with a pillow, or rolled towel, under the head. The therapist uses sliding fingertips to pushing the fascia in a direction from the area lateral to the eyes toward the occipital area (Fig. 10.18).

Lateral line

The lateral line (LL) travels, as the name implies, along the lateral aspect of the body (Fig. 10.19). The LL assists in balancing the anterior, posterior, and lateral aspects of the athlete's body. In addition, it stabilizes rotational movements in the trunk (Myers 2002).

Important myofascial structures of the LL (Myers 2002)

- Peroneal muscle group, starting at the insertion of the peroneus longus muscle at the first cuneiform bone.

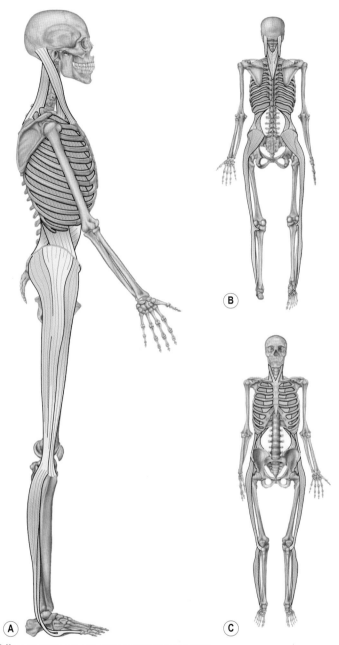

Figure 10.19 • Lateral line Reproduced with permission from Myers 2002

- Lateral aspect of the ankle.
- Lateral compartment of the lower legs.
- Anterior ligament of the head of fibula.
- Iliotibial tract.
- Tensor fasciae latae.
- Gluteus maximus.
- Abdominal obliques.
- External and internal intercostal muscles.
- Splenius capitis.
- SCM muscles.

Treatment of fascial structures of the lateral line in the lower leg

The athlete lies on the side with the knee flexed. The therapist places a flat fist just superior to the lateral aspect of the ankle joint (Stanborough 2004). The fascia of the lateral part of the lower leg, including the lateral compartment, is stretched as the fist slowly glides up toward the knee in sections of 5–7 in (Fig. 10.20). As the tissue softens the pressure can increase. The athlete can actively dorsiflex the foot during the stroke on the therapist's command.

Iliotibial tract

The athlete lies on the side with the knee flexed and hip joint slightly adducted. The therapist places a flat fist just inferior to the greater trochanter. The tissue is stretched as the fist slowly glides down toward the lateral aspect of the knee joint in sections of 8–12 in (Fig. 10.21).

Additional iliotibial tract release is described in Chapter 14.

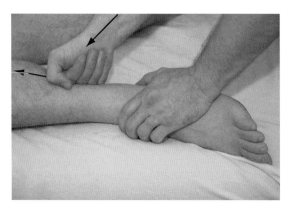

Figure 10.20 • Peroneal muscle group, lateral aspect of the ankle, and the lateral compartment of the lower legs

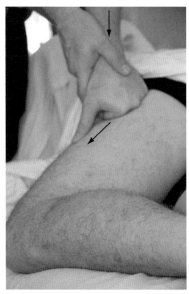

Figure 10.21 • Iliotibial tract

Tensor fasciae latae fascia

The therapist places a flat part of the elbow just posterior to the superior aspect of the muscle at the ASIS. As the stroke slowly moves anteriorly, transverse to the fiber direction, the elbow is gradually flexed to hook the tissue with the inferior part of the olecranon (Fig. 10.22). The process is repeated until the whole area of the TFL is treated.

Fascial structure of the gluteus maximus muscle

The athlete lies on the side with the knee and hip slightly flexed. The athlete's flexed knee should end up just outside the edge of the treatment table. The therapist uses either the fingertips or one elbow during the treatment. The stroke slowly slides toward the sacral area whilst the therapist gradually pushes the athlete's bent leg into further hip flexion (Fig. 10.23). The athlete can assist by

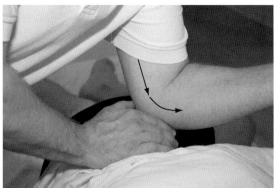

Figure 10.22 • Tensor fasciae latae fascia

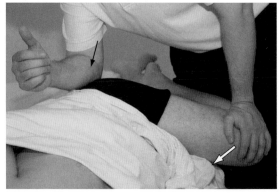

Figure 10.23 • Fascial structure of the gluteus maximus muscle

actively generating flexion in the hip joint upon the therapist's command.

Abdominal obliques

The athlete lies on the side with the hip and knee joints flexed. The therapist supports the athlete's sacrum and pelvis with the side of one hip. For the external obliques, the athlete's shoulder is slowly pressed toward the table, generating rotation of the trunk, as the fingertips slowly glide along the muscle. The internal abdominal obliques are treated from the same position, except the treated muscle area is on the opposite side of the athlete's body. Here, the therapist's fingertips will instead hook into the tissue, pulling the fascia in a medial direction (Fig. 10.24).

Release of the superficial fasciae of the lateral aspect of the chest

The athlete lies on the side with the hip and knee joints flexed to stabilize the body, and the arm reaching above the head (Fig. 10.25). The therapist places both forearms on the side of the chest and gently clasps the hands. The elbows are slowly pushed out as the hands are kept together, with forearms sliding along the chest wall. The athlete can assist by reaching the arm cranially, and inhaling and exhaling deeply.

External and internal intercostal muscles

The athlete lies on the side with the hip and knee joints flexed to stabilize the body. The therapist applies one or two fingertips that slowly glide

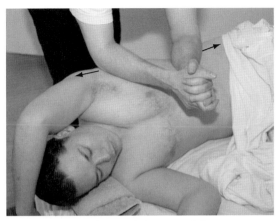

Figure 10.25 • Release of the superficial fasciae of the lateral aspect of the chest (Jenings 2003)

between the ribs, starting posteriorly and sliding anteriorly (Fig. 10.26). The client can assist by performing deep inhalations and exhalations during the stroke upon the therapist's command.

Splenius capitis

The athlete lies supine, with the neck rotated 30 degrees. The therapist uses a loose fist, particularly the second and third phalangeal bones. The stroke commences at the mastoid process and slides separately both under the occipital ridge and obliquely down along the lateral/posterior aspect of the neck (Fig. 10.27).

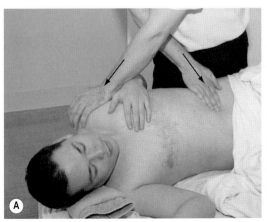
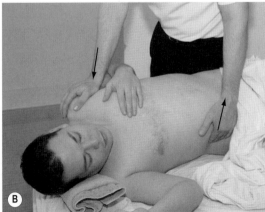

Figure 10.24 • Abdominal obliques • A External obliques B Internal obliques

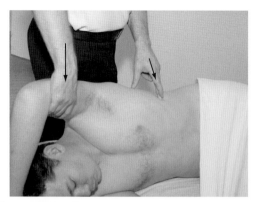

Figure 10.26 • External and internal intercostal muscles

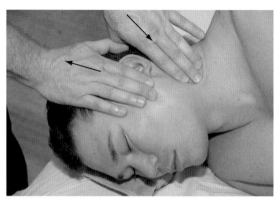

Figure 10.28 • SCM

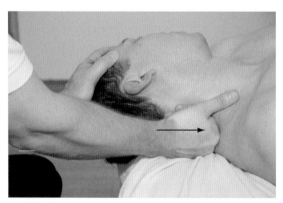

Figure 10.27 • Splenius capitis

SCM

The athlete lies on the side with the hip and knee joints flexed to stabilize the body. The neck is slightly extended and laterally flexed with a rolled towel under it for support. The therapist slides the fingertips along the muscle area, starting at the mastoid process and finishing at the sternum and medial third of the clavicle (Fig. 10.28).

Spiral line

The spiral line (SL) wraps around the body in a helix (a three-dimensional spiral) (Myers 2002), and assists in balancing every plane of the body (Fig. 10.29). It connects the pelvic angle with the arches of the feet and controls knee tracking in walking (Myers 2002). The SL commences on the side of the skull just superior to the nuchal line, continuing down via the splenius capitis muscle, linking the spinous process of C6–T5 (Myers 2002), connecting on the opposite side with the rhomboid muscles, serratus posterior superior, and the medial border of the scapula, and continues via infraspinatus to the serratus anterior that inserts to ribs 5–9. The SL continues down diagonally over the abdomen, down the lateral aspect of the opposite hip, leg, knee, and foot arch. It continues up on the posterior aspect of the body via biceps femoris and erector spinae, to reconnect with the fasciae of the skull. If dysfunctional, the SL creates, maintains, or compensates for rotational and lateral shifts in the body (Myers 2002).

Important fascial structures of the SL

- Splenius capitis and cervicis.
- Rhomboid major and minor.
- Serratus anterior.
- External oblique.
- Abdominal aponeurosis, including linea alba.
- Internal oblique.
- Tensor fasciae latae (TFL).
- Iliotibial tract.
- Peroneus longus.
- Biceps femoris.
- Sacrotuberous ligament.
- Sacrolumbar fascia.
- Erector spinae.

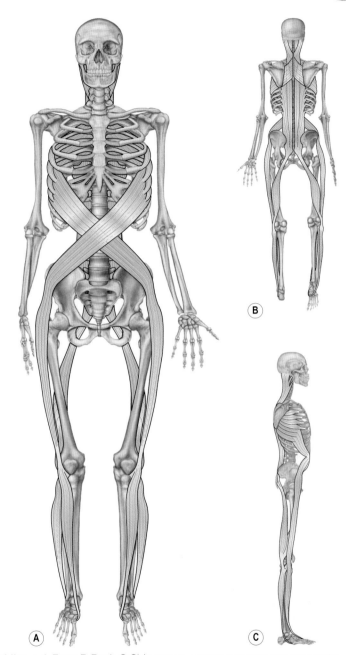

Figure 10.29 • Spiral line • A Front B Back C Side Reproduced with permission from Myers 2002

Arm lines

The arm lines (AL) consist of a superficial and deep line on both the anterior and posterior aspects of the arm (Fig. 10.30). Since the arms have a great ROM, the myofascial line pattern becomes slightly more complex, with a greater number of crossover linkages compared with areas with more stability (Myers 2002). Increased movement ability creates a need for more "lines of pull" (Myers 2002) to

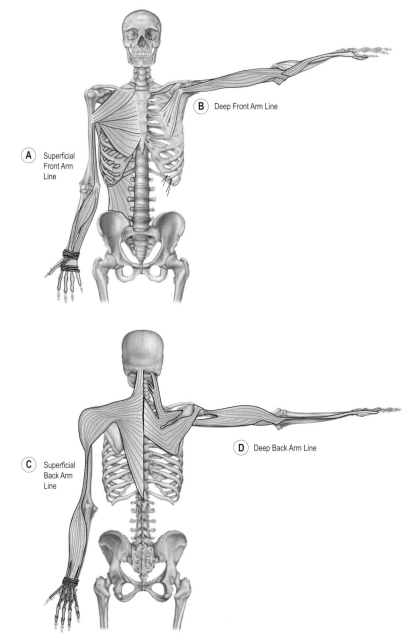

Figure 10.30 • Arm lines • A Superficial front AL B Deep front AL C Superficial back AL D Deep back AL Reproduced with permission from Myers 2002

generate the necessary tensile strength and stability in the area.

The AL has postural effects in that the elbow positions will affect the mid back, and shoulder positions will have consequences for areas like the ribs and neck.

Important myofascial structures of the AL (Myers 2002)

Superficial front AL

• Pectoralis major and latissimus dorsi.
• Medial intermuscular septum.

- Superficial and deep flexor group of the forearm and hand.
- Carpal tunnel.

Deep front AL
- Pectoralis major and clavipectoral fascia.
- Biceps brachii.
- Radial periosteum, anterior border, radial collateral ligaments.
- Thenar muscles.

Superficial back AL
- Trapezius.
- Deltoid.
- Lateral intermuscular septum.
- Deep and superficial extensor group of the forearm and hand.

Deep back AL
- Rhomboids and levator scapulae.
- Rotator cuff muscles, i.e. supraspinatus, infraspinatus, teres minor, subscapularis.
- Triceps brachii.
- Ulnar periosteum.
- Ulnar collateral ligaments.
- Hypothenar muscles.

Deep front line

The deep front line (DFL) is situated between both lateral lines and is surrounded by the spiral lines. It encompasses the "myofascial core" (Myers 2002) of the body. It commences in the deep layers of the plantar aspect of the foot, continues in the deep portion of the posterior lower leg, travels up the inside of the thighs, up the anterior aspect of the hip joint, the pelvis, and lumbar spine, and runs through the thoracic viscera, ending at the neuroviscero cranium (Myers 2002) (Fig. 10.31). The DFL occupies more volume than the other lines.

Posturally, the DFL raises the medial longitudinal arch of the feet, stabilizes the legs, and supports the lumbar spine. In addition, it stabilizes the chest to facilitate breathing, and balances both the neck and head.

Dysfunctions will lead to a general shortening, and trigger collapse in the spinal and pelvic core, causing compensatory distortions in the other lines.

Important myofascial structures of the DFL (Myers 2002)

- Tibialis anterior and the long toe flexors.
- Popliteus fascia and the local capsule of the knee joint.
- Posterior intermuscular septum.
- Adductor magnus muscle.
- Pelvic floor fascia, levator ani, obturator internus fascia, anterior sacral fascia.
- Anterior intermuscular septum, adductor brevis and longus.
- Psoas muscles, iliacus, pectineus, and the area of the femoral triangle.
- Anterior longitudinal ligament, longus colli and capitis muscles.
- Posterior diaphragm, crura of the diaphragm, central tendon.
- Pericardium.
- Fascia prevertebralis, pharyngeal raphe, scalene muscles, medial scalene fascia, mediastinum, parietal pleura.
- Anterior diaphragm, crura of the diaphragm.
- Endothoracic fascia, transversus thoracis.
- Infrahyoid muscles, fascia pretrachialis.
- Suprahyoid muscles.
- Jaw muscles.

Functional lines

Functional lines (FL) are extensions of the arm lines reaching the trunk and contralateral aspect of the pelvis and legs (Myers 2002) (Fig. 10.32). They are activated during movement, and so have relevance for athletes. They are superficial and have minimal postural function, and can be assessed by observing the athlete's movements. Treatment is aimed at restoring balance and removing unbalanced restrictions.

Important structures of the FL (Myers 2002)

The important structures of the FL are fascial structures of the back functional line and front functional line.

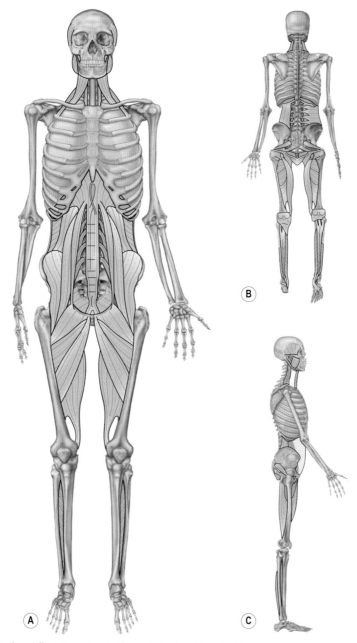

Figure 10.31 • Deep front line Reproduced with permission from Myers 2002

Back functional line

- Latissimus dorsi.
- Lumbosacral fascia.
- Sacral fascia.
- Gluteus maximus.

- Vastus lateralis.
- Subpatellar tendon.

Front functional line

- Lower part of pectoralis major muscle.
- Lateral sheath of rectus abdominis.
- Adductor longus muscle.

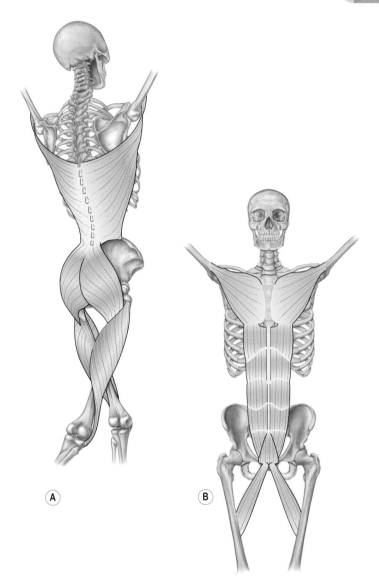

Figure 10.32 • Functional lines (FL) • A Front B Back Reproduced with permission from Myers 2002

Connective tissue massage

The German physiotherapist Elisabeth Dicke founded connective tissue massage ("Bindegewebs-massage") in 1929 (Ylinen & Cash 1993). It is indicated that manipulation of the skin and subcutaneous tissues can have favorable effects on tissues distant from the actual treatment area. It is believed that the effects are mediated by neural reflexes causing increased blood flow to the affected regions together with inhibition of pain (Goats & Keir 1991).

Connective tissue massage treatments focus on specific regions of the body, assigned in segmental order to internal organ systems and structures of the spinal cord, joints, and muscles. As a modality, connective tissue massage is considered to be an important element of physiotherapy (Michalsen & Bühring 1993), particularly in European countries like Germany.

Research that involved conducting a series of 15 connective tissue massage treatments over a 10-week treatment period on individuals with fibromyalgia, presented a gradual pain-relieving effect of 37%, a reduction in depression, decreased use of analgesics, and a generally perceived improvement in quality of life (Brattberg 1999).

Soft tissue can present palpable reflexive changes such as (Chaitow 2003):

- compressed areas of tissue
- drawn-in bands of tissue
- elevated areas of tissue that can be misinterpreted as localized swelling
- muscle hypertrophy or hypotrophy/atrophy
- bone deformation of the spinal column.

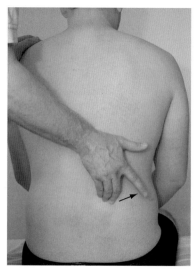

Figure 10.33 • Connective tissue massage stroke

Treatment technique

Connective tissue massage is usually conducted by pulling and stretching portions of the skin with the radial side of the long finger, braced by the 4th and 5th fingers (Fig. 10.33). The strokes are either short or long, with the shorter strokes presenting a slightly more intense stretch sensation. Emollient is not used, to guarantee enhanced effect in the cutaneous and subcutaneous tissues. Release of areas with restricted skin movement has been shown to produce stimulating effects on the body's circulatory system.

The treatment position is generally seated to take advantage of the gravitational effects placed on the soft tissue during the strokes. The amount of pressure and angle of the treating hand are adjusted to optimize the "grip" in the tissue. Connective tissue massage treatments normally start in the lumbar area and are gradually moved superiorly along the treatment patterns (Figs 10.34–10.36). An area is considered to be completed when the soft tissue restriction is released.

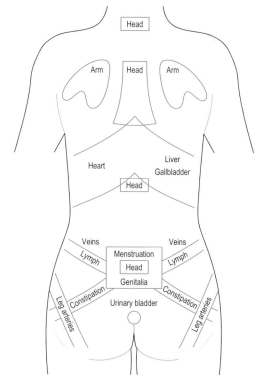

Figure 10.34 • Important reflex zones on the back

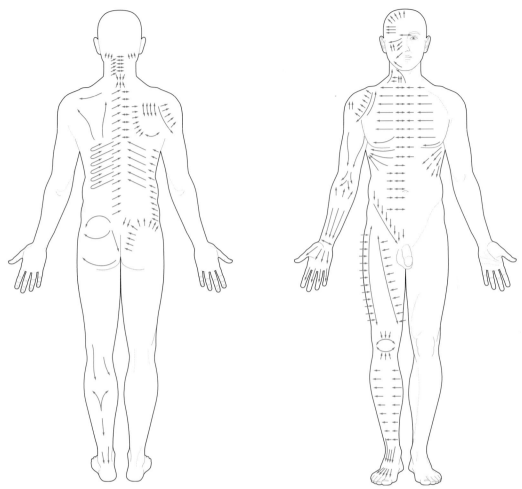

Figure 10.35 • Posterior treatment pattern

Figure 10.36 • Anterior treatment pattern

References

Archer, P., 2007. Therapeutic massage in athletics. Lippincott Williams & Wilkins, Baltimore, MD. 88–97.

Arroyo-Morales, M., et al., 2008. Effects of myofascial release after high-intensity exercise: a randomized clinical trial. J. Manipulative Physiol. Ther. 31 (3), 217–223.

Brattberg, G., 1999. Connective tissue massage in the treatment of fibromyalgia. Eur. J. Pain 3 (3), 235–244.

Chaitow, L., 2003. Modern neuromuscular techniques. second ed. Churchill Livingstone, Edinburgh, pp. 82–83.

Chikly, B.J., 2005. Manual techniques addressing the lymphatic system: origins and development. JAOA 105 (10), 457–464.

Di Fabio, R.P., et al., 1992. Effect of knee joint laxity on long-loop postural reflexes: evidence for a human capsular-hamstring reflex. Exp. Brain Res. 90 (1), 189–200.

Goats, G.C., Keir, K.A., 1991. Connective tissue massage. Br. J. Sports Med. 25 (3), 131–133.

Henley, C.E., et al., 2008. Osteopathic manipulative treatment and its relationship to autonomic nervous system activity as demonstrated by heart rate variability: a repeated measures study. Osteopath. Med. Prim. Care 2, 7.

Huijing, P.A., Baan, G.C., 2008. Myofascial force transmission via extramuscular pathways occurs between antagonistic muscles. Cells Tissues Organs. Mar 19 [Epub ahead of print].

Jenings, B., 2003. Myofascial release techniques.

Jones, T.A., 2004. Rolfing. Phys. Med. Rehabil. Clin. N. Am. 15 (4), 799–809, vi.

Konczak, C.R., Ames, R., 2005. Relief of internal snapping hip syndrome in a marathon runner after chiropractic treatment. J. Manipulative Physiol. Ther. 28 (1), e1–e7.

Langevin, H.M., Sherman, K.J., 2007. Pathophysiological model for chronic low back pain integrating connective tissue and nervous system mechanisms. Med. Hypotheses 68 (1), 74–80. Epub 2006 Aug 21.

Michalsen, A., Bühring, M., 1993. Connective tissue massage. Wien. Klin. Wochenschr. 105 (8), 220–227.

Myers, T.W., 2002. Anatomy trains. Churchill Livingstone, Edinburgh.

Smith, J., 2005. Structural bodywork. Elsevier, Edinburgh.

Smith, O., 1919. The connective tissue monograph. Chicago College of Naprapathy, Chicago.

Smith, O., 1932. Naprapathic genetics I. Smith, Chicago.

Smith, O., 1966. The autobiography of Doctor Oakley Smith. Chicago College of Naprapathy, Chicago.

Stanborough, M., 2004. Direct myofascial release technique. Churchill Livingstone, Edinburgh.

Sucher, B.M., 1993. Myofascial manipulative release of carpal tunnel syndrome: documentation with magnetic resonance imaging. J. Am. Osteopath. Assoc. 93 (12), 1273–1278.

Schleip, R., et al., 2005. Active fascial contractility: fascia may be able to contract in a smooth muscle-like manner and thereby influence musculoskeletal dynamics. Med. Hypotheses 65 (2), 273–277.

Ylinen, J., Cash, M., 1993. Idrottsmassage. ICA bokförlag, Västerås.

Watkins, J., 1999. Structure and function of the musculoskeletal system. Human Kinetics, Champaign, IL.

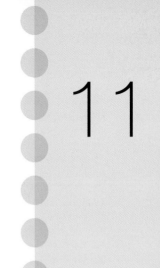

Myofascial pain syndrome— myofascial trigger points

11

Myofascial pain syndrome (MPS) is one of the most common causes of pain stemming from soft tissue dysfunction (Alvarez & Rockwell 2002), and can be described as pain from muscle tissue with surrounding fascia. Chronic myofascial pain is often a result of both physical and psychosocial influences that may complicate convalescence (Wheeler 2004). It is estimated that around 10–15% of the US population have some form of myofascial pain (Alvarez & Rockwell 2002; Wheeler 2004). The prevalent occurrence and effects also make it a valid concern for athletes. Myofascial trigger points (MTrPs) are considered to be the main cause of MPS (Bonci 1993; Dommerholt et al. 2006), and it is suggested that MTrPs can affect athletic performance in negative ways, even when not actively producing actual pain sensations (Bonci 1993). Several probable mechanisms can cause the formation of MTrPs, including direct trauma, low-level muscle contractions, uneven intramuscular pressure distribution, unaccustomed eccentric contractions, eccentric contractions in unconditioned muscles, and maximal or submaximal concentric muscle contractions (Dommerholt et al. 2006).

A myofascial trigger point can be described as a hypersensitive focal nodule in a taut band of skeletal muscle fibers. MTrPs generally present motor sensory (Alvarez & Rockwell 2002; McPartland 2004; Dommerholt et al. 2006) and referred autonomic symptoms (Simons et al. 1999; Dommerholt et al. 2006). Sensory disturbances may include local tenderness, allodynia, hyperalgesia (Box 11.1), and referred pain to a distant area and/or certain muscles unique for each MTrP (Dommerholt et al. 2006). Motor symptoms can manifest as disturbed motor function, muscle weakness from inhibition, limited range of motion, and muscle stiffness.

MTrP and taut band

The taut band "housing" the MTrP is found in an otherwise more relaxed muscle (Fig. 11.1). The band forms by tension generated from contracted and stretched sarcomeres relating to a more centrally located knot (Simons & Dommerholt 2006a). It is important to note that MTrPs will always be found in a taut band, but a taut band does not always contain a MTrP.

MTrPs are generally divided into active and latent MTrPs. Both active and latent MTrPs are normally painful upon compression. The pain referral zone is commonly projected to a distant area, sometimes without necessary spontaneous pain sensations at the actual site of the trigger point itself.

The exact etiology of MTrPs has yet to be fully established (Simons 2008), but different theories have been presented over the years.

MTrPs and trauma

It is suggested that some form of trauma initially damages the end sacs of the sarcoplasmic reticulum (SR) and the sarcolemma. The trauma is either acute or in the form of repetitive microtrauma caused by overuse or overload of local muscles, something heavily prevalent in the athletic community. This produces a substantial release, with increased intracellular concentration, of calcium ions (Ca^{2+}),

DOI: 10.1016/B978-0-443-10126-7.00011-3

Box 11.1

Useful definitions

- **Acetylcholine (ACh)**—neurotransmitter activating skeletal muscle contraction and the autonomic nervous system.
- **Acetylcholinesterase**—enzyme breaking down ACh.
- **Adenosine triphosphate (ATP)**—a "stored energy form" utilized by the cells.
- **Allodynia**—pain from a stimulus that does not normally provoke pain.
- **Ca^{2+}**—calcium ions that stimulate contraction of skeletal muscle cells.
- **Dorsal horn**—site of spinal cord receiving and processing incoming sensory information.
- **Hyperalgesia**—elevated reaction to a stimulus that is normally painful.
- **Hypothyroidism**—disease caused by insufficient production of certain hormones by the thyroid gland.

- **Motor endplate**—flat end part of a motor neuron transmitting nerve impulses to a muscle cell.
- **Nociceptive**—responding to a physiological pain stimulus.
- **Reversed T3 (rT3)**—a mostly inactive thyroid hormone that can still occupy receptors dedicated for the active T3 hormone.
- **Sarcolemma**—cell membrane of a muscle cell.
- **Sarcomere**—smallest contractile unit in a muscle cell, consisting of thin actin and thick myosin protein filaments.
- **Sarcoplasmic reticulum (SR)**—"tubular network" in the muscle cells. The end sacs of the SR store calcium ions vital for muscle contraction.
- **Vasoconstriction**—constriction of certain blood vessels.

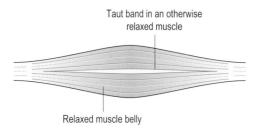

Taut band in an otherwise relaxed muscle

Relaxed muscle belly

Figure 11.1 • MTrP and taut band

triggering contractions of local sarcomeres in the affected muscle cells (Fig. 11.2).

More recent research has formed the generally adopted theory named "the integrated trigger point hypothesis" (Simons et al. 1999; Fig. 11.3). It suggests that an abnormal release of acetylcholine (ACh) from the motor endplates, even during rest, produces a sustained depolarization of the affected muscle cells.

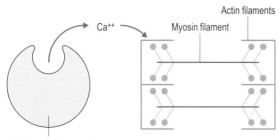

Actin filaments

Ca^{++} Myosin filament

Vesicle in SR, housing Ca^{++} ions
Ruptured due to trauma Ca^{++} 'leaks'
out causing contraction.

Figure 11.2 • MTrP and trauma

ACh triggers the calcium channels in the SR to start releasing Ca^{2+}. An impaired release of acetylcholinesterase is also found to play a role (Simons 2008).

The malfunctioning motor endplates form a "central MTrP" located at the innervation site of the muscle. MTrPs seems to begin in a region of multiple dysfunctional endplates with an abnormal release of ACh. The dysfunctional endplates are connected to a section of muscle fibers forming a contractile knot and taut band in an otherwise more relaxed muscle. The sustained contraction increases local metabolic demands and constricts local capillaries, which reduces available oxygen and nutrient levels in the area, limiting ATP production. An accumulation of metabolites triggers local vasoconstriction that further decreases blood circulation. This finally leads to a local energy crisis due to a lack of ATP. The calcium pump returning calcium into the end sacs of the SR is highly dependent on ATP. The sudden lack disrupts its function, potentially sustaining the localized contractile reaction (Simons et al. 1999). The energy crisis triggers release of substances, i.e. bradykinin, cytokines, serotonin, histamine, E-type prostaglandins, substance P, etc., causing increased pain sensation. It is thought likely that if the endplate dysfunction is allowed to continue for any length of time, chronic fibrotic changes may occur in the tissue (Hou et al. 2002).

Contributing additional factors to MTrP development are deficiencies in vitamins B1, B6, B12, C, D, and folic acid, magnesium, zinc, and iron (Dommerholt et al. 2006; Simons & Dommerholt 2006a) as well as

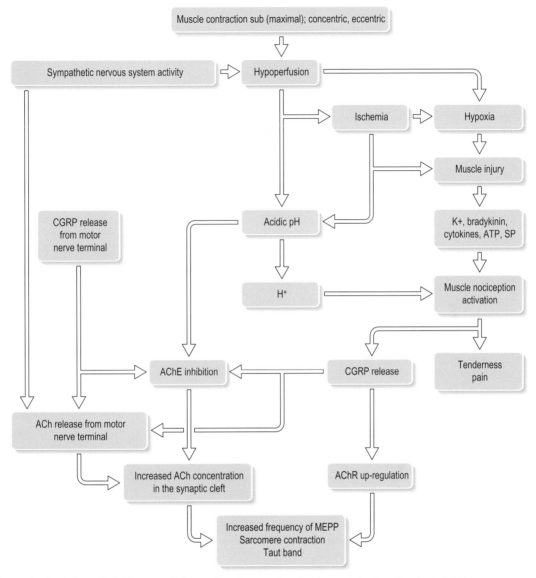

Figure 11.3 • Integrated trigger point hypothesis Reproduced with permission from Gerwin et al. 2004

hormonal dysfunctions like hypothyroidism, increased levels of reversed T3, and human growth hormone deficiency (Simons & Dommerholt 2006a). Depressive emotional states have also been shown to predispose people to MTrP formation (Simons et al. 1999).

Pain and myofascial trigger points

Because MTrP pain does not project along regular dermatomes, the exact explanation model for referred MTrP pain is still somewhat uncertain, although particular neural explanation models are favored. Some correlations between MTrPs and acupoints have also been mapped, and more recent investigations suggest the possibility that MTrPs and Ah Shi points could be the same phenomenon (Birch 2003; Simons & Dommerholt 2006b). It has also been shown that drawings by patients describing their pain pattern coincided to a high degree with the pathways of acupuncture channels (Baldry 1993).

Reproduction of the local or referred pain is possible through mechanical stimulation of a MTrP, either by focal compression or stretching. The pain may appear immediately or after a 10–15 s delay. Although distinctive referred pain patterns for each MTrP have been established, substantial variations exist (Dommerholt et al. 2006).

Convergence–projection

This theory is one of the more widely adopted models of explanation (Baldry 1993; Simons et al. 1999). It is considered that cutaneous, visceral, or skeletal muscle afferent nerve fibers converge in the same spinal neuron. The referred pain patterns from MTrPs are not automatically restricted to regular peripheral dermatome nerve distributions or single segmental pathways. MTrPs cause constant irritating stimulation, increasing both the size and number of receptive areas to which a single dorsal horn nociceptive neuron may respond, and this affects the referred pain sensation (Dommerholt et al. 2006). It is believed that the sensory cortex of the brain could possibly misinterpret a strong visceral or skeletal muscular input as stemming from the corresponding skin site.

Sympathetic hyperactivity

The referred pain area of MTrPs can have lowered skin temperature, induced by sympathetic hyperactivity causing constriction of superficial blood vessels (Baldry 1993). This may lead to the release of chemical sensory afferent sensitizing substances, which could generate pain in a local pain zone.

Classification of myofascial trigger points

Active MTrPs

Active trigger points refer pain, other paraesthesias (Dommerholt et al. 2006), and/or cause referred autonomic phenomena when the muscle is contracted, stretched, or during rest. Active MTrPs are always tender and prevent full lengthening of the muscle. One example of pain caused by active trigger points is tension-related headaches. During a treatment it is common that an active trigger point is reduced to a latent trigger point. The pain is

relieved, but the taut band with the MTrP still remains, and is considered completely cleared only when the taut band has dissolved.

Latent MTrP

Latent trigger points do not cause spontaneous referred pain or autonomic phenomena unless stimulated; however, they do still render the muscle shorter and weaker than normal since the taut band and dysfunction are present. Latent trigger points often shift into active trigger points when the muscle is overloaded.

Central MTrP

A central trigger point is closely associated with dysfunctional motor end plates and is located at or near the center of a muscle belly where the nerve innervates the muscle (Simons et al. 1999). Central MTrPs are generally treated first.

Attachment MTrP

Attachment trigger points arise near the musculotendinous junction and/or at the bony origin or insertion due to the strain at the attachments from the formed taut band (Simons et al. 1999). If the strain is more intense, two attachment trigger points may form at the site, with one at the musculotendinous junction and one at the tendon–bone junction.

Key trigger points

Key trigger points activate one or more satellite trigger points (Simons et al. 1999). Deactivating a key MTrP may automatically deactivate its satellite MTrPs.

Associated trigger points

Associated trigger points occur concurrently with a trigger point in another muscle (Simons et al. 1999). One may have induced the other, or they may both stem from the same mechanical or neurological origin.

Satellite trigger points

A satellite trigger point is a central trigger point formed in a muscle located within the referred pain zone of a key trigger point (Simons et al. 1999). Satellite trigger points can also appear in overloaded synergistic muscles compensating the trigger point muscle, or in an antagonistic muscle countering increased tension from the muscle with a key trigger point.

How to localize MTrPs

MTrPs are generally located by evaluation of the skin condition, presence of taut band, local or referred pain, reflex/reactions, and/or referred autonomic phenomena.

Increased skin moisture over the MTrP

By slowly and lightly dragging one finger across the skin over the troubled area, greater resistance is noted over a MTrP. This is caused by the increased skin moisture the MTrP induces (Chaitow & Delany 2000; Fig. 11.4).

Reduced skin motility over the MTrP

The skin and fascia over an area of dysfunction tend to be less mobile compared with a healthy site (Chaitow & Delany 2000). By gently pushing the skin in different directions, resistance can be noted at the dysfunctional site (Fig. 11.5).

Palpation

To localize the MTrP, the therapist also palpates the muscle in search of the taut band of muscle fibers. Pressure of the taut band in the affected muscle is often a sure diagnosis.

Locating the taut band

The taut band is located by moving the fingers transversally to the muscle fibers without sliding on the skin, or by grasping a muscle belly between the fingertips, gently rolling the tissue between the fingers (Fig. 11.6). Once located, the band is further carefully pressed or squeezed along its length in search of the hypertender trigger point, first centrally in the muscle belly, followed by pressure at the attachments. There are three common ways to palpate:

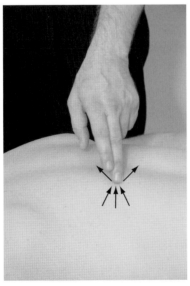

Figure 11.4 • Detecting skin resistance

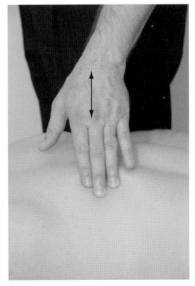

Figure 11.5 • Reduced skin motility

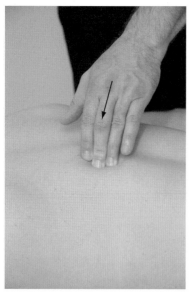

Figure 11.6 • Locating the taut band

- flat palpation
- pincer palpation
- deep/probing palpation.

Flat palpation

Flat palpation is executed with the fingertips, over muscles lacking a graspable edge, for example infraspinatus and erector spinae muscles (Fig. 11.7). Moving the skin, without sliding, perpendicular to the fiber direction helps locate the taut band.

Pincer palpation

Pincer palpation is implemented on a muscle with a palpable edge, for example latissimus dorsi, teres major, and the descending part of trapezius (Fig. 11.8). The muscle is gently squeezed and rolled

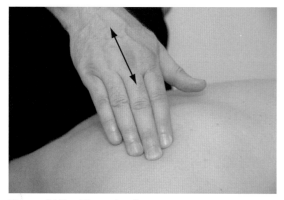

Figure 11.7 • Flat palpation

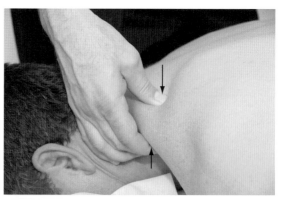

Figure 11.8 • Pincer palpation

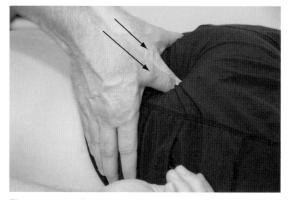

Figure 11.9 • Deep palpation

between the fingertips in the search for a taut band and the MTrP.

Deep/probing palpation

Deep/probing palpation is performed on more deeply situated muscles overlaid by other muscles, for example piriformis, supraspinatus, and pectoralis minor, or on adipose tissue (Fig. 11.9).

Referred pain

Referred pain from MTrPs generally presents with a dull and aching quality (Fig. 11.10). The pain can range from slight discomfort to being torture-like. If the trigger point is strongly active, the pain may exhibit a sharper quality.

Referred autonomic phenomena

MTrP-related referred autonomic phenomena occur either alone or in combination with other MTrP

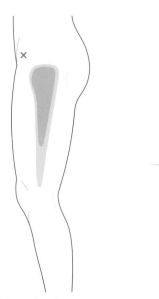

Figure 11.10 • Referred pain

symptoms (Simons et al. 1999). They generally arise within the referred pain pattern of a MTrP (Simons et al. 1999). Only a few muscles are known to generate referred autonomic phenomena, commonly the trapezius, sternocleidomastoid, and masseter muscles.

One perceived reason these muscles are able to cause referred autonomic phenomena is their relation or close proximity to the accessory nerve (cranial nerve XI). Referred autonomic phenomena are believed to stem from autonomic reflexes. Examples are:

- dizziness
- vertigo
- tinnitus
- loss of hearing
- blurred vision
- increased lacrimation
- dry eyes
- double vision
- vasoconstriction
- vasodilation
- sweating
- increased salivation
- pilomotor response.

Local twitch response

The local twitch response (LTR) is triggered by a sudden change in pressure over a MTrP. The presence of an LTR indicates the likelihood of a MTrP in the examined muscle. LTR is a rapid reflexive contraction of the muscle fibers in a taut band associated with a MTrP as the therapist's fingers snap perpendicularly across the taut band. It is noted as a twitch under the skin near the attachment of the taut band, and may also be palpated through the skin during examination. LTR can also be triggered by needle penetration of a trigger point, or by applying direct pressure on the MTrP itself.

Jump sign

As a MTrP is compressed, the client may respond with a forceful jerk caused by an intense pain response from the MTrP, but it can sometimes appear to be without a direct pain sensation.

Treatment

Even though the exact causatory mechanisms behind MTrP formation have still not been completely revealed (Simons 2008), effective treatment methods are well documented. Probably the most important aspect of treatment is to stretch the contracted muscle fibers to normalize their length. Different distraction methods are used to block the MTrP pain during the stretch. Other effective modalities include local heat or cold applications, dry or wet needling, etc. (Majlesi & Unulan 2010).

Manual massage techniques

Deep stroking massage

Deep stroking massage, or "stripping," is executed slowly along the muscle fibers (Simons et al. 1999; Fig. 11.11). The taut band is slowly massaged from

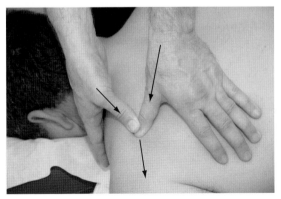

Figure 11.11 • Deep stroking massage

the origin to the insertion of the muscle, whilst passing over the trigger point nodule. The aim is to achieve a "milking" effect with a localized stretch effect of the MTrP and taut band. The slower pace ensures a better contact and stretch effect of the soft tissue. This technique is particularly effective on central MTrPs, which may clear from this treatment alone.

Strumming

Strumming has a similar effect to deep stroking massage except that the stroke runs perpendicularly across the muscle fibers at the site of the MTrP nodule without "snapping" over the taut band (Simons et al. 1999; Fig. 11.12). The stroke is applied alternately from one side of the band to the other until it softens. This is useful on shorter muscles and central MTrPs.

Ischemic muscle pressure

It has been suggested that ischemic compression therapy using either 90 s low pressure up to the pain threshold or 30 s stronger pressure up to pain tolerance can create immediate pain relief and MTrP sensitivity suppression (Baldry 1993; Simons et al. 1999; Hou et al. 2002). It is important to execute this technique correctly to avoid accidental activation of latent trigger points. For maximum benefit, some form of stretching should follow ischemic muscle pressure.

The pressure is performed with braced thumbs, long, or index fingers (Fig. 11.13). The muscle tissue and MTrP are slowly compressed until the athlete begins to experience identical referred pain. The

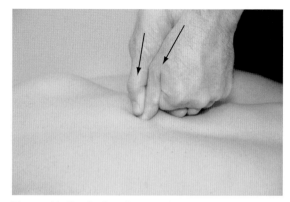

Figure 11.13 • Ischemic muscle pressure

pressure is maintained until the pain subsides. When the pain is relieved, the MTrP is compressed further until identical pain reappears. The process is repeated three or four times. The therapist slowly releases the pressure during a 10 s period. The pressure is not reduced unless it is too high, which is recognized by the pain either being uncomfortable to the athlete or not decreasing in intensity.

Skin rolling

Skin rolling (Fig. 11.14) is used to increase blood circulation by stretching the skin and "breaking up" or stretching adhesions or fibrosis between the skin and its underlying fascia. Skin rolling is also useful in the assessment and treatment of panniculosis. Releasing potential panniculosis in the shoulders, upper back, and gluteal region seems to relieve MTrPs in those areas (Simons et al. 1999).

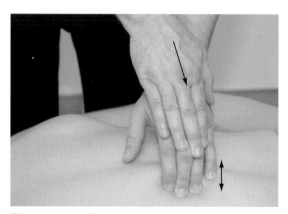

Figure 11.12 • Strumming

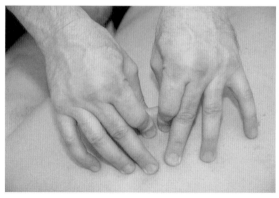

Figure 11.14 • Skin rolling

Muscle and connective tissue stretch techniques

Trigger point pressure release

This method sometimes replaces ischemic muscle pressure. The pressure must be light since the muscle at the trigger point is already in a state of local ischemia, and it is felt that no apparent benefit takes place from adding more (Simons et al. 1999). The treatment should be pain-free since the MTrP already is hypersensitive from released nerve sensitizing agents.

The muscle is gently lengthened to the point of increased resistance, where a mild stretch sensation is felt without pain (Fig. 11.15). A gentle gradual digital pressure is applied to the trigger point until a significant increase in tension is noted in the tissue. The pressure is held until the tissue softens under the finger, and the pressure increases further to the new resistance barrier. The pressure is gradually deepened a few times and then slowly released over about 10 s. The treated muscle should be in a "nonslacked" position during the whole trigger point pressure release treatment.

This technique can be applied to all the bands in a muscle housing MTrPs. Adding supplemental techniques within the pain barrier, like PIR or reciprocal inhibition, may further enhance this technique.

Spray and stretch/ice and stretch

The cold sensation from a vapocoolant spray effectively blocks MTrP pain as the muscle is stretched (Simons et al. 1999). Ethyl chloride is predominatly used today due to its superior availability. Fluori-Methane®, which used to be the spray of choice, has more or less been abandoned due to its negative impact on the planet's ozone layer.

During spray and stretch the "stretch is the action and spray is the distraction" (Simons et al. 1999). The muscle is gently lengthened to its end point. The vapocoolant is sprayed slowly and rhythmically over the area of the trigger point and its pain referral zone. The stretch should be mild and basically only take up the slack in the muscle. The function of the cooling sensation of the spray is merely to block the MTrP pain sensation as the muscle is stretched. It is important the muscle itself remains warm. The vapocoolant spray can be substituted by ordinary ice, i.e. the method known as "ice and stretch." The ice is placed in a plastic bag to keep the skin dry, and is otherwise applied identically to "spray and stretch" with a vapocoolant spray.

Stretch with "4-finger stroke"

The muscle is gently lengthened to its end point. The therapist slowly massages the muscle, back and forth, with four fingertips from origin to insertion along the fiber direction (Fig. 11.16). The skin contact efficiently blocks any referred MTrP pain through stimulation of cutaneous touch and pressure receptors, and generates a more specific stretch effect in the treated muscle and connective tissue.

Percussion and stretch

Finger percussion

A rubber mallet or braced fingers are used to tap the trigger point as the muscle is stretched (Fig. 11.17).

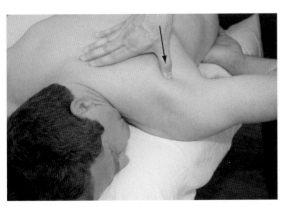

Figure 11.15 • Trigger point pressure release

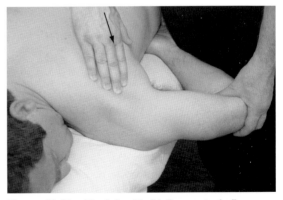

Figure 11.16 • Stretch with "4-finger stroke"

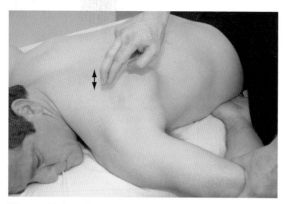

Figure 11.17 • Finger percussion

The treatment starts by lengthening the muscle to the end point as the trigger point is tapped ten times at the exact same location. The percussions should not be faster than one every second and not slower than one every five seconds (Simons et al. 1999).

Voluntary contraction and release methods

PNF and MET techniques are effective tools when treating MTrPs (Simons et al. 1999). The stretches should be gentle and preferably combined with other pain-distracting techniques. (See Chapter 6.)

Positional release technique

Positional release techniques can be an effective modality, particularly on active MTrPs, thanks to its sedative qualities. (See Chapter 8). Some form of stretching technique normally follows the PR treatment.

Integrated neuromuscular inhibition technique, INIT

Integrated neuromuscular inhibition technique (INIT), developed by Dr. Leon Chaitow (Chaitow & Delany 2000), combines ischemic pressure, positional release, stretch, and reciprocal inhibition to clear MTrPs.

Ischemic compression is applied to the MTrP in a continuous or alternating mode. As the referred or local pain subsides, the muscle housing the MTrP is placed in a "position of ease" for 20–30 s. This allows the nervous system to reset, reduces pain activity, and facilitates blood circulation.

A gentle isometric contraction of the muscle is initiated followed by a stretch of the whole muscle. The athlete assists the movement by activating the antagonistic muscle, triggering reciprocal inhibition to facilitate relaxation.

Myofascial release

Precise release of fasciae associated with the MTrP muscle is beneficial (Simons & Dommerholt 2006a), possibly from a stretch point of view as well as to enhance blood circulation by decompressing blood vessels. (See Chapter 10.)

Home stretching exercises

To accelerate the body's healing rate, gentle muscle-specific home stretching exercises may be prescribed (Simons et al. 1999).

Range of motion

Following the trigger point treatment, it is beneficial to move the treated muscles through the full range of motion (ROM) so as to help the nervous system and soft tissue return to their normal state.

Additional treatment methods

Moist heat

Moist heat is used to increase blood circulation and make the connective tissue more pliable. It penetrates more effectively than dry heat (Simons et al. 1999; Simpson 1983) and does not dehydrate the tissue.

Dry or wet needling

Dry needling or acupuncture can break the cycle perpetuating MTrPs, especially when a LTR is elicited during the insertion (Simons & Dommerholt 2006a). Wet needling with procaine, saline solution, or botuline toxin has also been shown to be effective (McPartland 2004).

Transcutaneous electric nerve stimulation

Transcutaneous electric nerve stimulation (TENS) is used for temporary pain management (Simons et al. 1999).

Microcurrent therapies

Frequency-specific microcurrent treatments (Fig. 11.18) have demonstrated beneficial effects during MTrP treatment.

Drug treatments

Prescribed for sleep disturbances, muscle relaxation, and pain relief (Simons et al. 1999).

Herbal remedies

Herbal remedies and essential oils may be used when treating MTrPs, especially herbs that contain linalool that limits ACh release (McPartland 2004). These include:

- lavender (*Lavandula angustifolia*)
- lemon balm (*Melissa officinalis*)
- rosemary (*Rosmarinus officinalis*)
- kava-kava (*Piper methysticum*)
- skullcap (*Scutellaria lateriflora*)
- passionflower (*Passiflora incarnata*)
- rose (*Rosa* spp.)
- valerian (*Valeriana officinalis*).

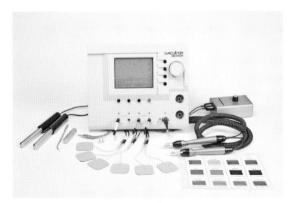

Figure 11.18 • Acutron Mentor

Example of a MTrP treatment

The treatment will vary depending on the athlete's needs but the following order of techniques can be used as a basic guideline:

1. The therapist locates the taut band. Light finger drags on the skin or gentle pressure along the taut band locates the MTrP. Signs like referred pain, referred autonomic symptoms, and LTR are noted.
2. Deep stroking massage or strumming is applied to the muscle and taut band.
3. Trigger point pressure release is used on the trigger point. Tissue response is closely monitored.
4. Further muscle stretching techniques are utilized.
5. The therapist performs soothing massage over the treated area.
6. The athlete slowly moves the treated body part through its full ROM.
7. Home exercises including moist heat and mild but specific muscle stretches are prescribed.

Common MTPs of the lower body

- Quadriceps femoris and adductor magnus (Fig. 11.19).
- Ischiocrural muscles (Fig. 11.20).
- Gastrocnemius and soleus (Fig. 11.21).
- Gluteus medius and minimus (Fig. 11.22).
- Piriformis (Fig. 11.23).
- TFL and tibialis anterior (Fig. 11.24).

Common MTPs of the upper body

- Supraspinatus, infraspinatus, and teres minor (Fig. 11.25).
- Subscapularis and biceps brachii (Fig. 11.26).
- Trapezius and levator scapulae (Fig. 11.27).
- Rhomboids (Fig. 11.28).
- Pectoralis major and minor (Fig. 11.29).
- SCM and scalenus anterior (Fig. 11.30).

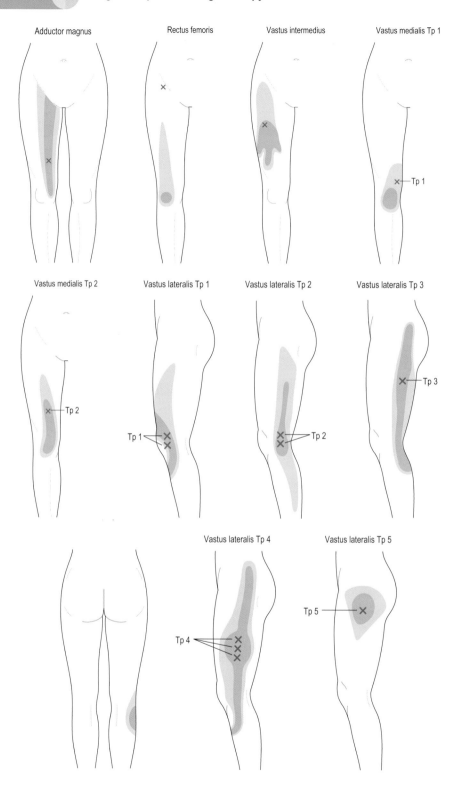

Figure 11.19 • Quadriceps femoris and adductor magnus

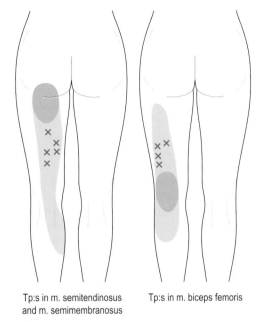

Tp:s in m. semitendinosus
and m. semimembranosus

Tp:s in m. biceps femoris

Figure 11.20 • Ischiocrural muscles

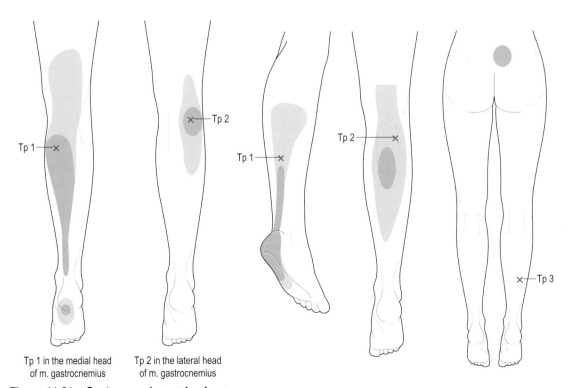

Tp 1

Tp 2

Tp 1

Tp 2

Tp 3

Tp 1 in the medial head
of m. gastrocnemius

Tp 2 in the lateral head
of m. gastrocnemius

Figure 11.21 • Gastrocnemius and soleus

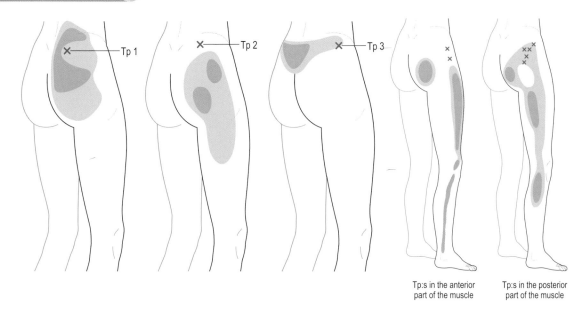

Figure 11.22 • Gluteus medius and minimus

Tp:s in the anterior
part of the muscle

Tp:s in the posterior
part of the muscle

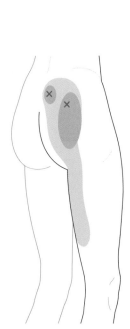

Figure 11.23 • Piriformis

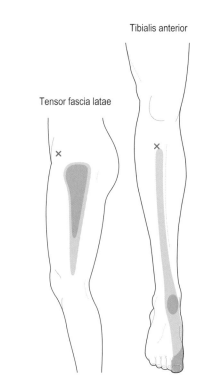

Tibialis anterior

Tensor fascia latae

Figure 11.24 • TFL and tibialis anterior

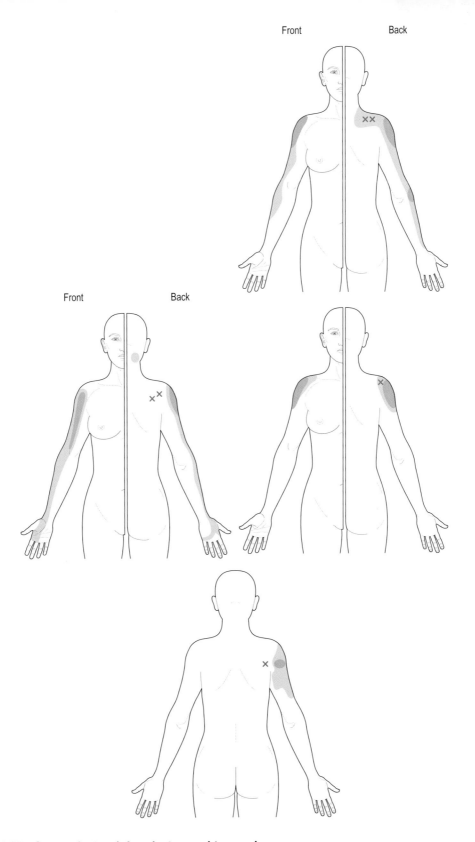

Figure 11.25 • Supraspinatus, infraspinatus, and teres minor

175

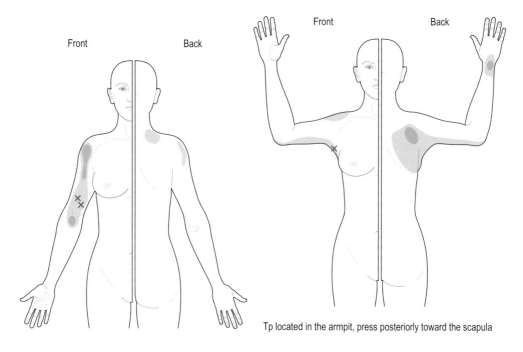

Tp located in the armpit, press posteriorly toward the scapula

Figure 11.26 • Subscapularis and biceps brachii

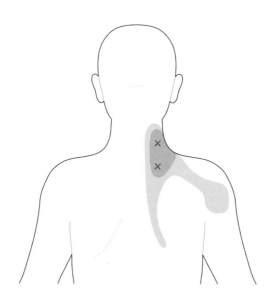

Figure 11.27 • Levator scapulae and trapezius

Continued

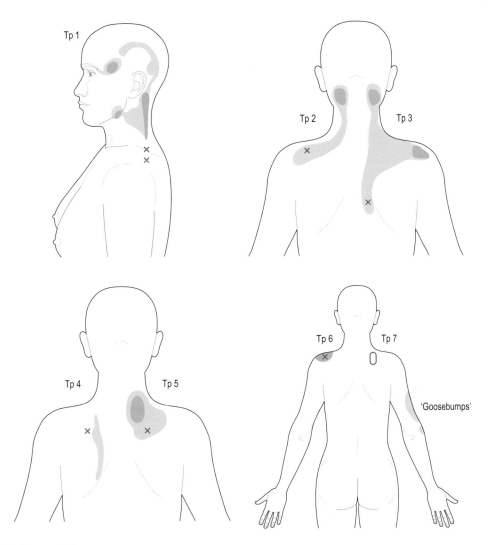

Tp 1

Tp 2   Tp 3

Tp 4   Tp 5

Tp 6   Tp 7

'Goosebumps'

Figure 11.27—cont'd

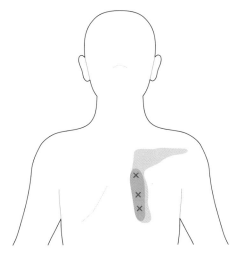

Figure 11.28 • Rhomboids

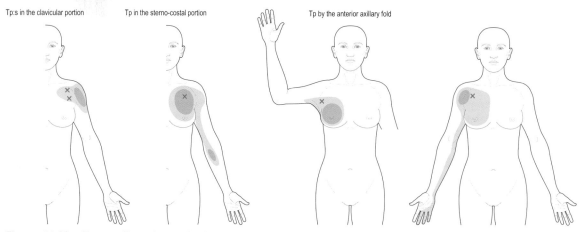

Tp:s in the clavicular portion   Tp in the sterno-costal portion   Tp by the anterior axillary fold

Figure 11.29 • Pectoralis major and minor

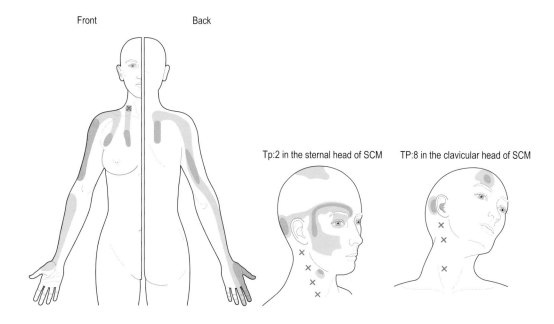

Front   Back

Tp:2 in the sternal head of SCM   TP:8 in the clavicular head of SCM

Figure 11.30 • Scalenus anterior and SCM

References

Alvarez, D., Rockwell, P., 2002. Trigger points: diagnosis and management. Am. Fam. Phys. 65 (4), 653–657.

Baldry, P.E., 1993. Acupuncture, trigger points and musculoskeletal pain, second ed. Churchill Livingstone, Edinburgh.

Birch, S., 2003. Trigger point–acupuncture point correlations revisited. J. Altern. Complement. Med. 9 (1), 91–103.

Bonci, A., 1993. Myofascial barriers to peak athletic performance. Dynamic Chiropractic 11 (1), 1.

Chaitow, L., Walker Delany, J., 2000. Clinical applications of neuromuscular techniques. Churchill Livingstone, Edinburgh.

Dommerholt, J., Bron, C., Franssen, J., 2006. Myofascial trigger points: An evidence-informed review. JMMT 14 (4), 203–221.

Gerwin, R.D., et al., 2004. An expansion of Simons' integrated hypothesis of trigger point formation. Curr. Pain Headache Rep. 8, 468–475.

Majlesi, J., Unulan, H., 2010. Effect of treatment on trigger points. Curr. Pain Headache Rep. 14 (5), 353–360.

McPartland, G.M., 2004. Travell trigger points—molecular and osteopathic perspectives. J. Am. Osteopath. Assoc. 104 (6), 244–249.

Simons, D.G., 2008. New views of myofascial trigger points: etiology and diagnosis. Arch. Phys. Med. Rehabil. 89 (1), 157–159.

Simons, D.G., Dommerholt, J., 2006a. Myofascial pain syndromes—trigger points. J Musculoskeletal Pain 14 (2), 59–64.

Simons, D.G., Dommerholt, J., 2006b. Myofascial trigger points and myofascial pain syndrome: a critical review of recent literature. JMMT 14 (4), E124–E171.

Simons, D.G., et al., 1999. Myofascial pain and dysfunction: the trigger point manual, second ed. vol. 1. Lippincott Williams & Wilkins, Baltimore, MD.

Hou, C.R., et al., 2002. Immediate effects of various physical therapeutic modalities on cervical myofascial pain and trigger-point sensitivity. Arch. Phys. Med. Rehabil. 83 (10), 1406–1414.

Simpson, C., 1983. Heat, cold, or both? Am. J. Nurs. 83 (2), 270–273.

Wheeler, A.H., 2004. Myofascial pain disorders: theory to therapy. Drugs 64 (1), 45–62.

Sports injuries

12

Dr. Kristjan Oddsson

Introduction

Regular physical activity can improve health in numerous ways. Several scientific studies indicate that it may reduce the risk of developing many diseases. This chapter presents some of the scientifically proven positive effects of physical activity (US Department of Health and Human Services 1996). These include:

- Reduced risk of dying prematurely.
- Reduced risk of dying from heart disease.
- Reduced risk of developing diabetes.
- Reduced risk of developing high blood pressure.
- Reduction in blood pressure in people who already have high blood pressure.
- Reduced risk of developing colon cancer.
- Reduced feelings of depression and anxiety.
- Helps control weight.
- Helps build and maintain healthy bones, muscles, and joints.
- Helps older adults become stronger and better able to move about without falling.
- Promotes psychological wellbeing.

During the 1990s several recommendations were published indicating the importance of physical exercise, with suggested guidelines. These recommended that every US adult should accrue at least 30 min of daily moderate physical activity (Pate et al. 1995). This has since evolved so that the current guidance is that healthy adults aged 18–65 need moderately intense aerobic physical activity, or a combination of moderate and intense exercise, for a minimum of 30 min a day for five days a week (Haskell et al. 2007).

People aged over 65 are additionally considered to benefit from flexibility and balance exercises to reduce the risk of falling (Nelson et al. 2007). Research has also indicated substantial benefits from strength training for older people (Pollock et al. 1999; Kryger et al. 2007).

Although the existing benefits of exercise are clear (Fig. 12.1), physical activity can also increase the risk of injury. Approximately seven million people a year are treated for injuries acquired from physical activity and/or sports, and 25% of the injured individuals are absent from work or school for at least one day due to the injury (Conn et al. 2003). Injuries are more frequent among younger individuals, and in men twice as often as in women. In the USA, some of the most frequent sports injuries are from contact sports like football, ice hockey, basketball, and soccer. Baseball and softball are sports with less frequent injuries (Hootman et al. 2007). In Europe, soccer and basketball are also among the most injury-frequented sports (Belechri et al. 2001).

It is important for the sports massage therapist to have basic knowledge of the most common sports injuries, their symptoms, and basic treatment protocols. A sports therapist is often asked questions by both coaches and athletes about how to avoid sports injuries and about basic rehabilitation advice.

Basically all tissues and musculoskeletal structures can be affected by sports injuries, i.e. bone, periosteum, joint cartilage, joint capsules, ligaments, menisci, discs, muscles, fasciae, tendons, bursae, blood vessels, and nerves. Properly executed physical exercise will increase the structural size and strength of all affected tissues; however, if the load exceeds the tissues' ability to adapt, injuries and pain may

© 2011, Elsevier Ltd.
DOI: 10.1016/B978-0-443-10126-7.00012-5

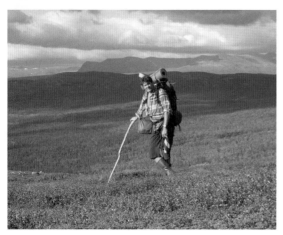

Figure 12.1 • Physical activity, in this case trekking, is good for physical and mental health

arise. This is true for both the "weekend warrior," who starts training at too high an intensity, and the elite athlete, who constantly trains at the upper level of what the body can handle.

During sports activity, the athlete's body is exposed to extreme stress. For sports with explosive movements, for example certain track and field disciplines (sprints, jump, and throwing events) and team sports (football, soccer, basketball, volleyball), the force between the athlete and surface can reach 1800–2200 lb. It is easy, therefore, to understand how different types of injury can arise during such circumstances, especially if the athlete's body is exposed to loads like this on a regular basis.

Sports injuries generally fall into two major categories: acute injuries and overuse injuries.

Pain and inflammation

Pain is defined by the International Association for the Study of Pain (IASP) as "An unpleasant sensory and emotional experience associated with actual or potential tissue damage, or described in terms of such damage" (Merskey et al. 1994).

Pain receptors in the form of free nerve endings, i.e. nociceptors, exist in almost all forms of tissue but they are extra prevalent in the skin, periosteum, fasciae, ligaments, and tendon synovial sheaths. The nociceptors can be stimulated by chemicals (for example, potassium ions, histamine, prostaglandins) or by mechanical deformation. When activated, the receptors transmit signals through afferent myelinated Aδ-fibers (approx 30 m/s) and even through unmyelinated C-fibers (approx 0.1–1 m/s), to the dorsal horn in the spinal cord.

The most important pain pathway is the spinothalamic tract. The nerve impulses reach the postcentral gyrus in the parietal lobe via the thalamus in the brain. There are also more diffuse subcortical areas in the brain where pain sensations are interpreted more emotionally.

Pain anatomy

Figure 12.2 shows how the pain signal travels from the peripheral nociceptors, through Aδ- and C-fiber axons to the nerve roots, then to the spinal cord, from there to the brainstem, to the thalamus, and finally to the cortex, which leads to an awareness of pain.

Pain may be classified in the following categories (Woolf 2004):

- **Nociceptive pain.** Transient pain in response to a noxious stimulus.
- **Inflammatory pain.** Spontaneous pain and hypersensitivity to pain in response to tissue damage and inflammation.
- **Neuropathic pain.** Spontaneous pain and hypersensitivity to pain in association with damage to, or a lesion of, the nervous system.
- **Functional pain.** Hypersensitivity to pain resulting from abnormal central processing of normal input.

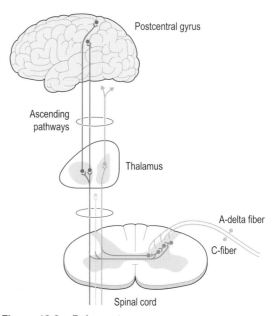

Figure 12.2 • Pain anatomy

Pain is also divided into acute or chronic pain. Pain with a duration of more than three months is medically classified as chronic.

In sports injuries, one of the purposes of the inflammatory pain experience is to promote healing of the injured tissues. The pain reduces movement of and contact with the injured body part to assist the body's healing efforts. There is generally an organic connection between an injury and the pain sensation. Most soft tissue injuries probably heal within 3–4 months. There are many theories about exactly why pain may be experienced long after the actual injury has healed. One theory is that pain receptors may acquire increased sensitivity during an injury due to chemical metabolites; another is that the brain misinterprets signals from "low-threshold" mechano-receptors, creating pain sensations instead of positional information.

Microscopically, as tissues are injured, the inflammatory process commences with the release of chemicals from damaged cells. Mast cells release histamine, which promotes vasodilatation of small blood vessels. White blood cells and other phagocytes also participate in the "inflammatory battle." The injured blood vessels, in conjunction with vasodilatation and increased capillary permeability, create an increased swelling in the area (Nisell et al. 1999).

Macroscopically, inflammation has five common signs:

- pain—dolor
- heat—calor
- redness—rubor
- swelling—tumor
- reduced function—functio laesa.

To reduce pain and inflammation, doctors or other healthcare providers sometimes recommend the patient takes nonsteroid antiinflammatory drugs (NSAIDs), such as aspirin, ibuprofen, ketoprofen, or naproxen sodium. For more severe pain, doctors may prescribe NSAIDs in prescription strengths. It should be noted, however, that the cause of pain and inflammation is never a deficiency of NSAIDs; instead the therapist must seek and treat the real cause of the ailment.

The body's different tissue types react forcefully to the inflammatory processes; however, tendons seem not to react with inflammation during tissue damage except in the acute stage. Instead, injuries to tendons seem to tend to develop into chronic, sometimes degenerative, conditions, i.e. tendinosis and tendinopathies.

Principles of rehabilitation

Rehabilitation is an integral part of the treatment of both acute injuries and overload traumas. Besides creating freedom from pain, the intention is to restore ROM, strength, endurance, coordination, and function.

The pain experience and degree of tenderness when using the body part should guide the duration and intensity of the training. Movement training should commence with gentle isometric exercises, initially without any external load, and gradually increase in intensity. When normal ROM and strength are achieved, rehabilitation training is gradually transferred to concentric–eccentric training at a higher speed and with smaller loads: the athlete's own body weight is often enough. Certain injuries, like chronic Achilles tendinitis, have been shown to respond well to heavier eccentric exercises.

Another specific type of strength training is isokinetic training, i.e. training with the same speed throughout the whole movement. This type of rehabilitation training is often used in postsurgical treatment of knee injuries, etc.

One very important part of rehabilitation training is balance and coordination exercises.

Balance boards

During rehabilitation of ligament and joint injuries, it is important to use different kinds of balance board to place stress on the proprioceptive system (Fig. 12.3). The body's neuromuscular functions are also affected by tissue damage. A balance board, spring board, rope jumping, etc., help to assist the athlete's proprioceptive system.

Acute injuries

Acute injuries include:
- fractures
- dislocations/luxations
- muscle injuries
- ligament injuries
- acute tendon injuries
- acute bursa injuries.

A sports injury can almost always be connected to a specific event, either internal or external violence to the body's structures, for example muscle strain or

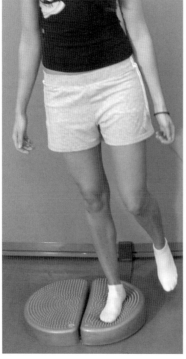

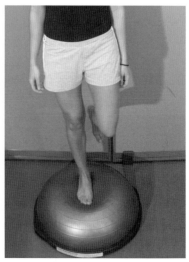

Figure 12.3 • Balance boards

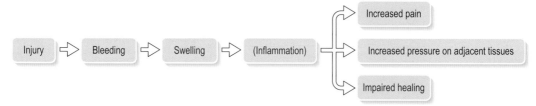

Figure 12.4 • Tissue injury

contusions, or a sprained ankle in conjunction with training or competitive sports activity. A severe hematoma is commonly present, which leads to further unwanted effects (Fig. 12.4).

Fractures

Acute fractures are emergencies and should be examined and treated in hospital. Fractures can be simple (closed) or compound (open) (Figs 12.5;12.6), and are commonly accompanied by soft tissue injuries. Contact sports have a higher incidence of bone fractures, and commonly affected areas are the fingers, clavicle, radius, and tibia.

The symptoms are pain, swelling, discoloration, and possibly misalignment. After a proper examination and diagnosis, the bone is either reduced or not, depending on the possible misalignment; more complex fractures may require surgical intervention. A cast or splint is often used for 3–12 weeks, depending on the location in the body, to immobilize the affected body part.

Avulsion—a complete tear of a ligament or tendon attachment—is more common among children and adolescents.

Fractures stemming from overload injuries, i.e. stress fractures, are described further in the section "Overuse injuries" below.

Dislocations (luxations)/subluxations

Dislocations are another emergency to be examined, diagnosed, and treated at hospital. They are often caused by external violence, for example a shoulder dislocation created by a fall with extended arms, and

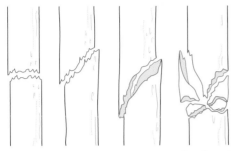

Figure 12.5 • Different types of fracture in a long bone

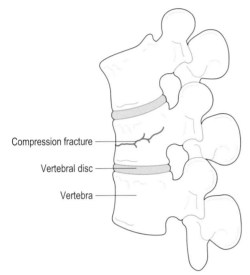

Compression fracture

Vertebral disc

Vertebra

Figure 12.6 • A compression fracture of a lumbar vertebra

sometimes cause fractures in addition. Dislocations may also be caused by internal violence, for example when an arm is hooked and the athlete forces through the movement, thus causing damage.

The most frequent dislocations are of the shoulders and finger joints. More stable joints like the hip, elbow, and ankle require greater forces to dislocate them. Dislocations are commonly associated with soft tissue damage to muscles, ligaments, joint capsules, and occasionally nerves.

Muscle injuries

Muscle injuries can be caused by internal forces, in which case they are called muscle strains. Muscles spanning two or more joints, for example the hamstrings, are more frequently exposed to this type of

muscle injury, which is common among track and field athletes in sprinting, jumping, or other events involving explosive muscle contractions. Muscle strains are often located at the musculotendinous junction and are thought to occur in the interplay between high-speed concentric and eccentric muscle contractions.

Muscle strains are classified as:

1. **Grade I.** Mild strain with damage to less than 5% of the muscle fibers, causing localized pain sensation without substantial strength impairment.
2. **Grade II.** Moderate strain, a substantially larger injury with notable pain during palpation and/or contraction attempt. A swelling is commonly noted.
3. **Grade III.** A complete tear of the muscle.

External forces may cause muscle injuries called muscle contusions, for example when one football player collides with another, and a knee crushes the quadriceps muscle toward the underlying femur, or through falling on a hard object. This type of muscle injury can potentially happen in any sport containing moments of contact, such as football, soccer, basketball, or ice hockey.

The symptoms of acute muscle injuries are commonly a sudden stabbing pain accompanied by difficulty contracting the injured muscle. Other symptoms are swelling, possible muscle cramping, and occasionally a palpable gap in the muscle tissue.

The bleeding caused by the injury can be either intermuscular or intramuscular. Intermuscular bleeding is localized between muscles due to a rupture of the muscle fascia. As the blood is spread over a larger area it causes a more visible hematoma, but it has a faster recovery time. An intramuscular hematoma remains within the muscle since the fascia is intact, and has a longer healing period since it is more difficult for the body to absorb the localized edema encapsulated within the muscle. It may additionally cause complications like severe scarring, impaired ROM and/or calcification or ossification of the scar tissue, i.e. myositis ossificans, which may require surgical intervention.

Muscle cramps may be defined as involuntary, often painful, muscle contractions. Their origin is still somewhat unclear, but Parisi et al. (2003) have divided muscle cramp into three categories, based on etiology:

1. paraphysiological cramps
2. idiopathic cramps
3. symptomatic cramps.

Muscle cramps relating to physical activity are categorized as paraphysiological cramps. It is suggested that this type arises from a hydroelectrolytic imbalance caused by hard, long-term, and sometimes repetitive activity leading to hyperexcitability of the terminal nerve branches in the area. Research has additionally indicated low magnesium levels (Klarkeson et al. 1995). Dehydration, glycogen depletion, salt deficiency, previous muscle bleeding, small muscle ruptures, or the athlete's general health are other possible causes.

The athlete should prevent cramping by adequate basic training, including warm-up routine, and ensuring proper nutrition and fluid, electrolyte, and glycogen deposit uptake (Peterson et al. 2001).

The sports massage therapist can perform cramp release using stretching, cryo-, and physiotherapy, for example strong effleurage and deep friction massage (Brukner et al. 2010). Another popular and effective method involves simultaneous relaxation, approximation, and compression of the cramping muscle combined with alternating isometric contractions of antagonistic muscles (Fig. 12.7). The athlete is asked to contract the antagonistic muscle for 4–5 s whilst the approximation/compression is maintained and further increased between every isometric muscle contraction.

Ligament injuries

A sprain is a stretch or a tear of a ligament, and commonly occurs in conjunction with acute

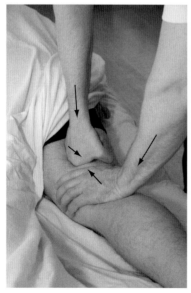

Figure 12.7 • Cramp release

violence toward the affected joint. Sprains are classified as:

1. **Grade I.** Mild injury involving microscopic tears and some tenderness.
2. **Grade II.** Moderate injury with partial ligament rupture, notable swelling, and tenderness.
3. **Grade III.** Serious injury with a complete tear of the ligament. Generates notable instability and intense pain.

Since the symptoms of ligament sprains in different joints vary, it makes the classifications more difficult to use clinically. The possibilities for healing vary depending on whether the ligament is extracapsular (for example, the calcaneofibular ligament in the ankle), intracapsular (for example, the cruciate ligaments in the knee joint), or capsular (for example, the anterior talofibular ligament in the ankle) (Figs 12.8; 12.9). Intracapsular ligaments do not heal after a complete tear, while a capsular ligament can have better possibilities of doing so (Bahr et al. 2004).

Ligaments located in the ankle and knee joints are most frequently injured during sports activity. It is estimated that about 20 000 ankle sprains/day occur in the USA. Of these 70% occur in the anterior talofibular ligament. In the knee, there are 200 000 anterior cruciate ligament injuries/year, 100 000 requiring surgical intervention (American Association of Orthopedic Surgeons 2008).

Acute tendon injuries

Almost every acute spontaneous rupture of tendons is preceded by pathological changes in the tendon (Peterson et al. 2001). Tendon injuries are classified similarly to ligament injuries. Ruptures commonly present where the tendon's blood supply is minimized, for example, for the Achilles tendon, almost 1 in above the calcaneus. Many tendons that are exposed to injuries (for example, Achilles tendon, supraspinatus tendon, patellar ligament) may show degenerative changes as early as in the third decade (Maffulli et al. 2005).

Rupture of the calcaneus/Achilles tendon

The calcaneus/Achilles tendon is the strongest tendon in the body. The load during walking is estimated to be 2.5 times the body weight, and running may increase this up to 6–12 times (Komi et al. 1992; Merskey et al. 1994). Men are more frequently exposed than women to complete ruptures of the

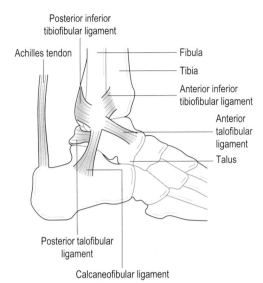

Figure 12.8 • **Ligaments in the ankle joint (lateral view of the ankle).** • There are three stabilizing ligaments: the anterior talofibular ligament, the calcaneofibular ligament and the posterior talofibular ligament. The first one is the most often injured in inversion ankle sprains

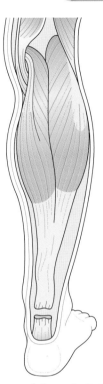

Figure 12.10 • **A complete rupture of the Achilles tendon**

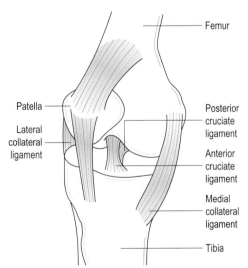

Figure 12.9 • **Ligaments in the knee joint** • Injury to the anterior cruciate ligament is common and one of the most controversial and difficult to treat sports injuries

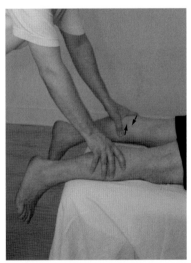

Figure 12.11 • **Thompson's test for total Achilles rupture** • Squeezing the calf muscle will result in a small plantar flexion of the foot. If not, the test is positive

calcaneus tendon (Fig. 12.10), which has an acute onset with sharp pain and impaired function. Thompson's test (Simmond's calf squeeze test) is positive as the foot fails to plantarflex as the calf muscle is squeezed (Brukner et al. 2001; Fig. 12.11).

Treatment of a complete rupture of the calcaneus tendon is either surgical or conservative

(for example, cast treatment for 8–10 weeks). Even though the evidence is not yet fully conclusive, it seems that the risk of a new rupture is somewhat larger after conservative treatment. Despite the inherent risks of surgery, it is therefore the preferred treatment for athletes thanks to the possibility of early motion, which is essential for effective rehabilitation (Brukner et al. 2001; Peterson et al. 2001).

Acute injuries to the bursa

Bursae reduce pressure and frictions over sensitive areas, for example protruding bone, between tendons and bone, close to joints, or under the skin. Bursae injured by acute violence may swell as a result of bleeding, a condition called hemobursitis, which is treated as for other acute soft tissue injuries. Common areas of bursitis are the subcutaneous areas such as the olecranon bursae, prepatellar bursae, and trochanteric bursae.

Treatment of acute sports injuries

The aim of acute sports injury treatment is to reduce bleeding and swelling, which may decrease pain sensation, and reduce rehabilitation time. The mnemonic PRICE is used to describe the acute treatment principles:

- **P**rotection
- **R**estricted activity/**R**est
- **I**ce
- **C**ompression
- **E**levation.

Protection and rest are applied to minimize the complications of the injury. Since the blood circulation in the muscles can be ten times higher compared with when they are at rest, it is important to reduce the blood supply to the injured body part. Ice treatment likely has less effect on the bleeding, but is important for pain relief. Studies have shown that a hematoma is established as early as 30 s after the injury occurrence. Compression bandaging, preferably combined with a foam rubber pad, can effectively stop the bleeding.

Ankle injury

The application of a compression bandage with a foam rubber pad on the ankle gives effective compression over the injured area (Fig. 12.12). A Cryo/Cuff (ice water in an insulated boot) in combination with compression bandage, gives effective results on both acute swelling and pain

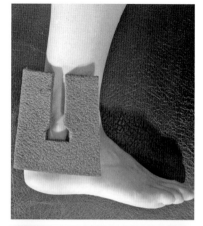
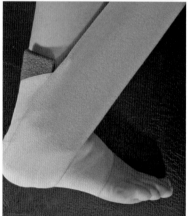
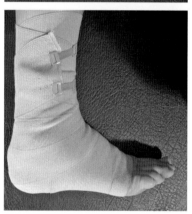

Figure 12.12 • Treatment of ankle injury

(Fig. 12.13). This may be applied either as a restrictive compression aid for 15–20 min, or intermittently with compression intervals (three 10 min intervals with a short rest between them). After application of the initial firm compression bandage, a supportive bandage is used over the days immediately following.

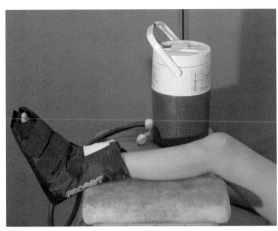

Figure 12.13 • Use of a Cryo/Cuff in ankle injury

Elevation reduces swelling and creates a reduced peripheral tissue pressure. Studies have shown that the blood flow in the leg decreases when elevation exceeds 30 cm. An injured body part should be elevated as high as possible for the first 30–60 min following a sports injury, and as often as possible during the following 48 h.

After the initial 48 h, treatment is given to increase blood circulation and healing, and heat falls into this category. The elasticity and plasticity of collagen fibers increases during heat treatment, which is beneficial for rehabilitation therapy. Examples of heat-producing modalities are massage, a heat lamp, heat pad, warm bath, sauna, shortwave, and ultrasound treatment.

Overuse injuries

Both young and older athletes are exposed to overuse injuries. This type of injury is often more difficult to treat as often the cause may be unknown.

Overuse injuries are divided into the following three categories:

1. inflammations
2. stress fractures
3. degenerative conditions.

Inflammations

- Apophysitis.
- Paratendinitis.
- Tendinitis.
- Periostitis.
- Bursitis.

Stress fractures

Degenerative conditions

- Arthrosis/osteoarthritis.
- Tendinosis/tendinopathies.

Overload injuries are cause by repeated loads over a long period of time. The symptoms initially present with mild pain and stiffness. Initial neglect often causes further tissue damage and a more chronic pain condition (Fig. 12.14).

Although there is a lack of scientific evidence to back this up, a large number of intrinsic and extrinsic factors may cause the formation of overload injuries.

Extrinsic factors

Training-related factors

- Monotonous training.
- New unfamiliar exercises.
- Increased training load and/or intensity.
- Poor technique.
- Insufficient warm-up.

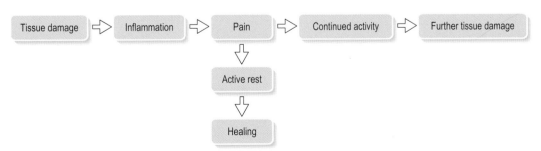

Figure 12.14 • Overuse injuries

Equipment-related factors

- Shoes.
- Other garments.

Environmental factors

- Surface.
- Cold, heat.

Intrinsic factors

- Malalignment
  - pes planus/varus
  - genu valgus/varus
  - increased q-angle
  - patella alta/baja
  - knee recurvatum
  - femoral neck anteversion
  - leg length discrepancy.
- Flexibility and strength
  - hypo-/hypermobility
  - muscle imbalance/weakness.
- Sex, size, body composition.
- Impaired balance/coordination.
- Psychological stress.
- Poor rehabilitation after injury.

Inflammation

Apophysitis

Apophysitis is when the attachment of a muscle or tendon is inflamed from overload. Most prevalent in growing adolescents, it is characterized by pain during activity, palpative tenderness, and possible swelling. Common areas of apophysitis are the calcaneus tendon (Sever-Haglund disease), tuberositis tibiae (Osgood-Schlatter disease), or the superior attachment of the patellar ligament (Sinding-Larsen's disease). It is important to reduce the load on the area to avoid chronic conditions.

Paratendinitis/peritendinitis/tenovaginitis

This is inflammation in the synovial sheath covering the tendon. Symptoms include pain during activity, swelling, and occasionally crepitations. Common areas are the wrists.

De Quervain's syndrome is a result of shear microtrauma resulting from repetitive gliding of the first

dorsal compartment tendons, abductor pollicis longus, and extensor pollicis brevis beneath the sheath of the first compartment over the radial styloid process (Rettig 2004). Golfers and those who play different racquet sports commonly suffer from this condition. It presents with local pain, swelling, and palpative tenderness. Finkelstein's test (pain when the athlete flexes the thumb into the palm whilst the examiner ulnarly deviates the wrist) is generally positive.

Tendinitis

The term "tendinitis" is used more seldom these days, and is instead replaced with tendinopathy or tendinosis, indicating a degenerative element rather than pure inflammation.

Biopsies have revealed that classic inflammatory signs are not always observed in chronic tendon pain conditions (Chard et al. 1994; Astrom et al. 1995). As tendon tissue contains a limited amount of blood vessels, the inflammatory process from overload injuries is limited. Histologically degenerative change is noted instead, with loss of collagen in the tendon tissue and local cell death.

Periostitis

This condition, which is a symptom rather than a diagnosis, has had many different names over the years: shin splints syndrome, medial tibial syndrome, tibial stress syndrome, posterior tibial syndrome, soleus syndrome, and periostitis.

Medial tibial stress syndrome is a more modern name for this very common condition, and some studies show it to be responsible for nearly 50% of all lower leg injuries reported in certain populations (Kortebein et al. 2000). Load and palpative pain along the medial tibial border are noted.

Shin pain is extremely common among athletes and generally involves one or more of three pathological processes; bone stress, inflammation, and raised intracompartmental pressure (Brukner et al. 2010). Manual treatments (massage, stretching), together with active rest, a complete analysis concerning which activities caused the condition, and examination of the tibialis posterior muscle are very important.

Bursitis

A bursa is a small, fluid-filled connective tissue sac located in areas of pressure and/or friction. Many bursae are close to the joints and may communicate with the joint cavity, for example the popliteal bursa, suprapatellar bursa of the knee, and the iliopectineal bursa that communicates with the hip joint.

An injury inside a joint, like a meniscus injury in the knee joint, may cause a swelling of a communicating bursa owing to increased fluid production inside the joint. Baker's cyst is just such a condition. Chronic bursitis may arise from external pressure and/or friction, for example prepatellar bursitis (housemaid's knee) and olecranon bursitis (student's elbow). Symptoms are local swelling, tenderness, and heat over the affected bursa.

The treatment aims to reduce the stress over the area to allow the inflammation to heal.

Stress fractures

Stress fractures may be called "the ultimate overload injury," where one of the body's hardest tissues breaks from the repeated and cumulative stress to which it is exposed. The causes can be summarized as "too much, too often, too quick, and too short rest." Athletes active in endurance-oriented sports, for example runners, and military personnel are most frequently exposed to this injury type (Bennell et al. 1996; Kaufmann et al. 2000).

The bones commonly affected are the tibia, metatarsals, tarsal navicular, femur, and the pelvis (Brukner et al. 2010). Symptoms are load-bearing and palpatory pain, and local swelling. Healing requires reduced stress in the bone, and most stress fractures heal within 6–8 weeks.

Degenerative conditions

Osteoarthritis/osteoarthrosis/arthrosis

The articular cartilage can be damaged through trauma or overuse. Repetitive small injuries can result in osteoarthritis, although osteoarthrosis or arthrosis is a more correct term for the condition (Peterson et al. 2001). The condition includes breakdown and wear of the joint cartilage.

Athrosis is generally divided into two categories: primary arthrosis with unknown etiology, and secondary arthrosis stemming from previous injury or wrong weight load. Genetic factors like old age, female gender, being overweight, and previous injuries are known factors causing arthrosis.

Symptoms can be insidious and may present as weight-bearing pain, swelling, morning stiffness, heat, and crepitations. The symptoms may indirectly cause muscular hypotrophy. Commonly affected areas are the hips, fingers, and/or joints of the spine.

Diagnosis is confirmed by radiologic investigation. Treatment is generally pain relief with NSAIDs, hyaluronic acid derivatives, modification of activity, and specific strength training. It is possible, but not yet scientifically proven, that manual techniques like massage and careful range of motion exercises can relieve some of the symptoms. New surgical treatments with autologous chondrocyte transplantation have shown promising long-term results for cartilage injuries in the knee (Peterson et al. 2001).

Tendinopathies/tendinosis

Overuse tendon injuries account for about 30–50% of all sports injuries (Kannus 1997). A commonly proposed name for tendon pain problems in general is "tendinopathy" (Peterson et al. 2001).

The most typical symptoms are a combination of local pain, swelling, and impaired performance (Paavola et al. 2002). The symptoms are more visible on superficial tendons. The pain is commonly sensed before and after physical activity. Morning stiffness in the area and crepitations are common occurrences. Symptoms present from 0–6 weeks can be described as acute, symptoms present from 6–12 weeks as subacute, and symptoms present for more than 3 months can be categorized as chronic (Fredberg et al. 2008).

Alfredson et al. (1998) showed very good results with eccentric exercises as a treatment for chronic Achilles tendinosis. When comparing the efficacy of eccentric vs. concentric exercises, it was shown that superior results were obtained by using eccentric contractions in rehabilitation of tendinopathies (Mafi et al. 2001; Jonsson et al. 2005).

Treatment of overload injuries

To determine if an overload injury is related to the muscle–tendon complex, specific stress tests are performed:

1. isometric contraction of the muscle
2. passive elongation of the muscle/tendon
3. palpation of the muscle/tendon.

If two of these tests are positive (generate pain), it is almost certain that the problem is related to the muscle–tendon complex.

Treatment aims to prevent further tissue damage and inflammation by avoiding activities and movements that cause pain, and should include active rest, i.e. physical activity without stressing the injured body part. Also beneficial are strength training with low weights and high repetitions, pool training (swimming, wet vest, etc.), stationary cycling, and other forms of training like fitness, yoga, Pilates, and BOSU training.

The sports massage therapist performs manual treatment (deep transverse friction and other massage techniques, PRT, and stretching). The scientific effects of deep friction massage are not well known but it is reasonable to assume that the technique and other soft tissue mobilization techniques can promote scar formation postacute, heal soft tissue lesions, reduce excessive adhesion and scar formation in chronic soft tissue lesions, reduce intramuscular tissue thickening, and reduce spasm secondary to pain (Davidson et al. 1997; Gehlsen et al. 1999; Brukner et al. 2001).

Pain can also be relieved by the "gate control theory" mechanism, where stimulation of thick nerve fibers (Aβ) from touch and pressure receptors activates interneurons in the dorsal horn of the spinal cord and thereby inhibits the signals from pain nerve fibers (Aδ, C) (Kandel et al. 2000). Release of oxytocine during and after sports massage treatments can be another possible cause of pain relief (Lund et al. 2002).

Cortisone injections are also used and may be very effective for some conditions, though less useful in others. It is important to note that cortisone tends to break down connective tissue and thereby make the treated tissue even more fragile. The load placed on the treated tissue should therefore be minimized for 2–3 weeks following the injection.

Some more serious cases require surgical intervention.

Some common sports injuries

Ankle distortion

Ankle distortion is a very common sports injury, especially in ball games like rugby, soccer, volleyball, handball, and basketball. In 70% of cases the anterior talofibular ligament is torn, partially or completely. A typical occurrence is landing after a jump on a foot which is supinated. Symptoms typically include acute pain, swelling, and tenderness. If a total ligament tear is suspected, the anterior drawer test can show instability in the ankle joint compared with the uninjured side (Fig. 12.15).

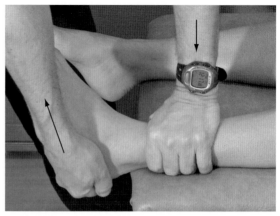

Figure 12.15 • Anterior drawer test for rupture of the anterior talofibular ligament (ankle joint in neutral position) • The test is performed by pulling the calcaneus forward (i.e., upward), in relation to the lower leg. Compare with the uninjured side

The acute injury is best treated with PRICE. After 48 h the rehabilitation phase starts with different kinds of thermotherapy, early motion, and careful weight-bearing activities. It is very important to remember the proprioception and balance exercises, because a ligament injury is not just an injury to a bundle of connective tissue fibers. Proprioceptors in the ligament and in the joint capsule are torn and so the rehabilitation program should include different kinds of balance exercise.

Rupture of the anterior cruciate ligament (ACL)

A tear of the ACL is the knee injury of greatest concern to the athlete. The injury is often caused by a rotation and/or a hyperextension/flexion trauma. Usually this is a high-energy injury with near dislocation of the knee. Acute pain and hearing a "popping" or "snapping" sound is typical. Swelling within a few hours is a result of hemarthrosis (blood in the knee). With time, the patient can develop "giving way" problems (instability). Tests are often difficult to perform in the acute phase because of the pain. The anterior drawer sign in 90 degrees of flexion (Fig. 12.16) and/or Lachman's test in 20–30 degrees of flexion (Fig. 12.17), pulling the tibia forward in relation to the femur, are positive diagnostics for an ACL tear (Brukner et al. 2010; Peterson et al. 2001).

The athlete must visit the hospital for further investigation if ACL or PCL injury is suspected.

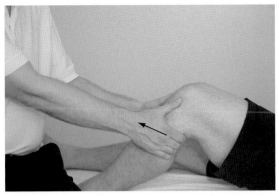

Figure 12.16 • Anterior drawer test in 90 degrees of flexion for testing the anterior cruciate ligament • The test is performed by pulling the tibia forward in relation to the femur. Compare with the uninjured side

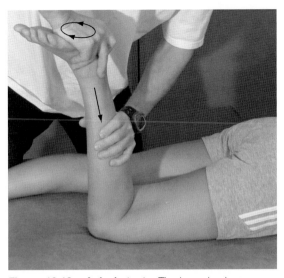

Figure 12.18 • Apley's test • The lower leg is compressed, with simultaneous gradual external and internal rotation. Perceived knee pain during external rotation may indicate an injury to the medial meniscus. If pain instead presents during internal rotation, an injury to the lateral meniscus may be existent.

Symptoms of meniscus injuries include "locking" phenomena, palpatory pain in the joint space, pain in maximal extension and flexion during loading, and sometimes an effusion of fluid in the joint. Apley's test can be positive (Fig. 12.18). The orthopedic surgeon may perform arthroscopy surgery by completely removing, resecting, or suturing the damaged part of the meniscus. It is very important to exercise the thigh muscles after such treatment to generate the necessary stability and support.

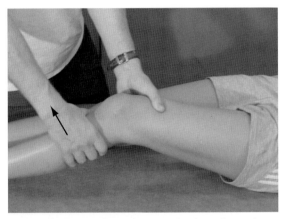

Figure 12.17 • Lachman's test • Lachman's test in 20–30 degrees of flexion. The test is performed by pulling the tibia forward in relation to the femur. Compare with the uninjured side

Scaphoid bone fracture

This fracture is common in contact sports, or after breaking a fall with extended arms. Since the pain can often be moderate, it is common for the injury to go undiagnosed for weeks after the incident. Radiologic investigation then reveals the condition, but pain and swelling in the "anatomical snuff box," located between the tendons of the extensor pollicis longus and the extensor pollicis brevis/abductor pollicis longus, is also common. Due to the fact that the blood supply to the scaphoid bone enters distally, a complete fracture can occasionally result in avascular necrosis.

Meniscus tear

The menisci serve as stabilizers and shock absorbers in the knee joints. Injuries can give rise to locking phenomena in the affected knee joint. The medial meniscus also attaches to the medial collateral ligament and joint capsule, and so is exposed to combination injuries with these structures. The injury mechanism is commonly torsional violence. A torsion where the lower leg is rotated laterally in relation to the femur may cause a medial meniscus injury. The opposite rotation can cause a tear of the lateral meniscus. During a "bucket handle injury," the meniscus causes an extension defect of the knee.

An x-ray, bone scan, and/or MRI will confirm the diagnosis, and the wrist and thumb are usually immobilized with a plaster cast for at least 3 months.

Overuse injuries

Achilles tendinopathy

One of the most common overuse conditions in sport is Achilles tendinopathy (Fig. 12.19). Morning stiffness in the tendon and before and/or after activity is typical. Sometimes a local swelling can be palpated. Initial treatment, if the condition presents over just a week or two, is "active rest" with cycling and swimming activities, with instructions to avoid movement that causes pain. The sports massage therapist may administer different manual treatment techniques, for example massage, deep friction, or stretching. If the problem still remains, it may be necessary to use eccentric exercises for the calf muscles. The original "Alfredson protocol" consists of eccentric strength exercises, 3×15 repetitions of inverted toe raises with straight leg, followed by 3×15 repetitions with the knee slightly bent. After each repetition the noninjured leg can be used to return to the starting position. The program is repeated twice a day, seven days a week (Alfredson et al. 1998), and the intensity is adjusted depending on fitness and motivation levels.

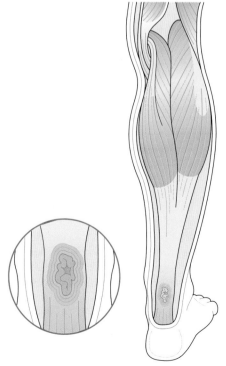

Figure 12.19 • Achilles tendinosis

Eccentric exercise of the calf muscles can often help if the Achilles tendon problem is chronic (Fig. 12.20). Start from maximal plantar flexion position and go slowly down to end position in maximum dorsal flexion. Repeat from maximum plantar flexion position.

Plantar fasciitis

Plantar fasciitis is an overload injury, often stemming from long-term monotonous load to the plantar aponeurosis. This leads to a local inflammation often in the origin at the calcaneus bone. Athletes with low (pes planus) or high (pes cavus) arches may be predisposed to plantar fasciitis. The condition may heal faster with active rest, orthotics, manual therapies (like PRT and deep friction), and supportive taping.

Painful heel pad

The fat pad at the heel may be pressed laterally and expose the underlying bone and bursa after repeated jumping or running on hard surfaces (Fig. 12.21). This may lead to severe heel pain and/or bursitis. This condition can be difficult to heal and the correct choice of shoes is important.

Chronic compartment syndrome

This is more of a symptom than a diagnosis/assessment. There are four compartments in the lower leg. The anterior houses tibialis anterior, extensor hallucis longus, extensor digitorum longus muscles, blood vessels, and nerves. The deep posterior contains tibialis posterior, flexor hallucis longus, and flexor digitorum longus muscles. The superficial posterior compartment accommodates gastrocnemius and soleus muscles. The lateral contains peroneus longus and brevis muscles. Physical activity leads to increased muscle volume, which increases the intracompartmental pressure. This may cause ischemic pain.

Medial tibial stress syndrome/"shin splints"

Exercise-related pain at the medial border of the tibia can stem from more than one factor. Posterior lower leg compartment syndrome, periostitis, tibial stress

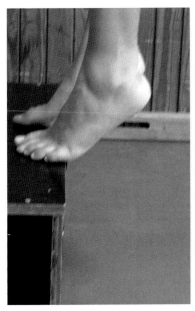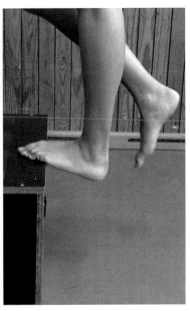

Figure 12.20 • Eccentric exercise for Achilles tendinosis

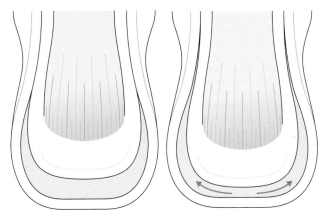

Figure 12.21 • Painful heel pad • Excessive heel strike with poor heel cushioning can result in pain right under the calcaneus bone. Good stable footwear and eventually heel pad taping can provide relief

reaction, or tendinopathy along the tibialis posterior tendon may generate this problem. "Toe running," hyper pronation, or change of running surface can contribute. Manual treatments like massage and stretching can be useful for the athlete. Orthotics, technique and/or equipment evaluation, and adequate warm-up may also help.

Patellofemoral pain syndrome

This is a collective name for pain in the patellofemoral part of the knee. Chondromalacia patellae, which often is associated with this condition, is instead a pathologic, anatomic diagnosis of changes in the joint cartilage of the patella. This is best diagnosed though arthroscopic investigation.

Iliotibial band friction syndrome/ "runner's knee"

This is the most common cause of lateral knee pain in runners. It may be caused by the friction that takes place as the iliotibial band repeatedly rubs against the lateral femoral condyle. The symptoms are very typically delayed onset of pain after

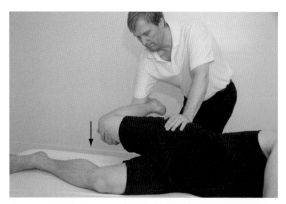

Figure 12.22 • Ober's test • Evaluation of tightness in the iliotibial band (ITB). The unaffected (lower) hip and knee are flexed, followed by 90 degrees flexion of the involved (upper) knee, and abduction and hyperextension of the leg. A positive test (i.e., tightness in the ITB) will prevent the extremity from dropping below the horizontal plane

a couple of minutes of running or sometimes cycling. It is a sharp, sometimes burning, pain, which disappears immediately after the patient stops the activity. Sometimes the region approximately 2–3 cm above the jointline may be painful to palpation.

Ober's test (Fig. 12.22) can show tightness in the iliotibial band. Manual treatment like massage and stretching of the iliotibial band, tensor fasciae latae, and the gluteus maximus muscles can be helpful.

Coxae saltans/"snapping hip"

This can be due to the same causes as "runner's knee," a friction condition with interference of hip muscles and iliotibial tract. Sometimes the trochanteric bursa is involved. Monotonous loading can produce a sudden snapping sound from the lateral hip, i.e. lateral snapping hip. Other somewhat less common causes are thickening of the anterior border of the iliotibial tract, when the iliopsoas tendon passes over the iliopectineal eminence (medial snapping hip) or when the biceps caput longum tendon passes over the ischial tuberosity. Manual treatment like massage and stretching of the iliotibial band, tensor fasciae latae, gluteus maximus, iliopsoas, and hamstring muscles can be helpful.

Impingement in the shoulder

The subacromial space is limited by the head of humerus, acromion, and the coracoacromial ligament. The three structures possibly impinged between this frame are the supraspinatus tendon, tendon of the long head of biceps brachii, and the subacromial bursa. Throwing athletes may have event-related swelling from tendinopathies in the supraspinatus tendon and/or biceps brachii tendon that may predispose for this condition. Bone spurs or a genetic anatomic limitation can also create problems. When the arm is moved in abduction and flexion, particularly with simultaneous lateral rotation, the soft tissues will be compressed and refer pain. Between 80–120 degrees abduction/flexion the pain is worse (this is also called painful arch). The empty can test (Fig. 12.23), full can test (Fig. 12.24), and Hawkins impingement test

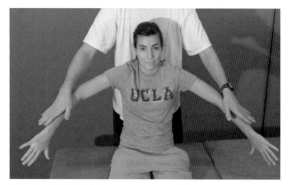

Figure 12.23 • Empty can test • The patient rotates the arm internally (thumbs down) and activates muscles isometrically, whilst the examiner puts downward pressure on the arms. The test is positive if there is significant pain or weakness on resistance

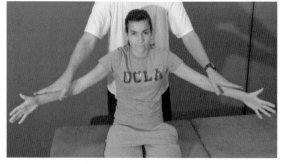

Figure 12.24 • Full can test • The patient rotates the arm externally (thumbs up), and activates muscles isometrically, whilst the examiner puts downward pressure on the arms. The test is positive if there is significant pain or weakness on resistance

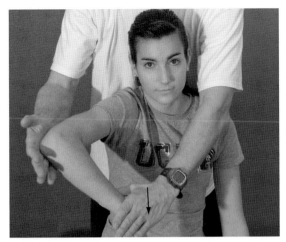

Figure 12.25 • Hawkins test • Forward flexion of the shoulder to 90 degrees and then forced internal rotation

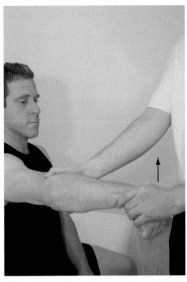

Figure 12.26 • Test for lateral epicondylalgia • Resisted muscle testing of the wrist extensors and simultaneous palpation of the muscle origins. A positive test provokes pain

(Fig. 12.25) are usually used to establish the diagnosis. It is possible that eccentric exercises combined with manual treatments like massage, PRT, and stretching techniques can be used by the sports therapist to treat this problem.

Lateral/medial epicondylitis/"tennis elbow"/"golfer's elbow"

This is commonly an overuse injury of the superficial extensor and flexor muscles of the hand, especially the extensor carpi radialis longus and brevis muscles. Microtears in the extensor aponeurosis attachment at the lateral humeral epicondyle cause edema and inflammation. The condition can evolve to a chronic degenerative pain condition similar to tendinosis. Symptoms are pain triggered by activity and palpation.

An isometric muscle contraction test combined with palpation may trigger identical pain (Fig. 12.26). Other possible causes of pain can be entrapment of the radial nerve, muscle strains, postexercise soreness, or myofascial trigger points in the shoulder and elbow region.

The sports therapist can treat this condition with manual therapies, for example massage techniques such as deep friction, PRT, and stretch techniques like lock and stretch, active release technique (ART), or active isolated stretching (AIS). Eccentric exercises may additionally be used during the rehabilitation.

References

Alfredson, H., et al., 1998. Heavy-load eccentric calf muscle training for the treatment of chronic Achilles tendinosis. Am. J. Sports Med. 26 (3), 360–366.

American Association of Orthopaedic Surgeons, 2008. http://www.aaos. org.

Astrom, M., et al., 1995. Chronic Achilles tendinopathy: a survey of surgical and histopathological findings. Clin. Orthop. 316, 151–164.

Bahr, R., et al., 2004. Förebygga, behandla, rehabilitera

Idrottsskador—en illustrerad guide. SISU Idrottsböcker, Stockholm.

Belechri, M., et al., 2001. Sports Injuries European Union Group. Sports injuries among children in six European union countries. Eur. J. Epidemiol. 17 (11), 1005–1012.

Bennell, K.L., et al., 1996. The incidence and distribution of stress fractures in competitive track and field athletes. Am. J. Sports Med. 24, 211–217.

Brukner, P., et al., 2010. Clinical sports medicine, third ed. McGraw-Hill, Sydney.

Chard, M.D., et al., 1994. Rotator cuff degeneration and lateral epicondylitis: a comparative histological study. Ann. Rheum. Dis. 53, 30–34.

Conn, J.M., et al., 2003. Sports and recreation related injury episodes in the US population, 1997–99. Inj. Prev. 9 (2), 117–123.

Davidson, C.J., et al., 1997. Rattendon morphologic and functional changes resulting from soft tissue mobilization. Med. Sci. Sports Exerc. 29 (3), 313–319.

Fredberg, U., et al., 2008. Chronic tendinopathy tissue pathology, pain mechanisms and etiology with special focus on inflammation. Scand. J. Med. Sci. Sports 8 (1), 3–15.

Gehlsen, G.M., et al., 1999. Fibroblast responses to variation in soft tissue mobilization pressure. Med. Sci. Sports Exerc. 31 (4), 531–535.

Haskell, W.L., et al., 2007. Physical activity and public health: updated recommendation for adults from the American College of Sports Medicine and the American Heart Association. Med. Sci. Sports Exerc. 39 (8), 1423–1434.

Hootman, J.M., et al., 2007. Epidemiology of collegiate injuries for 15 sports: summary and recommendations for injury prevention initiatives. J. Athl. Train. 42 (2), 311–319.

Jonsson, P., et al., 2005. Superior results with eccentric compared to concentric quadriceps training in patients with jumper's knee: a prospective randomised study. Br. J. Sports Med. 39 (11), 847–850.

Kandel, E.R., et al., 2000. Principles of neural science, fourth ed. McGraw-Hill, New York.

Kannus, P., 1997. Tendons—a source of major concern in competitive and recreational athletes. Scand. J. Med. Sci. Sports 53–54.

Kaufmann, K.R., et al., 2000. Military training-related injuries—surveillance, research and prevention. Am. J. Prev. Med. 18, S54–S63.

Klarkeson, P.M., et al., 1995. Exercise and mineral status of athletes: calcium, magnesium, phosphorus, and iron. Med. Sci. Sports Exerc. 27 (6), 831–843 Review.

Komi, P.V., et al., 1992. Biomechanical loading of Achilles tendon during normal locomotion. Clin. Sports Med. 11, 521–531.

Kortebein, P.M., et al., 2000. Medial tibial stress syndrome. Med. Sci. Sports Exerc. 32 (Suppl. 3), S27–S33.

Kryger, A.I., et al., 2007. Resistance training in the oldest old. Consequences for muscle strength, fiber types, fiber size, and MHC isoforms. Scand. J. Med. Sci. Sports 17, 422–430.

Lund, I., et al., 2002. Repeated massage-like stimulation induces long-term effects on nociception: contribution of oxytocinergic mechanisms. Eur. J. Neurosci. 16 (2), 330–338.

Maffulli, N., et al., 2005. Tendon injuries—basic science and clinical medicine. Springer, London.

Mafi, N., et al., 2001. Superior short-term results with eccentric calf muscle training compared to concentric training in a randomized prospective multicenter study on patients with chronic Achilles tendinosis. Knee Surg. Sports Traumatol. Arthrosc. 9 (1), 42–47.

Merskey, H., et al., 1994. Classification of chronic pain, second ed. IASP Press, Seattle.

Nelson, M.E., et al., 2007. Physical activity and public health in older adults: recommendation from the American College of Sports Medicine and the American Heart Association. Med. Sci. Sports Exerc. 39 (8), 1435–1445.

Nisell, R., et al., 1999. Smärta och inflammation. Fysiologi och terapi vid smärttillstånd i rörelseorganen. Studentlitteratur, Lund.

Paavola, M., et al., 2002. Achilles tendinopathy. J. Bone Joint Surg. Am. 84-A (11), 2062–2076.

Parisi, L., et al., 2003. Muscular cramps: proposals for a new classification. Acta Neurol. Scand. 107, 176–186.

Pate, R.R., et al., 1995. Physical activity and public health. A recommendation from the Centers for Disease Control and Prevention and the American College of Sports Medicine. JAMA 273, 402–407.

Peterson, L., et al., 2001. Sports injuries—their prevention and treatment, third ed. Martin Dunitz, London.

Pollock, M.L., et al., 1999. Resistance training for health and disease. Introduction. Med. Sci. Sports Exerc. 31, 10–11.

Rettig, A.C., 2004. Athletic injuries of the wrist and hand. Part II: Overuse injuries of the wrist and traumatic injuries to the hand. Am. J. Sports Med. 32, 262–273.

US Department of Health and Human Services, 1996. Physical activity and health: a report of the surgeon-general. US Department of Health and Human Services, Centers for Disease Control and Prevention. National Center for Chronic Disease Prevention and Health Promotion, Atlanta, GA.

Woolf, C.J., 2004. Pain: moving from symptom control toward mechanism-specific pharmacologic management. Ann. Intern. Med. 140, 441–451.

Taping for sports injuries

13

Dr. Kristjan Oddsson

Introduction

Taping is used to treat and prevent different musculoskeletal conditions, for example ankle sprains (Thacker et al. 1999), patellofemoral pain (Gigante et al. 2001), and wrist sprains (Rettig et al. 1997). It can *prevent* injuries in sports where the risk of certain acute injuries is greater, for example ankle distortions in basketball and football, or *protect* and stabilize a body part during rehabilitation after an injury. The purpose of athletic taping is to support joints and ligaments by preventing unwanted movements.

There are multiple mechanisms that may explain the effects of athletic taping, and different variables have been studied scientifically: range of motion, kinesthesia, neuromuscular response, joint velocity, ground reaction forces, and postural control. Of these variables, the most common mechanism proposed for effective taping and bracing is limitation of joint motion (Arnold et al. 2004).

Athletic taping works best on areas of the athlete's body where the skin cannot move too freely around the joint, i.e. where there is less soft tissue between the tape and the treated joint (Brukner et al. 2001; Peterson et al. 2001). Ankle and hand or finger joints are examples where taping works well. Taping the knee and groin areas can be more difficult, and these areas are often treated with a combination of nonelastic tape, elastic tape, and elastic bandaging for more lasting support, particularly for use during sports activity. Athletic taping should be applied with common sense; it should not replace injury rehabilitation (which contains ROM, strength, balance, and coordination training), but instead support the rehabilitation process.

Tape for general use, sometimes called "coach tape" or "zinc oxide tape," does not stretch, and should therefore never be used on acute injuries due to the risk of serious circulatory impairment. Nonelastic tape is normally 1.5 in (38 mm) wide and is designed to stabilize and prevent undesired joint movement. It works well for hand and ankle taping. For finger and toe taping, half the width is used. It is important that the injured ligament is kept in a shortened position while the tape is applied (Brukner et al. 2001).

Basic rules of taping

There are a few basic rules for sports taping:

1. The therapist should have clean, dry hands.
2. Either the treated area should be shaved or a specific underwrap should be used in combination with glue spray. The tape adhesive can cause allergic skin reactions and the underwrap helps prevent this.
3. All folds or creases should be smoothed out, and the tape must cover the entire treated area to ensure that no spaces or gaps are present. It often helps to use the other hand to closely follow the applied tape to smooth out any potential wrinkles during application.
4. Athletic taping normally starts from the uninjured part, spans over the injured or weak portion, and finishes on an uninjured part. It is crucial to preplan which movement needs to be restricted to achieve effective structural support from athletic taping.

DOI: 10.1016/B978-0-443-10126-7.00013-7

5. The therapist should use as little tape as possible, and not make the application unnecessarily complex: simple but stable is best.

6. The sports therapist should never tape an acute injury due to the high risk of circulatory impairment. If taping of an acute injury is required, it is best to have a sports doctor carry it out.

7. The tape must be removed carefully, often with a pair of taping scissors, so as not to damage the athlete's skin. If hair is present, the tape should be removed along the direction of hair growth to avoid unnecessary pain.

8. The taped athlete is always right. If the applied taping does not feel good, it should be reapplied.

Injury to the lateral ligaments, i.e. talofibular ligaments— "standard" taping technique

One of the most common injuries where athletic taping can have positive effects is ankle distortion. It is mostly one or more of the lateral ligaments of the foot that requires additional support.

1. The ankle is kept at 90 degrees. One anchor is applied around the lower leg, just below the muscle belly of the triceps surae muscle (Fig. 13.1A).

2. Stirrups are applied, starting on the medial side of the upper anchor. The first one (middle), covers the medial malleolus, goes right under the heel

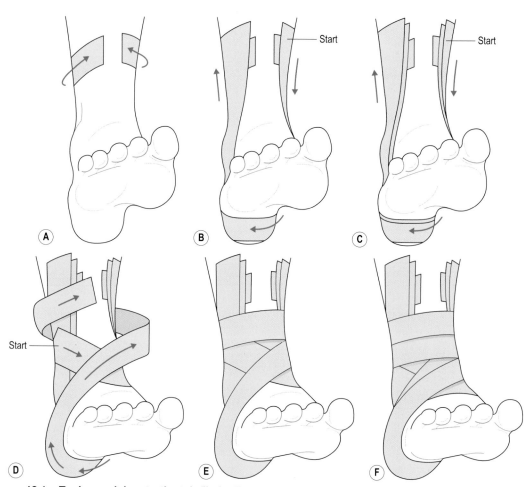

Figure 13.1 • Taping an injury to the talofibular ligaments—standard technique

and up to cover the lateral malleolus. The second stirrup starts from the same place but 2 cm in front of the first one, goes under the heel over the first one, and then ends 2 cm behind the first one. The third stirrup starts 2 cm behind the first one, goes over the two others under the heel, and ends 2 cm in front of the first one. Now you have three stirrups covering both malleoli (Fig. 13.1B&C).

3. Starting on the outside, tape is applied down the medial side, under the arch to the outside of the foot, and pulled up over the dorsal part of the foot around the ankle, finishing on the anchor.

4. Step 3 may be repeated if necessary (Fig. 13.1D&E).

5. The tape is finished with a fixation anchor as in Figure 13.1A (Fig. 13.1F).

Injury to the talofibular ligaments—easier variant

1. An anchor is placed around the lower leg, just distal to the muscle belly of the triceps surae (Fig. 13.2A).

2. Two or three strips are placed from the base of the 5th metatarsal bone, obliquely and posterior to the anchor (Fig. 13.2B).

3. The tape is applied in figure of eight loops from the lateral ligaments, up over the dorsal aspect of the foot, down over the longitudinal arch, and up the lateral side toward the anchor. The tape is pulled more on the lateral side to generate additional support for the ligament (Fig. 13.2C). The tape loops are fixated with another anchor as in Figure 13.2A.

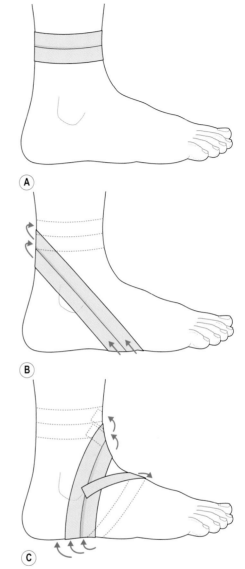

Figure 13.2 • Taping an injury to the talofibular ligaments—easier variant

Plantar fasciitis

1. An anchor is placed around the anterior aspect of the foot. A tape strip is applied from the anchor by the medial aspect of the 1st toe, along the foot, around the heel, and pulled up over the arch and toward the medial side of the 1st toe (strips 1–2) (Fig. 13.3A).

2. The tape is pulled from the anchor along the lateral side of the foot. It is then pulled around the heel, down the arch, and up along the

lateral side toward the 5th toe (strip 3) (Fig. 13.3B).

3. Tape strips are pulled from the medial and lateral side of the foot alternately, starting from the back of the foot and going forward until the last one reaches the anchor (strips 4–8) (Fig. 13.3C).

4. Two anchors are placed to secure the tape, one over the first anchor and one around the heel (strips 9–10) (Fig. 13.3D).

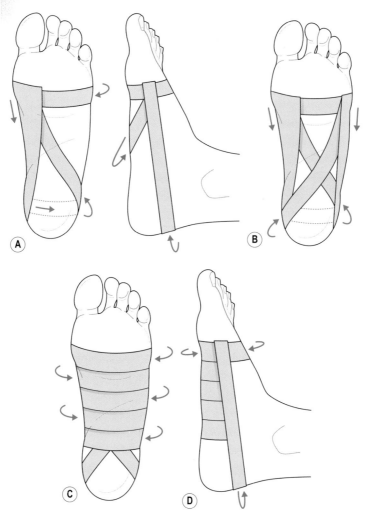

Figure 13.3 • Taping for plantar fasciitis

Painful heel pad

1. A horizontal stirrup is applied over the half malleolus, and a vertical stirrup directly in front of the malleolus (strips 1–2) (Fig. 13.4A).
2. Vertical stirrups are alternately applied from the inside to the outside (posterior to anterior) (strips 3–6) (Fig. 13.4B).
3. Two horizontal stirrups are applied to half of the previous area (strips 7–8) (Fig. 13.4C).

Stabilization of the thumb

1. Two anchors are applied around the wrist, and one anchor around the thumb (strips 1–3) (Fig. 13.5A).
2. One strip of tape is applied from the dorsal side of the thumb up to the wrist, another one from the thumb to the wrist, and finally one strip from the palmar side of the thumb up to the wrist (strips 4–6) (Fig. 13.5B–D).

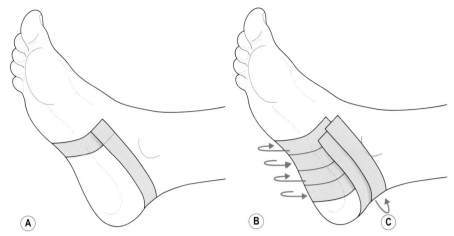

Figure 13.4 • Taping for a painful heel pad • A Strips 1–2 B Strips 3–6 C Strips 7–8

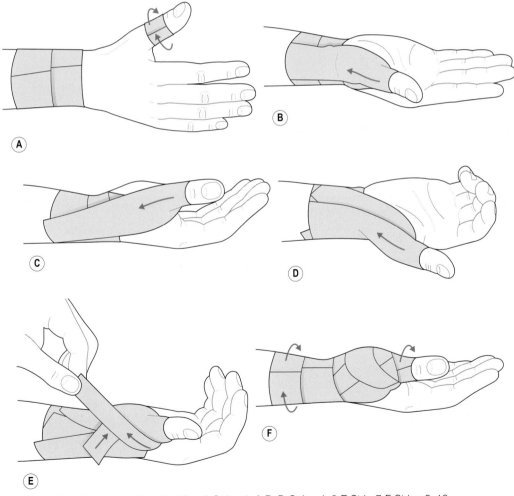

Figure 13.5 • Stabilization of the thumb • A Strips 1–3 B–D Strips 4–6 E Strip 7 F Strips 8–10

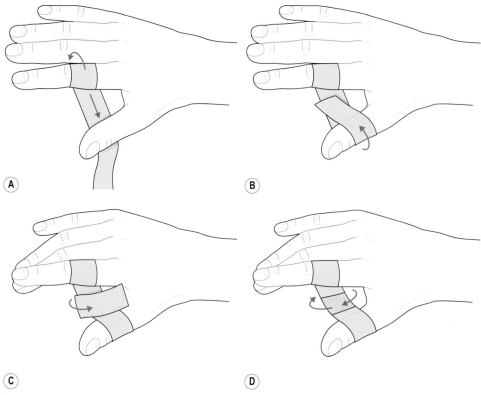

Figure 13.6 • Prevention of hyperextension of the thumb

3. Two turns of tape are applied and crossed over the joint, further attached to the anchors (the tape is split and used at half width) (strip 7) (Fig. 13.5E).

4. The tape is fixated by additional anchors placed over the previous anchors (strips 8–10) (Fig. 13.5F).

Prevention of hyperextension of the thumb

1. The tape is split and applied halfway around the index finger and further around the thumb with a little "slack" between the finger and thumb (Fig. 13.6A).

2. The tape is attached between the finger and thumb (Fig. 13.6B).

3. A short piece of tape is used to "lock" the slack part (Fig. 13.6C&D).

Finger stabilization/"Buddy" taping

A piece of foam rubber is placed between the two fingers (strip 1). The tape is split and one strip is applied proximal to, and the other distal to, the affected joint (strips 2–3) (Fig. 13.7).

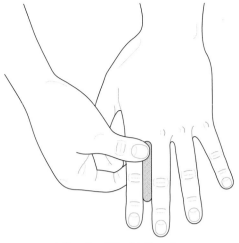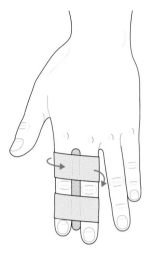

Figure 13.7 • Finger stabilization/"Buddy" taping

References

Arnold, B.L., et al., 2004. Bracing and rehabilitation—what's new. Clin. Sports Med. 23 (1), 83–95.

Brukner, P., et al., 2001. Clinical sports medicine, second ed. McGraw-Hill, Sydney.

Gigante, A., et al., 2001. The effects of patellar taping on patellofemoral incongruence. A computed tomography study. Am. J. Sports Med. 29 (1), 88–92.

Peterson, L., et al., 2001. Sports injuries—their prevention and treatment, third ed. Martin Dunitz, London.

Rettig, A.C., et al., 1997. Effects of finger and wrist taping on grip strength. Am. J. Sports Med. 25 (1), 96–98.

Thacker, S.B., et al., 1999. The prevention of ankle sprains in sports. A systematic review of the literature. Am. J. Sports Med. 27 (6), 753–760. Review.

Soft tissue treatment techniques for maintenance and remedial sports massage

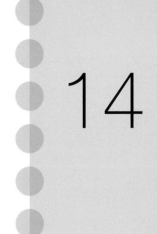

Restorative, maintenance, and remedial massage

Following the immediate postevent period, i.e. around 12–48 h, the initial "nonevent" massage treatment may often consist of a thorough restorative full body massage aimed at supporting the athlete's general recovery process. This treatment can normally last 1–2 h, depending on the current need, and is followed later by treatments of specific body sections to facilitate optimization of athletic biomechanical and physiological function, healing after injury, and/or individual rehabilitation (within the therapist's scope of practice).

Maintenance massage follows the restorative massage, and is performed during the interval between training and competition with the overall objective of helping to maintain the athlete's optimal physical performance during the training sessions (Benjamin & Lamp 1996). When the massage is focused on affected areas of the athlete's body in a problem-solving approach, assisting in healing and rehabilitation of injuries, the sports massage treatments are generally referred to as remedial sports massage (Benjamin & Lamp 1996; Cash 1996) (Box 14.1).

Remedial sports massage

The treatment techniques used in remedial massage cover a broad range, and the strokes are commonly applied deeper into the muscles and fascial structures, providing there is no acute injury in the area. All the strokes and techniques presented in this book may be used for remedial massage, and the choice of strokes with their inherent benefits is based upon the athlete's current need and the objective at hand. Remedial sports massage is tailored to each athlete treated, and will therefore consist of a vast amount of treatment combinations that will also change as the series of treatments progresses.

It is important to maintain ongoing communication and teamwork between the athlete, coach, trainer, and team doctors, since this will increase the value of each sports massage treatment. This includes staying informed of the athlete's current habits and training routines to more completely understand their specific problems and needs.

Remedial sports massage is aimed at reducing or eliminating pain and/or dysfunction, and is normally performed by a qualified, trained sports massage therapist (Benjamin & Lamp 1996). It may address a number of issues that do not require more involved medical attention (Benjamin & Lamp 1996), following an initial diagnostic evaluation by a medical professional. Examples of conditions often treated with remedial sports massage therapy are muscle and fascial imbalances, strains, spasms, tension, sprains, tendinitis, periostitis, and bursitis.

Remedial massage treatments should include some form of biomechanical and technique assessment to strive to find the root cause of the problem. It is suggested that about 50% of all sports injuries result from overuse and result from repetitive microtrauma causing local tissue damage. Sports injuries are often a product of biomechanical abnormalities

DOI: 10.1016/B978-0-443-10126-7.00014-9

Box 14.1

The differences between restorative, maintenance, and remedial massage

Restorative massage

- Commonly a full body massage that supports the athlete's general recovery process.

Maintenance massage

- Is more area specific compared with restorative massage.
- Aimed at maintaining the athlete's physical performance ability during training.

Remedial massage

- Treats specific areas of the athlete's body in a problem-solving approach, with the overriding goal of assisting in healing and rehabilitation of sports related injuries.
- Often has a stronger application, with deeper massage strokes and techniques.
- Any treatment technique, within the therapist's scope of practice, which can produce a favorable result, may be utilized.

not uncommonly at a distance from the specific injury area, requiring evaluation of the athlete's entire kinetic chain (Wilder & Sethi 2004). The sports therapist's initial assessment is of the athlete's whole body to seek the root cause of the injury or recurring problem.

It may be beneficial to start assessing the feet for the presence of restricted ankle dorsiflexion, pes cavus, pes planus, or increased inversion of the calcaneus, talus, navicular and/or cuboid bones. Joint mobilization techniques, good orthotics, and proper shoes may help address these issues.

The therapist must also note possible hypo- or hypermobility in joints, anterior/posterior, and/or medial/lateral strength or tensile muscle imbalances, etc. One-sided repetitive movements may additionally cause local tissue stress, and necessary ROM and function should be restored if lacking. As soft tissue restrictions limiting required ROM need to be eliminated, insufficient muscular support around hypermobile joints is generally balanced through strengthening and coordination exercises. It can be said that the sports therapist's overriding goal in remedial massage is to assist the athlete establish balance around the joints, including facilitating sufficient strength and flexibility in the tissues surrounding them.

The sports massage therapist may assist in the healing process of the athlete's sports injuries, and other conditions, either directly or indirectly, by:

- reducing tissue tension
- increasing blood circulation
- minimizing dysfunctional muscular strength and/ or tensile imbalances
- normalizing function, including ROM, or
- stimulating and/or facilitating the body's overall healing process.

A good understanding of the body's anatomy, physiology, and basic kinesiology, and the athlete's training methods (including sports-specific techniques), are important for helping a good sports massage therapist improve their ability to assess particular problems presented by the athlete. Reduced soft tissue flexibility and tension is one common cause of athletic problems and may arise from a number of reasons. Examples of more common causes are: previous immobility, scar tissue, and adhesion/fibrosis formation in the muscle and fascial structures; edema (swelling from fluid accumulation); fascial hypertrophy arising from long-term tissue stress; compensatory pain-induced muscle tension; proprioceptive dysfunction; focalized chronic muscle spasm; and muscular pain with shortening, stemming from myofascial trigger points (see Chapter 11). The sports massage therapist strives to restore muscle and joint function including other affected soft tissue structures, to support optimal injury-free athletic performance. Correctly executed remedial sports massage therapy can very often serve as one important tool available to the athlete to reach this goal.

When substantial muscle tension or spasm is present, it is beneficial to initiate the remedial treatment with applied positional release techniques (PRT). This will help normalize local proprioception before deeper strokes begin, otherwise there is a risk that dysfunctional muscle activity will resist the treatment by contracting further due to increased action from the local muscle spindles (see Chapter 8).

Lymphatic drainage massage (LDM)

Lymphatic drainage massage techniques may help to reduce swelling in the treated area, and can frequently have substantial value in remedial sports massage. It is indicated that complete decongestive physiotherapy is a highly effective treatment for both primary and secondary lymphedema (Ko et al. 1998).

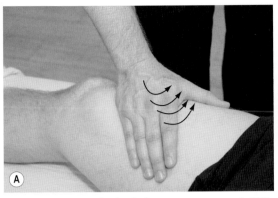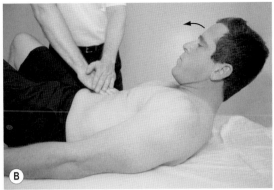

Figure 14.1 • Lymphatic drainage massage • A Of the legs B Of the abdomen. Athlete exhales in top position

During lymphatic drainage massage, the therapist moves the athlete's skin along the body part, horizontally and/or diagonally (French 2004) (Fig. 14.1). Moving across the direction of flow is considered to open lymphatic vessels, pushing along the lymphatic flow moves fluid, and finally allowing the stretched skin to "snap back" will accordingly close the vessels (Archer 2007). This generates a pumping effect as the lymphatic strokes are repeated a specific number of times or until tissue effect, i.e. reduced edema, is noted (French 2004; Archer 2007). The pressure is always light, since the treated lymphatic vessels are mostly located superficially, with the overall aim of moving excessive interstitial fluid into lymphatic vessels for further transportation, through lymphatic nodes, back into the venous blood stream. The strokes can often start distally to the edema, and gradually move toward larger vessels in the groin, armpits, and neck area. Some basic LDM strokes are listed below.

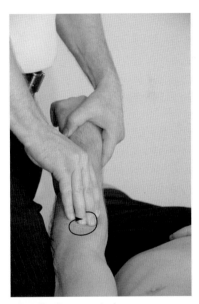

Figure 14.2 • Stationary circles

Stationary circles (Fig. 14.2)

1. One of the most fundamental LDM strokes is stationary circles, so named because they are performed 5–20 times (Archer 2007) in one location before moving to a new, adjacent area.
2. The therapist places the flat part of the fingers on the athlete's skin, and performs a light compression at the beginning of the stroke and a stretch of the skin in a circular movement at the end (French 2004). Some therapists also consider it important not to complete a full circle, but to massage more in an L-shape initially, transverse to the lymph flow, which opens the

initial vessels, and then finish the stroke along the flow to move the fluid in the proper direction (Archer 2007).

The pump (Fig. 14.3)

This stroke is effectively used on the extremities.

1. The therapist places a thumb on one side of the extremity, and the remaining four fingers flat on the athlete's skin.
2. The therapist compresses the surface lightly and moves the skin in a scooping motion toward adjacent lymph nodes.
3. The stroke is repeated in the area until a palpable change is noted in the treated tissue.

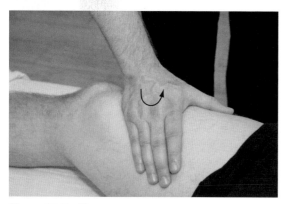

Figure 14.3 • The pump

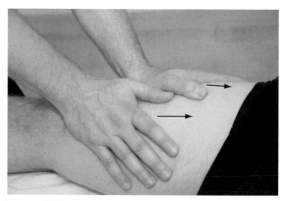

Figure 14.5 • Long strokes

J-stroke (Fig. 14.4)

This stroke is used on the torso, back, and the anterior or posterior aspect of the thighs.

1. The therapist lightly compresses the skin with the flat of the hand.
2. The skin is then twisted and pushed in a "J-shape" toward adjacent lymph nodes.

Long strokes (Fig. 14.5)

These are sliding strokes on the skin, similar to basic effleurage strokes.

1. The therapist places the flat hands lightly on the athlete's skin distally to the edema.
2. The hands are then pushed in a sliding motion toward larger vessels in the groin, armpit, and neck areas.
3. It is considered that the long strokes must initially stretch the skin to open the lymphatic vessels, with maintained tissue stretch during the complete stroke (Archer 2007).

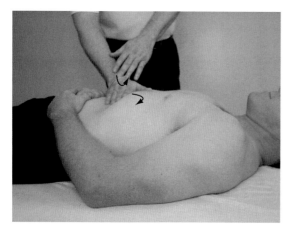

Figure 14.4 • J-stroke

Additional deep tissue strokes used in remedial sports massage

Deep gliding strokes

Additional deep tissue massage and myofascial release strokes used in remedial massage not already covered in Chapters 2 and 10 may be called deep gliding strokes. A few look similar to strokes presented in Chapter 10, but the execution is slightly different. These strokes can effectively release shortenings in both muscle tissue and fascial layers. They may additionally, to a certain extent, move blood and lymph thanks to their sliding quality. The effect in the tissue is further enhanced when the strokes are simultaneously combined with a stretch of the treated muscle. This is similar to the "lock and stretch" method described previously, but where a slow, deep, gliding movement replaces the stationary fixation of the soft tissue. As a general rule, if the stretch is applied prior to the gliding stroke, more superficial fibers will receive the major effect. For deeper fibers, the tissue is firstly locked down with the stroke, and the gradual specific stretch immediately follows the start of the deep gliding stroke.

Deep gliding strokes can reach deep into the soft tissue, and so it is important that the treated soft tissue is thoroughly warmed up prior to using these strokes. Massage strokes described in Chapter 2 and/or a 20 min premassage heat application can prepare the soft tissue.

A common rule is that the deeper the massage is performed, the slower the strokes are executed. This gives the athlete's body a better chance of adapting to the level of pressure, and gives the tissue time to stretch more effectively. The deep gliding strokes start superficially, and increase in depth as the tissue relaxes. They are virtually always reinforced with the other hand, not only to generate leverage, but also to create full stability and control.

The strokes are executed as long as there is "grip," i.e. resistance, in the soft tissue. When the therapist notes that the resistance is lost, the stroke is reapplied halfway from the previous starting point. In this way the strokes will overlap each other and the full effect of the stroke is transferred through the treated tissue.

Longer gliding strokes, whether superficial or deep, are generally performed in a direction toward the heart. This is especially important on the extremities due to the valves in the veins. Deep gliding strokes are occasionally performed in the opposite direction, however, for example when working by the ischial tuberosity at the origin of the hamstrings muscles. When massaging against the venous flow, the strokes are shortened to only 1–2 in to reduce potential stress on the venous valves and walls (Cash 1996).

Planar glide

The therapist uses four fingers on one hand re-inforced with the other hand grasping over the fingers. The treating fingers are slightly flexed to facilitate depth in the stroke (Fig. 14.6).

Thumb glide

1. Thumb glides work well in areas with less space, or when a more focal effect is desired.
2. Thumb glides are performed with the whole side of one thumb, along the thumb's natural movement pattern, where the other hand is placed over the treating thumb as a reinforcement and mover (Fig. 14.7A). It is the reinforcing hand that performs the actual stroke, whilst the treating thumb is acting passively.

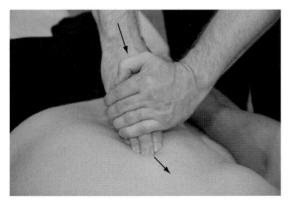

Figure 14.6 • Planar glide/reinforced 4-finger glide

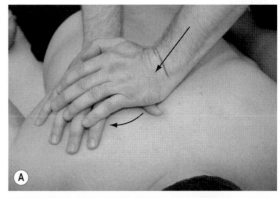

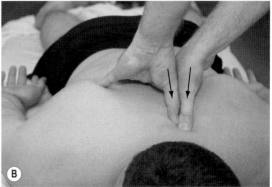

Figure 14.7 • Thumb glides

3. The tip of a reinforced thumb may slowly glide either along or across the fiber direction. Both hands are firmly pushed together to generate stability and reduce stress on the thumbs (Fig. 14.7B).

Fist glide

1. The therapist uses the flat part of a fist with the thumb facing forward. This minimizes stress on the wrist. The other hand may grasp around the treating wrist and hand for reinforcement, or hold the fist between the thumb and index finger to stabilize the stroke (Fig. 14.8).
2. The stroke starts with the main pressure level with the 2nd and 3rd knuckles, but shifts slightly as a radial deviation is added for increased depth.

Palm glide (Fig. 14.9)

1. The therapist uses the palm with the majority of the pressure on the palm heel. The angle of the wrist should not exceed 45 degrees extension.
2. The other hand may grasp around the treating wrist and hand for reinforcement.

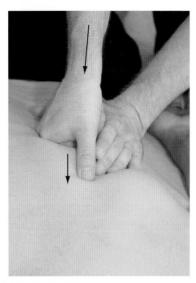

Figure 14.8 • Fist glide

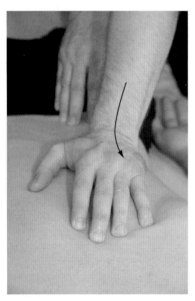

Figure 14.9 • Palm glide

Forearm glide (Fig. 14.10)

1. The therapist uses the muscular anterior part of the forearm.

2. The forearm is initially semisupinated and gradually pronates during the progression of the stroke.

3. This stroke covers a larger area but with slightly less depth due to its larger contact surface.

4. Forearm glides work very well on rounded surfaces like the arms and legs.

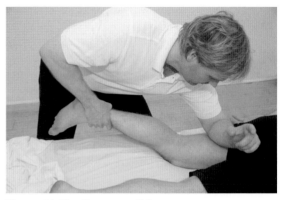

Figure 14.10 • Forearm glide

Elbow glide

1. The therapist places the flat part of one elbow, superior to the olecranon process, on the treated tissue whilst the fingers gently hold the therapist's neck for stability. The thumb and index or long finger of the other hand grasp around the elbow to steer the stroke during execution (Fig. 14.11A).

2. The therapist uses the flat part of one elbow, inferior to the olecranon process, during the stroke. The thumb and index finger of the other hand grasp around the elbow to steer the stroke during execution, whilst the long finger of the same hand palpates the tissue to avoid bone structures during the stroke (Fig. 14.11B).

3. The therapist uses the inferior part of the olecranon process. The elbow of the treating arm is initially semiextended and slowly moves into flexion during the stroke. This "hooks" the soft tissue on the inferior aspect of the olecranon process and greatly enhances the stroke's effect. The other hand rests flat on the athlete with the thumb gently pushing on the superior part of the olecranon (Fig. 14.11C).

4. The therapist uses the superior part of the olecranon process of one elbow. The elbow of the treating arm is initially semiflexed and slowly moves into further extension during the stroke. This "hooks" the soft tissue on the inferior aspect of the olecranon process and greatly enhances the stroke's effects. The other hand clasps the hand of the treating arm for additional power (Fig. 14.11D).

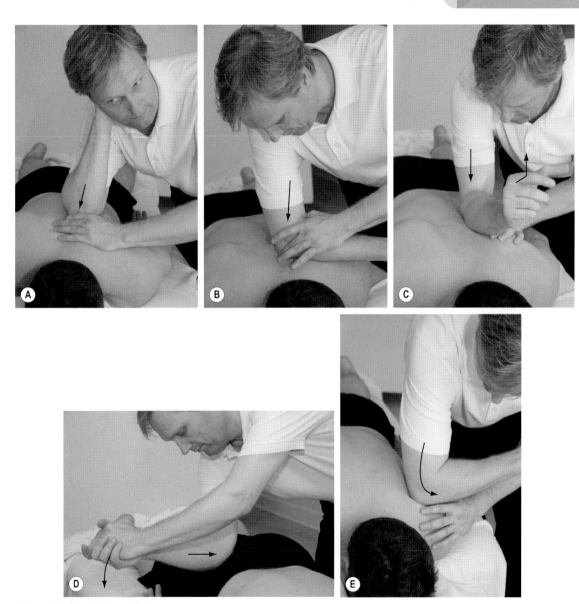

Figure 14.11 • Elbow glides

5. The therapist uses the tip of the olecranon process of one elbow. The arm is rotated medially 45 degrees to move the most prominent part of olecranon into position for treatment, and the elbow is positioned in 90 degree flexion. The thumb and index or long finger of the other hand grasp around the elbow to stabilize the stroke (Fig. 14.11E). This stroke may be used for gliding between muscular and/or fascial layers, or as focal ischemic pressure.

Rhythmic lock and stretch, variation

1. To effectively treat chronic spasm, adhesions, and adaptive shortenings of the connective tissue, the restricted area is compressed with a fist, reinforced thumb or elbow.
2. The therapist then instructs the athlete to continuously, initially with small increments, alternately move the joint in opposite directions, whilst the therapist maintains focal pressure (Fig. 14.12).

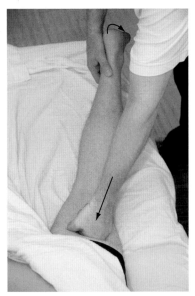

Figure 14.12 • Rhythmic lock and stretch variation

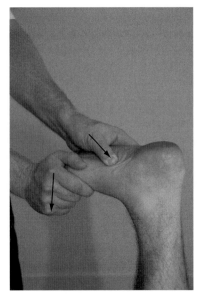

Figure 14.13 • Focal stretching and thumb glide of the plantar aponeurosis

Soft tissue release in the feet and lower legs

The feet and ankles

The feet carry a heavy load during most athletic activity, and are subsequently important to treat due to the large stress they suffer. Ankle sprains are a common occurrence in sports, and reduced dorsal flexion during walking combined with chronic ankle instability may be a risk factor for repeated ankle sprains (Drewes et al. 2008). Edema and reduced passive ROM are associated with overall dysfunction and limitations in sports activities. Exercises promoting increased dorsal flexion for ankle mobility are suggested to generate full recovery as early as 1 month after the moment of injury (Aiken et al. 2008).

Plantar fasciitis is considered to be the most common cause of heel pain, and is effectively treated with nonsurgical intervention for 90% of patients (Neufeld & Cerrato 2008). The sports massage therapist can treat the problem with positional release, cross frictions, contrast treatment, and focal stretching of the plantar aponeurosis. This may be particularly effective when the athlete performs home exercises, for example the athlete rolls the plantar surface of the foot on a tennis or lacrosse ball to successively stretch the plantar aponeurosis.

Focal stretching and thumb glide of the plantar aponeurosis (Fig. 14.13)

1. The therapist fixates the plantar aponeurosis distal, but yet fairly close, to the inflamed origin.
2. The fixating thumb will push both into the tissue and toward the inflamed site to effectively "slacken" the locally inflamed soft tissue. The plantar aponeurosis may thus firmly stretch without additional stress in the inflamed area. The fascia is stretched by extending each toe separately, assessing the "true line of stretch" (see Chapter 7). The lock and stretch may successively convert into a thumb gliding stretch.

Medial tibial stress syndrome

Medial tibial periostitis, i.e. shin splints, presents with pain along the medial border of the tibia, where the superficial posterior compartment housing the triceps surae muscle inserts in the bone.

Chronic Achilles tendinitis

Achilles tendinitis often stems from overuse, friction, or a partial tear of the calcaneus tendon. An acutely inflamed tendon is often red, painful, and swollen, whereas chronic inflammation often presents with a duller pain and an increased width of the affected tendon (Fig. 14.14).

The sports massage therapist aims to reduce the strain on the compartment and tendon by relaxing

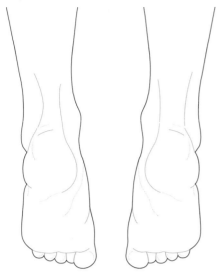

Figure 14.14 • Chronic Achilles tendinitis

the affected muscles along with their fascial components. The intention is also to break up or stretch potential scar tissue with adhesions both locally at the tendon and additionally along the whole length of the muscles and the fascial compartment. Eccentric exercises of the calf muscles have been shown to improve Achilles tendinitis (de Jonge et al. 2008).

Gastrocnemius muscle release (Fig. 14.15)

1. The athlete lies prone with the feet over the end of the treatment table.
2. The therapist uses a reinforced fist, or thumb glide, to slowly slide in a straight line, directed proximally. The depth of the stroke gradually increases as the tissue softens. The two muscle bellies, and the area between, are worked separately.

3. Additionally, the therapist places one knee on the ball of the athlete's foot to enable dorsal flexion. As the fist or thumb "grips" the tissue, the athlete is instructed to perform a slow complementary dorsal flexion in the ankle joint, utilizing antagonistic muscles and thus activating the reciprocal inhibition reflex.
4. The deep gliding strokes are performed in sections to ensure good stretch effect.

Soleus muscle release (Fig. 14.16)

1. The athlete lies prone with one knee flexed.
2. The therapist grasps the heel with one hand and places the forearm on the ball of the athlete's foot.
3. The other hand grasps the soleus muscle from the side, underneath the gastrocnemius muscle.
4. As the muscle is compressed, the athlete is instructed to execute a slow dorsal flexion in the ankle joint, assisted by the therapist's forearm pressure on the ball of the athlete's foot.

Patients with stenosing tenosynovitis of the flexor hallucis longus tendon frequently demonstrate overlapping signs and symptoms of flexor hallucis longus tendinitis, plantar fasciitis, and tarsal tunnel syndrome (Schulhofer & Oloff 2002). This condition may be treated with transverse frictions, myofascial release of the fascia, muscle, and tendon, and focalized "lock and stretch" techniques.

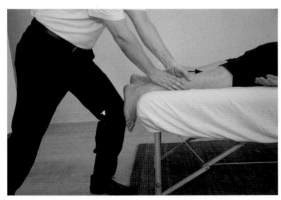

Figure 14.15 • Gastrocnemius muscle release

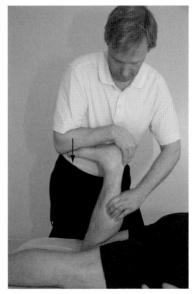

Figure 14.16 • Soleus muscle release

Peroneus longus and brevis

Peroneal muscle release (Fig. 14.17)

1. The athlete lies prone with one knee flexed.
2. The therapist grasps the ball of the athlete's foot. The other hand fixates the tensed section of the treated peroneal muscle.
3. As the muscle is compressed with one thumb, and simultaneously pushed toward the origin, the foot is pushed into a dorsal flexion and inversion by the therapist. The athlete is instructed to execute a slow dorsal flexion in the ankle joint, utilizing antagonistic muscles and thus activating the reciprocal inhibition reflex, assisted by the therapist's pressure on the ball of the athlete's foot.
4. After each repetition, the therapist compresses the muscle in a slightly different area, repeating the procedure.
5. A slow glide can be substituted for the fixation to help separate the fascial layers and push fluids through the treated tissues.

Tibialis anterior

The tibialis anterior muscle is housed within the anterior compartment of the lower leg, and plays a part in causing anterior compartment syndrome, generating pain and severe discomfort in the front of the lower leg and at, or next to, the lateral border of tibia. This condition should be differentiated from medial tibial stress syndrome, i.e. shin splints, which instead presents with pain along the medial border of the tibia, where the superficial posterior compartment housing the triceps surae muscle inserts in the bone.

It is important that the sports massage therapist works with the tibialis anterior muscle, due to its strong activity in most sports. It is one of the muscles working eccentrically during walking and running as it helps control the foot impact after the heel strike.

Tibialis anterior release (Fig. 14.18)

1. The athlete lies supine with the feet over the end of the table.
2. The therapist dorsal flexes the athlete's foot to relax the tissue.
3. One palm heel fixates the muscle by obliquely compressing the muscle in a posterior/superior direction.
4. The therapist slowly pushes the athlete's foot into plantar flexion and eversion mainly by pressing on the first metatarsal bone of the foot.
5. As the muscle stretches, the fixating pressure on the muscle is increased accordingly.
6. As the muscle softens, the lock and stretch is substituted by a gliding myofascial release stroke, with a palm, planar, or thumb glide.

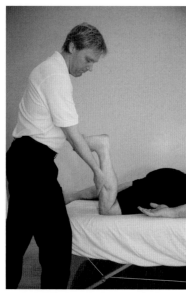

Figure 14.17 • Peroneal muscle release

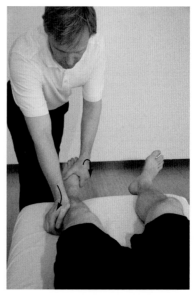

Figure 14.18 • Tibialis anterior release

Soft tissue release in the thighs, groin, and knees

The thighs and groin are frequently exposed to strains, and the knees are closely affected as regards muscular imbalance in the thighs. It is indicated that strength imbalances are a factor that increases the risk of hamstring injury (Croisier et al. 2008).

It is suggested that patellofemoral pain and instability are responsible for 25% of knee problems stemming from sports activity (Pagenstert & Bachmann 2008). It has been indicated that a substantial number of people with patellofemoral pain syndrome (PFPS) may experience considerable recovery in pain and function through quadriceps femoris muscle training, either with or without separate intentional activation of the vastus medialis oblique (VMO) fibers (Syme et al. 2008)—this although the VMO is considered responsible for countering the lateral movement from the vastus lateralis muscle and the Q-angle, i.e. the angle between the femur and tibia. Patellar taping, i.e. McConnell taping improving patellar tracking, appears additionally to reduce pain levels from PFPS (Aminaka & Gribble 2008).

Inflammation of the pes anserinus on the superior/medial aspect of tibia involves the sartorius, gracilis, and semitendinosus muscles. A shortened iliotibial tract may commonly cause pain at the lateral condyle of femur, i.e. runner's knee, or generate trochanteric bursitis from a lateral snapping hip syndrome, with associated pain over the greater trochanter area.

The iliopsoas tendon may cause a medial snapping hip. In this case, the medial aspect of the hip joint will feel painful and "locked." This is followed by an audible snapping sound as the joint is moved into further abduction and lateral rotation, with a release of the movement restriction in the groin as the tendon releases. Adductor strains generally also present with groin pain, and it is suggested that manual therapy treatment may prove effective for chronic adductor-related groin pain in athletes (Weir et al. 2008).

Research also indicates the importance of neuromuscular training programs in preventing acute noncontact injuries of the legs for floorball players (Pasanen et al. 2008).

The sports therapist can release unnecessary tension generating muscle imbalance, to reduce the level of stress on the knees and groin, and to lessen the risk of local muscle strains, particularly when the treatments are combined with rehabilitative strength and coordination training. Releasing tension in the rectus femoris and vastus lateralis muscle may reduce stress on the patella. PRT for ligamentous and meniscus injuries can be another safe, pain-reducing treatment modality.

Rectus femoris C-release

Rectus femoris C-release, pushing *(Fig. 14.19A)*
1. The therapist places the flat part of one elbow, inferior to the olecranon, on the lateral part of the athlete's rectus femoris muscle.

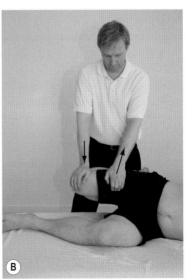

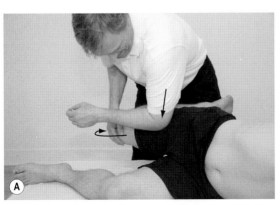

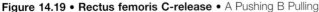

Figure 14.19 • Rectus femoris C-release • A Pushing B Pulling

2. The therapist pushes the elbow slowly cross-fiber, without slipping over the muscle belly, to force the muscle into a C-shape.

3. The elbow is concurrently slowly flexed to push the muscle to the end point, and the therapist enhances the stretch effect by gradually increasing flexion in the knee joint and extension in the hip joint by pushing the athlete's ankle with the hip.

Rectus femoris C-release, pulling (Fig. 14.19B)

1. The therapist pulls the rectus femoris muscle with the fingertips of one hand to force the muscle into a C-shape.

2. The other hand is used to fixate the leg.

3. The therapist enhances the stretch effect by gradually increasing flexion in the knee joint and extension in the hip joint by pushing the athlete's ankle with the hip.

Rectus femoris elbow C-release, athlete supine (Fig. 14.20)

1. The athlete lies supine.

2. The therapist pushes the muscle sideways as the elbow glides up along the rectus femoris muscle.

3. The therapist's elbow should slowly bend to gradually increase the power of the stroke.

Rectus femoris palm C-release, athlete supine (Fig. 14.21)

1. The athlete lies supine.

2. The muscle is pushed cross-fiber at a 45 degree angle with the palm heel.

Vastus lateralis release (Fig. 14.22)

1. The athlete lies prone.

2. The therapist grasps the athlete's ankle and flexes the knee joint to 90 degrees.

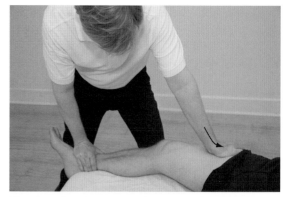

Figure 14.21 • Rectus femoris palm C-release, athlete supine

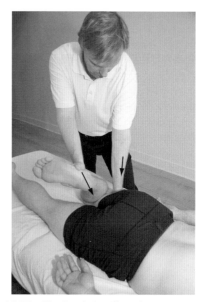

Figure 14.22 • Vastus lateralis release

3. The therapist's palm heel pushes on the muscle anteriorly/superiorly at a 45 degree angle, as the knee is further flexed by pushing the athlete's foot toward the opposite gluteus maximus muscle.

4. The stroke is repeated over different sections of the muscle and as the tissue softens, it is changed into a palm glide.

Iliopsoas release (Fig. 14.23)

The iliopsoas muscle is the prime hip flexor and shortening may affect the lower back, pelvis, and/or hip joint. Caution should be taken during

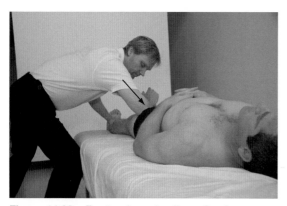

Figure 14.20 • Rectus femoris elbow C-release, athlete supine

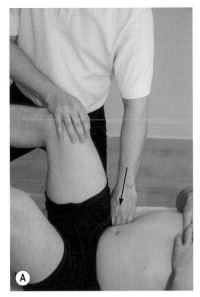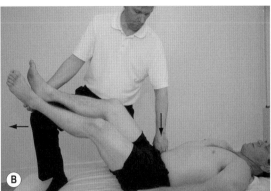

Figure 14.23 • Iliopsoas release

this release due to the sensitive area in which the therapist's hand pushes, i.e. proximity to the appendix, possible abdominal aortic abnormalities, potential tissue weaknesses predisposing to inguinal hernias, ovarian conditions, or general irritation/inflammation of the gastrointestinal system; hence, this release may occasionally be replaced by the regular therapeutic stretch presented in Chapter 7 (see Fig. 7.14).

1. The athlete lies supine with the hip joint placed in maximum flexion, and lateral rotation, with the calcaneus tendons resting on the therapist's thigh (see Fig. 14.23A).
2. The therapist slowly fixates the psoas major muscle in a direction toward the spine medial to and level with the anterior superior iliac spine (ASIS) with four fingers.
3. The muscle is then slowly stretched as the therapist slowly extends the athlete's hip joint (see Fig. 14.23B).
4. The procedure is repeated over the muscle until ROM improves.

Iliacus release (Fig. 14.24)

1. The athlete lies on one side.
2. The therapist locks the iliacus muscle medial to the ASIS with the long and index finger when the hip joint is in maximum flexion to relax the muscle.

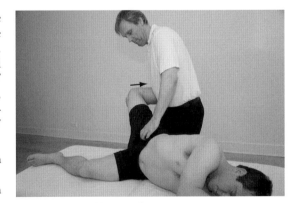

Figure 14.24 • Iliacus release

3. The muscle is further stretched as the therapist slowly extends the athlete's hip joint.
4. The procedure is repeated until the ROM is improved.

Hamstring release

Hamstring release, fist (Fig. 14.25A)

1. The athlete lies prone.
2. The therapist uses the flat part of the fist to glide superiorly along the hamstring muscles. The knee joint is slowly extended to increase the stretch effect of the stroke.

Hamstring release, elbow (Fig. 14.25B)

For added power elbow glides can replace the fist glide.

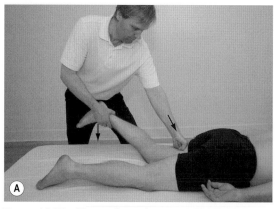
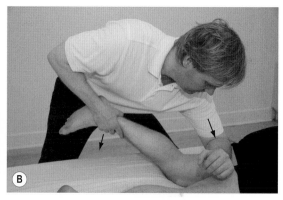

Figure 14.25 • Hamstring release • A Fist B Elbow

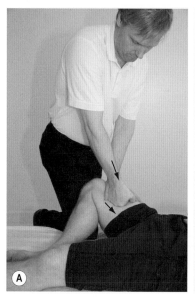
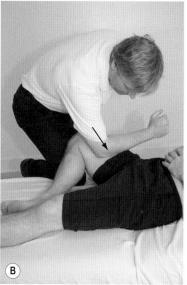

Figure 14.26 • Adductor muscle release • A Fist B Elbow

Adductor muscle release

Adductor fist release *(Fig. 14.26A)*

1. The athlete lies supine with the hip joint flexed.
2. The therapist uses the flat part of the fist to slowly glide superiorly along the adductor muscles.
3. The athlete's hip joint is slowly abducted to increase the stretch effect and power of the stroke.

Adductor elbow release *(Fig. 14.26B)*

The therapist may substitute the fist glide with an elbow glide for additional focal pressure.

Gracilis muscle release (Fig. 14.27)

1. The athlete lies supine.

2. The therapist extends the athlete's knee joint and moves the hip joint to 90 degrees flexion. From this position the athlete's leg is abducted close to the muscle's end point.
3. The therapist performs a palm glide at 45 degrees across the muscle fibers. The therapist may also use a slow fist glide along the muscle toward the groin area.

Iliotibial band (ITB) release

This version of iliotibial band (ITB) release has been presented by Dr. Leon Chaitow, and commonly generates marked results.

Step 1 *(Fig. 14.28A)*

1. The athlete lies on one side.

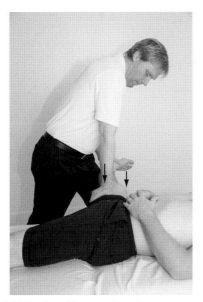

Figure 14.27 • Gracilis muscle release

2. The therapist grasps the athlete's ITB with both hands and bends it rapidly sequentially into a C-shape.

3. Moving the bent elbows in toward the body generates the main force in the stroke.

4. The therapist continues the stroke up and down the posterior aspect of the ITB for 1–2 min. The stroke is then repeated on the anterior aspect of the band.

Step 2 *(Fig. 14.28B)*

1. The athlete lies on one side.

2. The therapist grasps one edge of the ITB with the palm heel of one hand and the other edge of the ITB with the fingertips of the other hand.

3. The ITB is rapidly alternately pushed and pulled for an effective stretch.

4. The therapist continues up and down the entire ITB for 1–2 min.

Step 3 *(Fig. 14.28C)*

1. The athlete lies on one side.

2. The therapist pushes the lower part of the ITB with the thumb of one hand and index/long finger of the other hand.

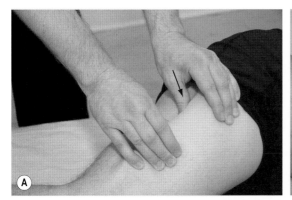

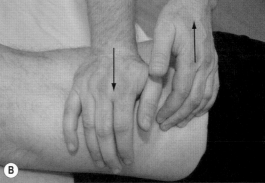

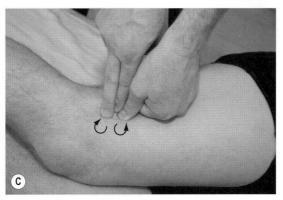

Figure 14.28 • Iliotibial band (ITB) release

3. The therapist generates a stretch by simultaneously pushing and twisting both hands, in opposite directions, over the inferior part of the ITB.

4. Moving the bent elbows in toward the body in a rapid motion generates the force in the stroke.

5. The stroke is continued for up to 1–2 min.

Soft tissue release in the hips and gluteal area

Gluteus maximus release (Fig. 14.29)

1. The athlete lies on one side.

2. The therapist flexes the athlete's knee joint and semiflexes the hip joint.

3. The therapist uses an elbow glide whilst pushing the athlete's leg toward the opposite shoulder with the side of the hip.

4. For larger athletes, the therapist may stand behind the athlete to massage the muscle as the athlete moves the treated leg him/herself.

Gluteus medius/minimus release (Fig. 14.30)

1. The athlete lies on one side.

2. The therapist flexes the athlete's knee joint and semiflexes the hip joint.

3. The therapist uses the flat part of one elbow for an elbow glide, starting at the greater trochanter, whilst simultaneously pushing the athlete's leg toward the floor.

4. For larger athletes, the therapist may stand behind the athlete to massage the muscle as the athlete moves the treated leg him/herself.

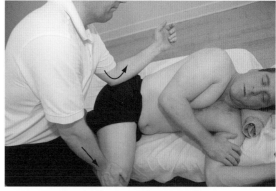

Figure 14.30 • Gluteus medius/minimus release

Greater trochanter release (Fig. 14.31)

1. The athlete lies on one side with the knee joint flexed and hip joint semiflexed.

2. The therapist places the pointed part of one elbow by the greater trochanter, with the elbow reinforced by the other hand to control the movements.

3. The therapist slowly glides with the elbow across the superior, anterior, and posterior tendon segments adjacent to the greater trochanter, to stretch the fascial and tendon structures in the area.

Tensor fasciae latae release (Fig. 14.32)

1. The athlete lies on one side.

2. The therapist places the inferior part of one elbow by the posterior edge of the tensor fascia latae muscle, just inferior to the ASIS.

3. The therapist slowly and methodically glides with the elbow across the tensor fasciae latae

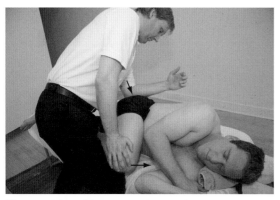

Figure 14.29 • Gluteus maximus release

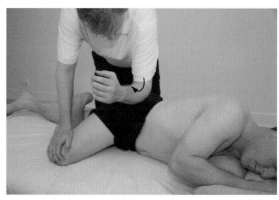

Figure 14.31 • Greater trochanter release

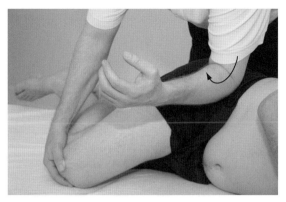

Figure 14.32 • Tensor fasciae latae release

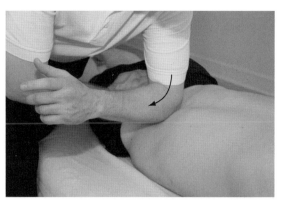

Figure 14.33 • Quadratus lumborum release

muscle at a 45 degree angle, while gradually flex the elbow joint to increase the treatment effect.

Soft tissue release in the lower and upper back

The back is exposed to large amounts of stress during sports activity, with complications like lower back pain, tendinitis, and/or strains of the local soft tissue. It is indicated that multiple modality treatments including massage therapy may serve as options in rehabilitation for athletes with lower back pain (LBP) (Ambartsumov 2001). Research has additionally shown that patients with subacute lower back pain benefit from massage therapy (Preyde 2000). It is suggested that there is a direct relationship between neuromuscular imbalance and LBP in athletes (Renkawitz et al. 2006), and core strengthening, also described as lumbar stabilization, is commonly used as a therapeutic exercise treatment regimen for conditions presenting LBP (Akuthota et al. 2008).

Quadratus lumborum release (Fig. 14.33)

1. The athlete lies prone, with the body laterally flexed on the table.
2. The therapist uses an elbow glide transverse to the muscle fibers, medially to laterally.
3. It is important to ensure that the 12th rib is not compressed, and starting just superior to the iliac crest helps the therapist ensure the correct area is treated. The reinforcing hand will also palpate the tissue during the execution of the stroke.

Erector spinae C-release (Fig. 14.34)

1. The athlete lies prone.
2. The therapist places the flat part of one elbow, inferior to the olecranon, on the medial edge of the athlete's erector spinae muscle.
3. The therapist leans over the athlete to enforce lateral stretch, and pushes the elbow slowly further laterally, without slipping over the muscle belly, by pointing the hand toward the opposite side, forcing the muscle into a C-shape.
4. The elbow is concurrently slowly flexed to push the muscle to the end point.
5. The stroke is repeated along the muscle and can be combined with slow gliding movements.

Latissimus dorsi and teres major release
Latissimus dorsi (Fig. 14.35A)

1. The athlete lies on one side. To increase the effect when treating the lower part of the muscle, a pillow is placed just superior to the hip to generate lateral flexion of the trunk.

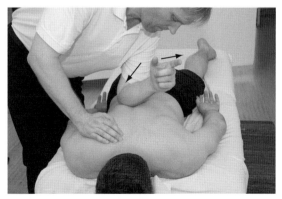

Figure 14.34 • Erector spinae C-release

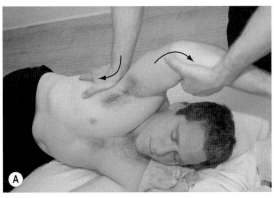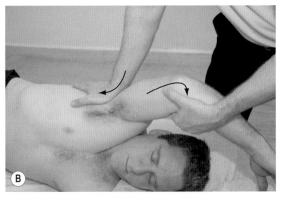

Figure 14.35 • Latissimus dorsi and teres major release • A Latissimus dorsi B Teres major

2. The therapist grasps around the athlete's elbow on the treated side.

3. The therapist applies a palm, planar, or fist glide to the muscle as the athlete's arm is simultaneously abducted over the athlete's head.

Teres major *(Fig. 14.35B)*
The athlete is treated from the identical position, with exception of the lateral flexion of the trunk. The strokes are executed between the humerus and the inferior angle of scapula.

Rhomboid major and minor release *(Fig. 14.36)*

1. The athlete lies prone with one arm fully abducted.

2. The therapist grasps under the elbow and places the palm heel over the muscles next to the spine.

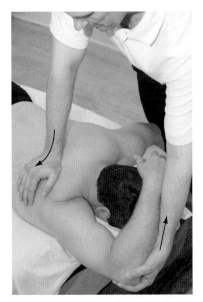

Figure 14.36 • Rhomboid major and minor release

3. As the therapist's palm heel slowly begins gliding along the rhomboid muscles, the athlete's arm is further abducted until the end point is reached.

4. Caution should be taken regarding generating the athlete's glenohumeral joint too much flexion during the stretch. It is more imperative for the therapist to focus on the glenohumeral abduction and palm heel pressure.

5. The stroke is repeated until increased soft tissue relaxation occurs.

Trapezius release

Descending part *(Fig. 14.37A)*

1. The athlete sits on the treatment table or in a chair.

2. The therapist uses the flat part of the elbow, inferior to the olecranon, to slowly glide along the fibers of the descending part of trapezius, as simultaneously the head is laterally flexed toward the opposite side, flexed, and mildly ipsilaterally rotated.

Transverse part *(Fig. 14.37B)*
This part of the trapezius muscle is treated in a similar way to the rhomboid muscles but without moving the athlete's arm. The focus is instead on using a palm glide on the muscle and pushing the scapula laterally. If pain is sensed in the athlete's shoulder during this movement, a rolled towel is placed on the anterior aspect of the shoulder.

Ascending part *(Fig. 14.37C)*

1. The athlete lies on one side with one arm over the head.

2. The therapist pushes the inferior angle in a superior/lateral direction whilst simultaneously executing a fist, palm, or planar glide along the muscle fibers.

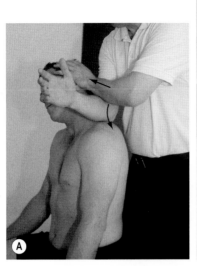
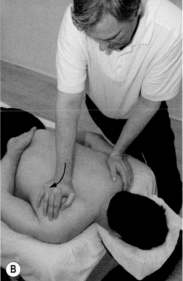
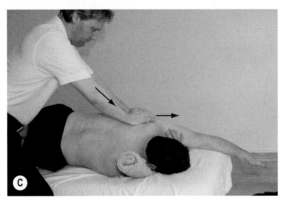

Figure 14.37 • Trapezius release • A Descending part B Transverse part C Ascending part

Soft tissue release in the chest region

The pectoral muscles are strong especially compared with the lateral rotators of the rotator cuff muscles. To help avoid overload injuries to the rotator cuff, the medial shoulder rotators, including the pectoralis major muscle, are treated.

Pectoralis major release (Fig. 14.38)

1. The athlete lies supine with one arm horizontally abducted.
2. The therapist grasps the athlete's arm and sets up a fist, palm, or elbow glide for the pectoralis major muscle.
3. As the stroke begins to glide, the therapist increases the horizontal abduction, lateral rotation, and traction in the athlete's glenohumeral joint.

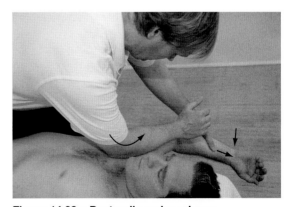

Figure 14.38 • Pectoralis major release

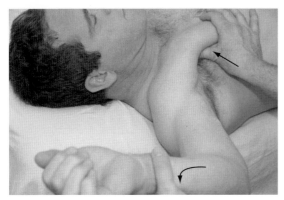

Figure 14.39 • Pectoralis minor release

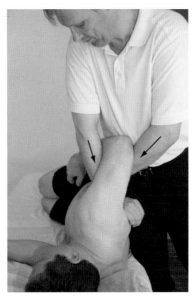

Figure 14.40 • Serratus anterior release

Pectoralis minor release (Fig. 14.39)

1. The athlete lies supine with the arms by the sides.
2. The therapist gently places the padded part of the thumb in the athlete's arm pit, pushing in horizontally just under the pectoralis major muscle, bending the pectoralis minor muscle into a C-shape.
3. The therapist pushes the thumb until the muscle is stretched to its end point.
4. As the muscle is fixated in a C-shape, the therapist flexes the athlete's glenohumeral joint by slowly lifting the athlete's arm towards the head.
5. The thumb pressure is released, the athlete's arm moved back half way, and the stroke is slowly and rhythmically repeated until increased tissue softening is noted.

Serratus anterior release (Fig. 14.40)

1. The athlete lies on one side.
2. The therapist stands behind the athlete and supports the athlete's back with the side of one hip.
3. The therapist pushes the lateral border of the scapula medially/superiorly and simultaneously performs planar glides with the other hand.
4. The scapular pressure is released and the stroke is slowly and rhythmically repeated until increased scapular ROM and/or tissue softening is noted.

Soft tissue release in the shoulders

The shoulders possess great mobility, partly from the substantial ROM of the glenohumeral joint, but also from supplementary movement in the rest of the pectoral girdle, i.e. scapulothoracic joint of the scapula, clavicle, acromioclavicular joint, sternoclavicular joint, and the 1st rib. The increased ROM of the glenohumeral joint additionally means less ligamentous support, which produces greater involvement and physical stress on the associated muscles in the area.

Sports including throwing events, or repeated overhead arm activity, such as swimming, may often generate injuries from strains or impingement of the rotator cuff muscle tendons, and/or the subacromial bursa, biceps tendons, pectoralis major tendon, and/or the tendons of the latissimus dorsi and teres major muscles. The superior size and strength of the larger medial rotators, i.e. pectoralis major and latissimus dorsi, can also cause increased stress on the weaker lateral rotators of the glenohumeral joint.

Other injury factors include association between the lesser tuberosity, bicipital sulcus and/or degenerative changes in the glenohumeral joint, with a pathologic progression from the subscapularis tendon to the long head of biceps brachii tendon, further on to glenohumeral joint involvement (Roberts et al. 2007).

It is suggested that most injuries stemming from overhead throwing appear in the shoulder and elbow. Throwing athletes are exposed to rotator cuff tears from tensile overload and lateral or medial impingement (Ouellette et al. 2005). Subscapularis involvement during shoulder pain should not be overlooked and soft tissue release of this muscle has been shown empirically to increase pain reduction and shoulder ROM.

The sports massage treatment often aims to ensure full sports-specific ROM in the shoulders, including associated structures like the scapulae, to break up or stretch adhesions/fibrosis, and focus on eliminating tension and/or adaptive shortening generating muscle imbalance in affected joints. Combined with the

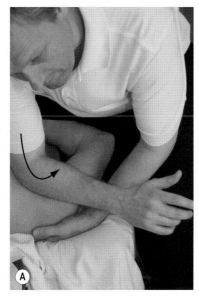
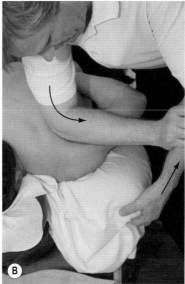

Figure 14.41 • Infraspinatus and teres minor release • A Elbow glide B Alternate reinforced elbow glide

athlete's specific training and/or rehabilitation regime, this can assist in rehabilitating or potentially reducing sports injuries in the shoulders.

Infraspinatus and teres minor release

Elbow glide for infraspinatus and teres minor *(Fig. 14.41A)*

1. The athlete lies prone with one arm on the back. If this is not possible either from pain or restricted scapular and glenohumeral movement, the arm may hang off the treatment table to generate a mild traction in the soft tissue.

2. The therapist can utilize an initial palm heel glide that is replaced with an elbow glide as the tissue softens. Starting on the muscle next to the medial border of the scapula, the stroke slowly glides all the way to the humerus. An elevated pressure on the elbow simultaneously pushes the arm into a gradually increased medial rotation and/or traction in the glenohumeral joint. The infraspinatus and teres minor muscles are treated separately.

3. The muscles are slowly and rhythmically massaged as the arm is pushed into increased medial rotation or traction.

Alternate reinforced elbow glide *(Fig. 14.41B)*

1. For athletes with more developed muscle mass, the elbow glide may be used exclusively.

2. The therapist can reinforce the stroke and generate more power by simultaneously grasping around the forearm or elbow with the hand of the treating arm, and grasping the treatment table with the other hand.

Supraspinatus release *(Fig. 14.42)*

1. The athlete lies on one side with the treated arm in a 90 degree flexion at both the glenohumeral joint and the elbow joint. The athlete's wrist is placed on the therapist's thigh.

2. The therapist initially lifts the athlete's elbow to relax the supraspinatus tendon, and the shoulder is gently pushed superiorly to disengage the descending part of the trapezius muscle.

3. With two fingers, normally the index and long finger, or one thumb, the therapist fixates the supraspinatus muscle. This is done by initially pushing away the relaxed trapezius muscle's anterior edge.

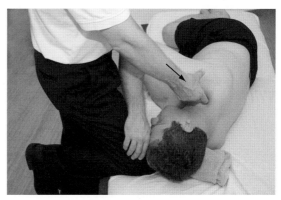

Figure 14.42 • Supraspinatus release

4. As the muscle is fixated, the therapist slowly lowers the athlete's elbow toward the treatment table. The fixating fingers will automatically start gliding in the opposite direction of the stretch.

5. The stroke is systematically repeated over the supraspinatus muscle and its tendon until tissue softening and increased ROM are noted.

Subscapularis release (Fig. 14.43)

1. The athlete lies supine with the arm by the side.

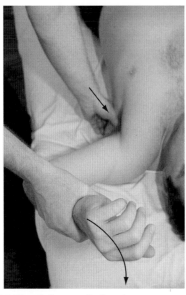

Figure 14.43 • Subscapularis release

2. The therapist fixates the muscle on the anterior aspect of the scapula. To find the correct position, it helps to follow the ribcage down to the scapula. The fixating pressure is initially applied close to the inferior border of the scapula.

3. As the muscle is fixated, a lock and stretch sequence along the muscle begins by lifting the athlete's arm toward the head. Caution should be taken in the upper part of the arm pit because of the lymphatic nodes.

4. Additional relaxation in the treated muscle is achieved when the athlete participates actively by lifting the arm against the therapist's manual resistance. This activates the reciprocal inhibition reflex.

Deltoid muscle release
Deltoid anterior (Fig. 14.44A)

1. The athlete lies prone.

2. The therapist is positioned at the top of the table, by the athlete's head, lightly extending the athlete's shoulder to the muscle's end point.

3. The therapist performs a planar glide as the shoulder is moved into additional extension.

4. The stroke is repeated until tissue relaxation and increased ROM are noted.

Deltoid intermedius (Fig. 14.44B)

1. The athlete lies on one side with the arm on the back.

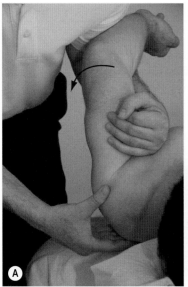 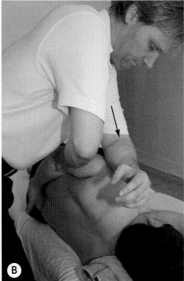 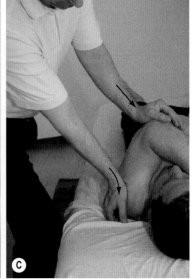

Figure 14.44 • Deltoid muscle release • A Anterior B Intermedius C Posterior

2. The therapist performs an elbow or planar glide as the athlete's arm is pushed into traction and adduction.

3. The stroke is repeated until tissue relaxation and increased ROM are noted.

Deltoid posterior (Fig. 14.44C)

1. The athlete lies supine

2. The therapist performs a palm glide as the athlete's arm is moved into horizontal adduction.

Soft tissue release in the neck area

Levator scapulae release (Fig. 14.45)

1. The athlete sits on the treatment table or in a chair.

2. The therapist locks the muscle with the flat part of one elbow, and commences an elbow glide as the athlete's head and neck are moved into lateral flexion toward the opposite side, flexion, and contralateral rotation. Essentially, this means moving the athlete's nose toward the opposite nipple area.

3. The stroke is repeated over different parts of the muscle until tissue relaxation and increased ROM are noted.

General neck muscle release
Step 1 (Fig. 14.46A)

1. The athlete lies prone with the head in a face cradle.

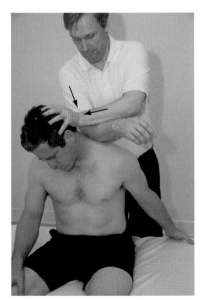

Figure 14.45 • Levator scapulae release

2. The therapist uses one thumb to slowly and methodically perform transverse thumb glides, medially to laterally, over the neck muscles.

3. The massage ranges from C7 level all the way up to the suboccipital muscle group.

4. The stroke is systematically repeated over different areas of the muscles until tissue relaxation and increased ROM are noted.

Step 2 (Fig. 14.46B)

1. The athlete lies prone with the head in a face cradle.

2. The therapist "hooks" the fingertips over the anterior aspect of neck fascia, the anterior scalene, and descending trapezius muscle.

3. The therapist lowers the body so the arms are almost horizontal, and leans backward to very slowly pull the fingers through the soft tissue. This is an effective myofascial release technique of this area.

4. The stroke is repeated until tissue relaxation is noted.

Step 3 (Fig. 14.46C)

1. The athlete lies supine. The therapist lifts the athlete's head off the table with one hand and uses the fingertips of the other hand to "hook" the neck muscles just lateral to the athlete's spinous process.

2. As the therapist slowly starts to pull the muscles laterally with bent fingertips, the athlete's head is simultaneously slowly lifted into further flexion, lateral flexion, and contralateral rotation, to increase the stretch effect in the stroke.

3. The stroke is repeated until tissue relaxation is noted.

Soft tissue release in the arms

Like other areas of an athlete's body, the arms too are exposed to overload injuries. Strains, tears, contusions, ligamentous sprains, tendinitis, tendinosis, etc., are fairly common occurrences. Inflammation of the tendon and/or synovial membrane of the long head of the biceps brachii muscle may cause incapacitating pain on the front of the shoulder.

Elbow pain is commonly caused by lateral or medial epicondylitis, where the superficial layer of the extensor, and flexor muscles of the wrist and hand originate. Even though the exact origin of lateral epicondylitis is not fully clear, it is suggested that the extensor carpi radialis brevis tendon has an anatomic location that renders its inferior surface vulnerable to abrasion against the lateral edge of the capitulum of

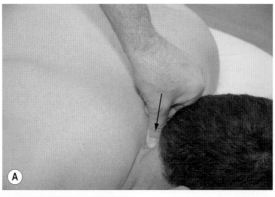

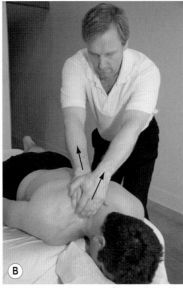

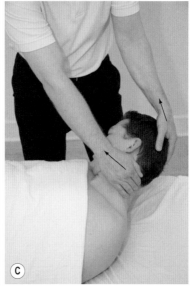

Figure 14.46 • General neck muscle release

humerus during elbow motion (Bunata et al. 2007). It is suggested that athletes with lateral epicondylitis may also have pain created by active myofascial trigger points (Fernández-Carnero et al. 2007). Medial epicondylitis of the elbow involves similar pathologic changes in the musculotendinous origins at the medial epicondyle of humerus (Ciccotti & Ramani 2003).

Remedial sports massage may focus on relieving stress on the inflamed area by performing massage and isolated stretching techniques to reduce muscle tension, in combination with other treatments like contrast treatment (i.e., ice massage), local heat treatment, transverse friction of local scarring and adhesions, myofascial trigger point treatments, myofascial and positional release techniques, or medically administered antiinflammatory medication. It is also suggested that adapted eccentric

training exercises in the treatment of chronic lateral epicondylar tendinopathy produces improvements (Croisier et al. 2007).

Biceps brachii release (Fig. 14.47)

1. The athlete lies prone
2. The therapist is positioned at the top of the table, by the athlete's head, lightly extending the athlete's shoulder and elbow, with an additional pronation of the hand to the muscle's end point.
3. The therapist initially locks the muscle by squeezing it with one hand, immediately followed by moving the athlete's arm into additional extension, and finally fine-tuning the stretch with a pronation of the hand.
4. As the muscle starts to soften, the therapist performs a planar glide along the remaining more

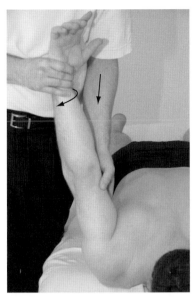

Figure 14.47 • Biceps brachii release

tensed segments of the muscle, with concurrent extension and pronation of the athlete's arm and hand.

5. The stroke is repeated until tissue relaxation and increased ROM are noted.

Brachialis release (Fig. 14.48)

1. The athlete lies supine with the arm resting on the therapist's leg.

2. The therapist flexes the athlete's elbow joint to slacken the muscle, and further fixates the muscle from either side by squeezing the muscle together.

3. The muscle is stretched at its end point after which the pressure is released.

4. The complete movement is continued over the rest of the muscle until tissue relaxation is noted in the area.

Triceps brachii release (Fig. 14.49)

1. The athlete lies supine with the palm placed over the spinous process of the 7th cervical vertebra.

2. The therapist grasps the athlete's elbow and commences a palm, fist, and/or planar glide as the arm is pushed into further flexion.

3. As the stretch is released, the stroke is rhythmically repeated over the three heads of the muscle until tissue relaxation and increased ROM are noted.

Brachioradialis release (Fig. 14.50)

1. The athlete lies supine with the treated forearm semisupinated.

2. The therapist commences a palm, forearm, or planar glide whilst simultaneously pronating the forearm and extending the athlete's elbow.

3. The stroke is repeated until tissue relaxation is noted.

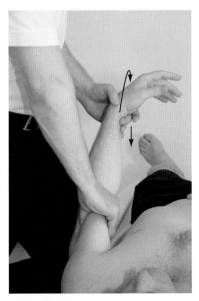

Figure 14.48 • Brachialis release

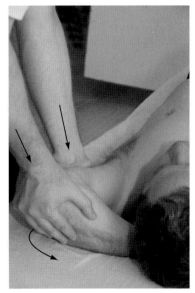

Figure 14.49 • Triceps brachii release

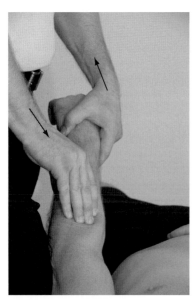

Figure 14.50 • Brachioradialis release

Superficial forearm extensor muscle release (Fig. 14.51)

1. The athlete lies supine with the elbow extended, the arm resting slightly elevated, and the hand lightly clenched.
2. The therapist locates a shortened section in the forearm and commences a thumb glide toward the origin, whilst simultaneously flexing the athlete's wrist and gently turning it toward the 5th finger.
3. The movement is repeated until tissue relaxation is noted.

Deep forearm extensor muscle release (Fig. 14.52)

The treatment is identical to the superficial layer with the difference that the elbow is flexed to relax the superficial layer.

Superficial forearm flexor muscle release (Fig. 14.53)

1. The athlete lies supine with the elbow extended, the arm resting slightly elevated, and the hand opened.
2. The therapist locates a shortened section in the forearm and commences a thumb or planar glide toward the origin, whilst simultaneously extending the athlete's wrist and fingers and gently turning the hand toward the 5th finger.
3. The movement is repeated until tissue relaxation is noted.

Deep forearm flexor muscle release (Fig. 14.54)

The treatment is identical to that for the superficial layer with the difference that the elbow is flexed to relax the superficial layer.

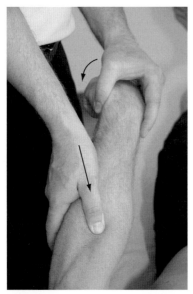

Figure 14.51 • Superficial forearm extensor muscle release

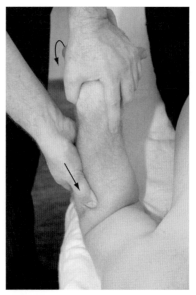

Figure 14.52 • Deep forearm extensor muscle release

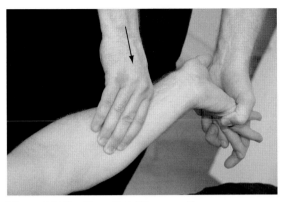

Figure 14.53 • Superficial forearm flexor muscle release

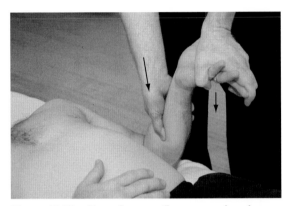

Figure 14.54 • Deep forearm flexor muscle release

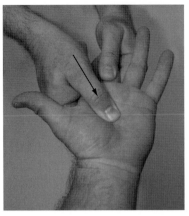

Figure 14.55 • Palmar hand muscle release

Soft tissue release in the hands

The muscles and fascial structures in the hand, mostly on the palmar side, are generally treated with thumb glides and/or lock and stretch variations.

Palmar hand muscle release (Fig. 14.55)

1. The therapist compresses the muscle with one thumb, and uses the other hand to extend the finger corresponding to the treated area as the thumb naturally commences gliding.
2. The movement is repeated until tissue relaxation is noted.

References

Aiken, A.B., et al., 2008. Short-term natural recovery of ankle sprains following discharge from emergency departments. J. Orthop. Sports Phys. Ther. 38 (9), 566–571. Epub 2008 Sep 1.

Akuthota, V., et al., 2008. Core stability exercise principles. Curr. Sports Med. Rep. 7 (1), 39–44.

Ambartsumov, R.M., 2001. Changes of the locomotor system in sportsmen with back pain. Lik. Sprava (1), 120–123.

Aminaka, N., Gribble, P.A., 2008. Patellar taping, patellofemoral pain syndrome, lower extremity kinematics, and dynamic postural control. J. Athl. Train. 43 (1), 21–28.

Archer, P., 2007. Therapeutic massage in athletics. Lippincott Williams & Wilkins, Baltimore, MD.

Benjamin, P.J., Lamp, S.P., 1996. Understanding sports massage. Human Kinetics, Champaign, IL.

Bunata, R.E., et al., 2007. Anatomic factors related to the cause of tennis elbow. J. Bone Joint Surg. Am. 89 (9), 1955–1963.

Cash, M., 1996. Sports & remedial massage therapy. Ebury Press, London.

Ciccotti, M.G., Ramani, M.N., 2003. Medial epicondylitis. Tech. Hand Up. Extrem. Surg. 7 (4), 190–196.

Croisier, J.L., et al., 2007. An isokinetic eccentric programme for the management of chronic lateral epicondylar tendinopathy. Br. J. Sports Med. 41 (4), 269–275. Epub 2007 Jan 15.

Croisier, J.L., et al., 2008. Strength imbalances and prevention of hamstring injury in professional soccer players: a prospective study. Am. J. Sports Med. 36 (8), 1469–1475. Epub 2008 Apr 30.

de Jonge, S., et al., 2008. One-year follow-up of a randomised controlled trial on added splinting to eccentric exercises in chronic midportion Achilles tendinopathy. Br. J. Sports Med. Oct 6. [Epub ahead of print].

Drewes, L.K., et al., 2008. Dorsiflexion deficit during jogging with chronic ankle instability. J. Sci. Med. Sport Oct 1. [Epub ahead of print].

Fernández-Carnero, J., et al., 2007. Prevalence of and referred pain from myofascial trigger points in the forearm muscles in patients with lateral epicondylalgia. Clin. J. Pain 23 (4), 353–360.

French, R.M., 2004. Milady's guide to lymph drainage massage. Thomson Delmar Learning, Clifton Park, NY.

Ko, D.S., et al., 1998. Effective treatment of lymphedema of the extremities. Arch. Surg. 133 (4), 452–458.

Neufeld, S.K., Cerrato, R., 2008. Plantar fasciitis: evaluation and treatment. J. Am. Acad. Orthop. Surg. 16 (6), 338–346.

Ouellette, H., et al., 2005. Imaging of the overhead throwing athlete. Semin. Musculoskelet. Radiol. 9 (4), 316–333.

Pagenstert, G.I., Bachmann, M., 2008. Clinical examination for patellofemoral problems. Orthopade 37 (9), 890–903.

Pasanen, K., et al., 2008. Neuromuscular training and the risk of leg injuries in female floorball players: cluster randomised controlled study. BMJ 337 (Jul 1), a295 doi: 10.1136/ bmj.a295.

Preyde, M., 2000. Effectiveness of massage therapy for subacute low-back pain: a randomized controlled trial. CMAJ 162 (13), 1815–1820.

Renkawitz, T., Boluki, D., Grifka, J., 2006. The association of low back pain, neuromuscular imbalance, and trunk extension strength in athletes. Spine J. 6 (6), 673–683.

Roberts, A.M., et al., 2007. New light on old shoulders: palaeopathological patterns of arthropathy and enthesopathy in the shoulder complex. J. Anat. 211 (4), 485–492 Epub 2007 Aug 15.

Schulhofer, S.D., Oloff, L.M., 2002. Flexor hallucis longus dysfunction: an overview. Clin. Podiatr. Med. Surg. 19 (3), 411–418 vi.

Syme, G., et al., 2008. Disability in patients with chronic patellofemoral pain syndrome: A randomised controlled trial of VMO selective training versus general quadriceps strengthening. Man. Ther. Apr 22. [Epub ahead of print].

Weir, A., et al., 2008. A manual therapy technique for chronic adductor-related groin pain in athletes: a case series. Scand. J. Med. Sci. Sports Aug 5 [Epub ahead of print].

Wilder, R.P., Sethi, S., 2004. Overuse injuries: tendinopathies, stress fractures, compartment syndrome, and shin splints. Clin. Sports Med. 23 (1), 55–81, vi.

Self-massage and myofascial release techniques for the athlete

15

Self-massage techniques are beneficial for the athlete since this modality can be administered whenever the need arises, independent of the presence of a sports massage therapist. Massage in different forms has demonstrated a reduction of the intensity of soreness after workout (Ernst 1998; Hilbert et al. 2003), and it is believed that massage in combination with other modalities can assist in the healing of repetitive strain injuries (Sheon 1997). The various benefits generated from massage can also fall under the category of self-massage, provided it is performed in an effective manner. Although self-massage has some limitations (Cash 1996), the techniques may serve as a good supplement to regular sports massage sessions. Self-massage is beneficially utilized during pre-, post- (Pozenik 2003), and interevent scenarios if no therapist is present, but the techniques also have a place in the remedial phase.

Tools

General self-massage is commonly performed with the hands, but correct usage of specific tools is very useful to enhance the effects, particularly for athletes with a more substantial muscle mass. A firm foam roll (Fig. 15.1A), or a massage device like The Stick (Fig. 15.1B), etc., may successfully increase the massage effects and additionally generate self-myofascial release for the athlete. Tennis or lacrosse balls can generate a similar result, especially when placed stationary (Fig. 15.1C), and a smaller soft exercise ball serves a similar purpose when used over more sensitive areas (Fig. 15.1D).

The following examples offer very basic suggestions for self-massage using the hands, foam rolls, balls, and/ or The Stick. The hand massage can additionally, like regular muscle massage, expand to utilize numerous variations on strokes, based on effleurage, compressions, petrissage, frictions, stripping, edging, special frictions, etc., discussed in Chapter 2.

Feet

Self-massage of the plantar aspect of the feet

1. The athlete can use a tennis ball, baseball, lacrosse ball, or a foot wheel (Fig. 15.2), to massage the plantar aspect of the foot. The massage is performed in circles, straight lines, or as compression, and should range from the heel to the plantar aspect of the toes. The pressure should generally increase as the tissue relaxes.
2. Thumb frictions on the dorsal part of the foot works between the metatarsal bones and the toes (Fig. 15.3).

Lower legs

Self-massage of the anterior lower leg

1. **Thumbs.** The athlete sits comfortably and relaxes the muscles in the lower leg. Using reinforced thumb stripping, the athlete massages

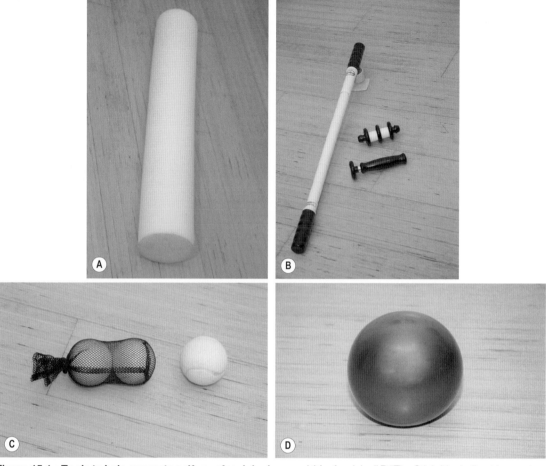

Figure 15.1 • **Tools to help generate self-myofascial release** • A Myofascial roll B "The Stick," including trigger wheel (used for smaller and/or specific areas), and foot wheel C Lacrosse and tennis balls D 8 lb soft exercise ball

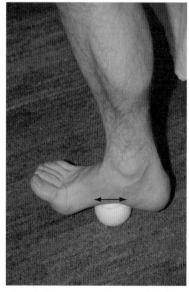

Figure 15.2 • **Self-massage of the plantar aspect of the foot**

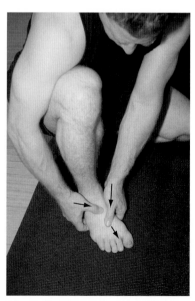

Figure 15.3 • **Self-massage of the dorsal aspect of the foot**

the tibialis anterior muscle, including the muscle belly and fascial structures, in short strokes (Fig. 15.4A).

2. **The Stick.** The athlete sits in the same position and systematically rolls The Stick along the tibialis anterior and peroneal muscles, with the majority of the pressure in the direction of the heart (Fig. 15.4B).

Self-massage of the posterior lower leg

1. **Thumbs.** The athlete sits with bent legs. The thumbs edge the lateral and medial aspect of each muscle belly along the muscle's length (Fig. 15.5A).
2. **The Stick.** The athlete sits in the same position and rolls The Stick along the length of the muscle, with the majority of the pressure in the direction of the heart (Fig. 15.5B).

Thighs

Self-massage of the anterior aspect of the thigh

1. **Hands.** The athlete sits with the legs relaxed and clasps the hands, performing double palm compressions of the quadriceps femoris muscle along its whole length (Fig. 15.6A).
2. **Reinforced thumb cross frictions.** This is followed by reinforced thumb cross frictions on tensed and/or fibrotic areas of the muscle (Fig. 15.6B).
3. **Foam roll.** The athlete lies on the ground with one leg on a foam roll, and slowly moves the body to have the roll massage along the thigh (Fig. 15.6C). To enhance the depth, the athlete initially performs an isometric muscle contraction of the quadriceps femoris muscle for 10 s, followed by relaxation and continued foam roll massage of the muscle. The athlete can also increase the amount of flexion in the knee joint to gradually increase the stretch effect during the treatment.

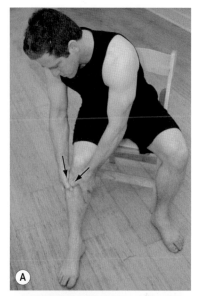

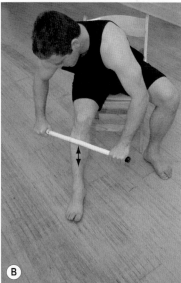

Figure 15.4 • Self-massage of the anterior lower leg

4. **The Stick.** The athlete either sits on the edge of a seat or stands, using The Stick to slowly massage the quadriceps femoris and adductor muscles along their length, with the majority of the pressure applied on the upward stroke toward the groin. To additionally increase the stretch effect, the leg is gradually flexed at the knee joint for the quadriceps femoris muscle, or abducted for the

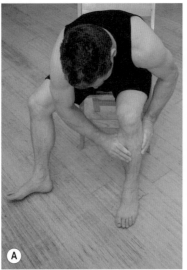

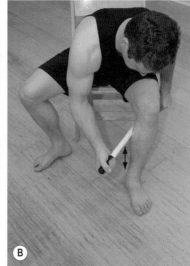

Figure 15.5 • Self-massage of the posterior lower leg

adductor muscles, to the end point for each stretch as the soft tissue relaxes (Fig. 15.6D).

Self-massage of the posterior aspect of the thigh

1. Fingertips. The athlete sits with the legs bent to access the hamstring muscles. The muscle is

edged and stretched with the fingertips, pushing into the mid part of the posterior thigh, stretching the soft tissue first medially, then laterally along the entire length of the muscles (Fig. 15.7A).

2. Foam roll. The athlete sits on the floor with a foam roll under one or both thighs, and slowly moves the body so that the foam roll massages along the thigh (Fig. 15.7B). To enhance the depth, the athlete

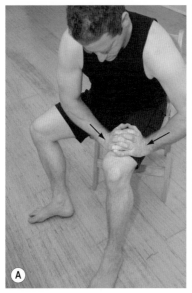

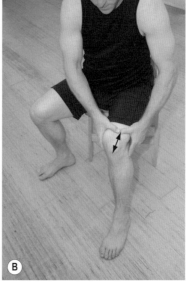

Figure 15.6 • Self-massage of the anterior aspect of the thigh

Continued

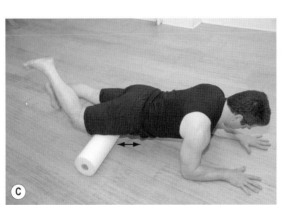

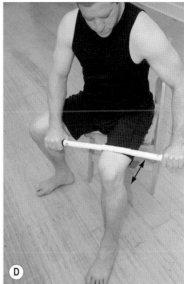

Figure 15.6—cont'd

initially performs an isometric muscle contraction of the quadriceps femoris muscle for 10 s, followed by relaxation and continued foam roll massage of the muscle.

3. The Stick. The athlete either sits on the edge of a seat or stands, using The Stick to slowly massage the muscles along their length, with the majority of the pressure applied on the upward stroke toward the ischial tuberosity. To additionally increase the stretch effect, the knee is gradually extended to the end point for each stretch as the soft tissue relaxes (Fig. 15.7C).

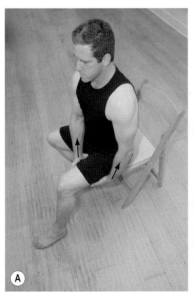

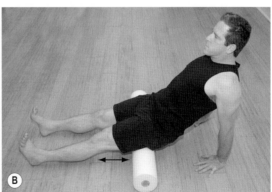

Figure 15.7 • Self-massage of the posterior aspect of the thigh

Continued

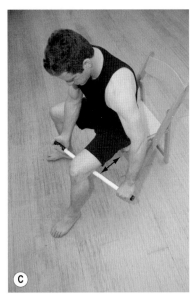

Figure 15.7—cont'd

Self-massage of the medial aspect of the thigh

1. **Hands.** The athlete sits with the legs relaxed. One hand grasps the adductor muscles and kneads them with palm heel petrissage strokes (Fig. 15.8A).
2. **The Stick.** The athlete sits in the same position, using The Stick to massage the muscles along their length, with the majority of the pressure

applied on the upward stroke in the direction of the groin (Fig. 15.8B).

Self-massage of the lateral aspect of the thigh, hips, and gluteal area

1. **Fingertips.** The athlete sits with the legs relaxed. Reinforced fingertips are used to perform cross frictions along the iliotibial tract and tensor fasciae latae muscle (Fig. 15.9A).
2. **Palm heel.** The gluteus medius and minimus muscles are massaged with palm heel petrissage (Fig. 15.9B).
3. **Foam roll.** The athlete lies on the ground and slowly moves the body so that the foam roll massages along the lateral aspect of the thigh and hip (Fig. 15.9C). The same area is also effectively massaged with The Stick, even whilst standing.

Back

Self-massage of the lower back

1. **Foam roll.** The athlete lies on the ground with bent knees. With the foam roll under the lower back, the athlete slowly moves the body so that the roll massages bilaterally along the lower back muscles (Fig. 15.10A). For a more unilateral effect, the athlete shifts the body weight to one side.

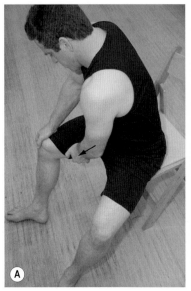

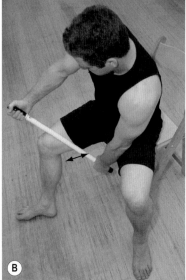

Figure 15.8 • Self-massage of the medial aspect of the thigh

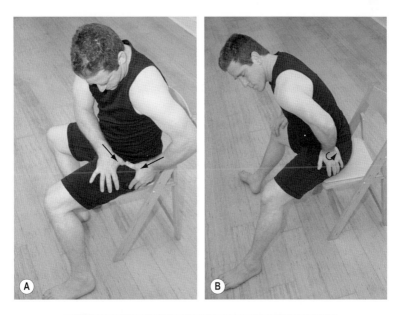

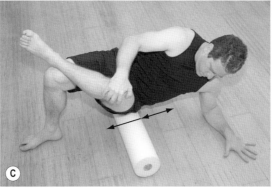

Figure 15.9 • Self-massage of the lateral aspect of the thigh, hips and gluteal area

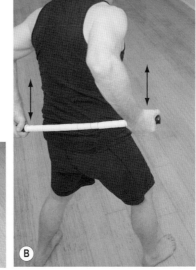

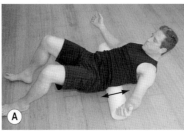

Figure 15.10 • Self-massage of the lower back

2. **The Stick.** The athlete stands with The Stick placed horizontally in the small of the back just superior to the sacrum. The Stick is rolled up and down each side on the lower back muscles, avoiding pressure on the vertebral spinous processes, to massage the local soft tissue (Fig. 15.10B).

Self-massage of the mid and upper back with tennis or lacrosse balls

Two tennis or lacrosse balls are either taped together or placed firmly together in a sock that is tied at the end. The athlete lies on the ground with the two balls placed on either side of the spine, starting at the first thoracic level (Fig. 15.11). It is important the balls do not glide apart under pressure, since this would present the risk of excessive pressure on the costovertebral joints. The pressure is kept stationary at each vertebral segment for 30 s to 3 min to achieve an effective stretch of the paravertebral muscles adjacent to the spine. For pressure massage of more laterally located muscles, such as rhomboids, trapezius, infraspinatus, and teres minor, the same set of balls or a single ball may be used for focal compression.

A foam roll is normally used for a broader, more general back massage.

Self-massage of the latissimus dorsi and teres major muscles

1. **Fingers.** The athlete can grasp the muscle belly with the fingers, kneading the muscles with petrissage strokes. The effect is increased if the athlete performs simultaneous abduction in the glenohumeral joint (Fig. 15.12A).

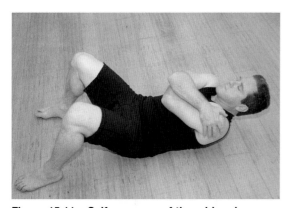

Figure 15.11 • Self-massage of the mid and upper back with tennis or lacrosse balls

2. **The Stick.** The athlete can also use The Stick, where one hand rests behind the back, holding the device stationary, whilst the other hand alternately moves The Stick® superiorly and inferiorly to massage the muscles (Fig. 15.12B).
3. **Foam roll.** When using a foam roll, the athlete lies on one side with the arm on the treated side over the head. The athlete uses the legs to move the body repeatedly over the roll for effective release of tensed soft tissue. To support the integrity of the glenohumeral joint, and induce reciprocal inhibition, the arm is actively reaching cranially (Fig. 15.12C).

Neck

Self-massage of the anterior aspect of the upper neck muscles

1. **The Stick.** The athlete uses The Stick to massage the upper portion of the trapezius muscle (Fig. 15.13A).
2. **Thumbs.** For the very upper part of the neck, the athlete clasps the fingers and compresses and stretches the muscles into a C-shape with one thumb, or uses both thumbs to treat the neck bilaterally (Fig. 15.13B). The thumbs can also perform an S-stroke from the same position, if the stroke is applied unilaterally.

Abdominal area

Abdominal and iliopsoas self-myofascial release technique

The athlete lies prone on the ground with a smaller (9 in), soft exercise ball under the abdomen (Fig. 15.14). The ball is moved to an area of elevated tissue tension. While resting on the ball, the athlete's body weight will generate the desired stretch effect. The pressure remains in the area for 30 s to 3 min, while the athlete passively relaxes on the exercise ball and continuously breathes using the diaphragm. To reach the iliopsoas muscle, the ball is moved to the lower abdominal area just below the umbilicus, lateral to the mid line, and down to the lesser trochanter in the groin.

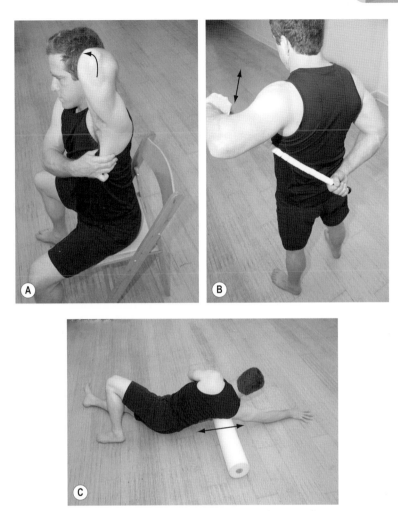

Figure 15.12 • Self massage of the latissimus dorsi and teres major muscles

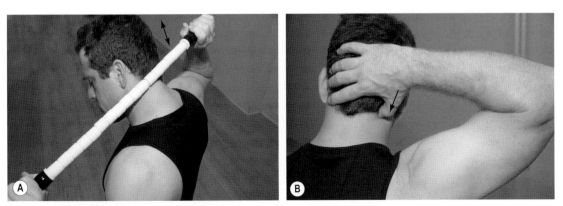

Figure 15.13 • Self-massage of the upper neck muscles including upper trapezius, levator scapulae, and the splenius muscle group

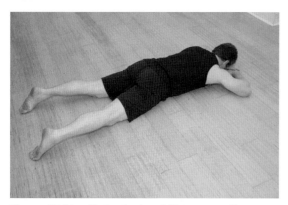

Figure 15.14 • Abdominal and iliopsoas self-myofascial release technique with a smaller soft exercise ball

Chest

Self-massage of the anterior aspect of the pectoral muscles

The athlete uses the fingertips to massage the pectoralis major and minor muscles using circular frictions. The fingertips are slightly bent and actively push and pull the soft tissue during the massage to enhance the stretch effect (Fig. 15.15).

Shoulders

Self-massage of the deltoid muscle

The athlete grasps the muscle with the fingertips, and rhythmically performs lifting petrissage strokes (Fig. 15.16).

Arms

Self-massage of the flexor and extensor muscles of the upper arm

1. The athlete grasps the biceps brachii muscle with the fingertips, including the web between the index finger and thumb, and rhythmically performs lifting petrissage strokes of the muscle, as the elbow is simultaneously extended. The brachialis muscle is reached by grasping immediately under the biceps brachii muscle (Fig. 15.17A).
2. The athlete places the palm over the spinous process of the 7th cervical vertebra and grasps the triceps brachii muscle with the fingertips, including the web between the index finger and thumb. The muscle is rhythmically massaged with lifting petrissage strokes (Fig. 15.17B).

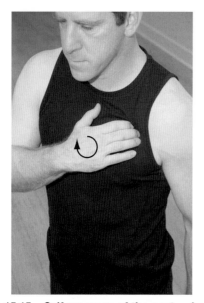

Figure 15.15 • Self-massage of the pectoral muscles

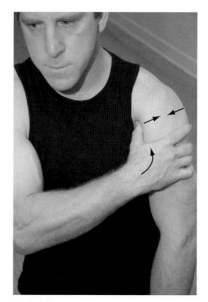

Figure 15.16 • Self-massage of the deltoid muscle

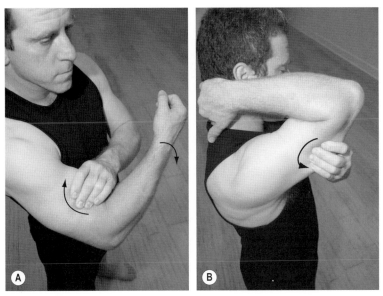

Figure 15.17 • Self-massage of the flexor and extensor muscles of the upper arm

Self-massage of the flexor and extensor muscles of the forearm and hand

1. Thumb. The athlete grasps around the forearm and uses the thumb or fingertips to massage the flexor and extensor muscles of the forearm with circular frictions (Fig. 15.18A). As the fingers massages the muscle, the hand can actively extend (for the flexor group) or flex (for the extensor group) to enhance the stretch effect.

2. The Stick. One end of The Stick is placed on a table at a 45 degree angle. While one hand holds the other end of The Stick, the flexor and extensor muscles of the free forearm are massaged separately. To enhance the stretch effect in the soft tissue, the hand is actively extended (for the flexor muscles) or flexed (for the extensor muscles) using the antagonistic muscles (Fig. 15.18B).

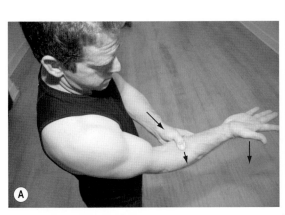
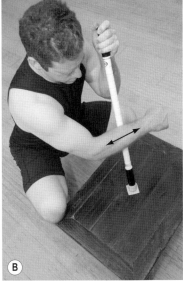

Figure 15.18 • Self-massage of the flexor and extensor muscles of the forearm and hand

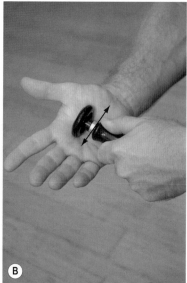
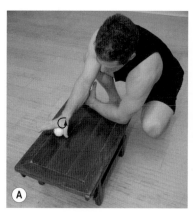

Figure 15.19 • Self-massage of the hand

Hands

Self-massage of the hand

1. Ball. The athlete may use a tennis or lacrosse ball to massage the muscles of the palm of the hand. The ball is moved in both small circles and straight lines to effectively treat tensed soft tissue on the palmar aspect of the hands (Fig. 15.19A).

2. Trigger wheel. A trigger wheel may also be used to effectively massage between the metacarpal bones (Fig. 15.19B).

References

Cash, M., 1996. Sports & remedial massage therapy. Ebury Press, London.

Ernst, E., 1998. Does post-exercise massage treatment reduce delayed onset muscle soreness? A systematic review. Br. J. Sports Med. 32 (3), 212–214.

Hilbert, J.E., et al., 2003. The effects of massage on delayed onset muscle soreness. Br. J. Sports Med. 37, 72–75.

Pozenik, R., 2003. Massage for cyclists. Vitesse Press, North Middlesex, VT.

Sheon, R.P., 1997. Repetitive strain injury, diagnostic and treatment tips on six common problems. The Goff Group. Postgrad. Med. 102 (4), 72–78 81–85.

Index

Note: Page numbers followed by *b* indicate boxes and *f* indicate figures.

A

abdomen, 109
  stretch of external and internal
    abdominal oblique, 109, 110*f*
  stretch of rectus abdominis muscle,
    109*f*
abdominal and iliopsoas self-myofascial
  release, 242–243, 244*f*
abdominal obliques, myofascial release,
  151, 151*f*
accessories, use of, 98–99
Achilles tendinitis, 122, 183, 214–215,
  215*f*
Achilles tendinopathy, 194, 194*f*
Achilles tendinosis, 191
  eccentric exercise for, 194, 195*f*
Achilles tendon
  rupture of, 186–188, 187*f*
  strain counterstrain, 124–125, 124*f*,
    125*f*
  tender points, 125*f*
Active Isolated Stretching (AIS), 87–89
  of ischiocrural/biceps femoris
    muscles, 89, 89*f*
  of ischiocrural/semitendinosus and
    membranosus muscle, 88, 89*f*
  use of strap, 88, 88*f*
Active Release Technique (ART), 90
acupressure, 130
  digital pressure, 130
  thumb pressure with simultaneous
    massage along the channels, 130,
    131*f*
acupuncture channels, 127, 128*f*
acupuncture points (acupoints), 127

Ah Shi points, 127, 130
  extraordinary points, 127
  regular, 127, 130
acute injuries, 183–188
  to bursa, 188
acute pain, 183
acute sports injuries, treatment of,
  188–189
acute tendon injuries, 186–188
acutron monitor, 171*f*
adductor magnus, 171, 172*f*
adductor muscle group, stretch, 101,
  104*f*
adductor muscle release, 220
  elbow, 220, 221*f*
  fist, 220, 220*f*
Ah Shi points, 127, 130
Alfredson protocol, 194
anatomical snuff box, 193
anatomy train lines, 141
anatomy trains, 140
ankle distortion, 192
ankle injury, treatment, 188–189, 188*f*
ankle joint, ligaments in, 187*f*
ankle sprains, 186
anterior cruciate ligament (ACL)
    injuries, 186
  rupture of, 192
anterior drawer sign, 192
anterior drawer test, 192, 192*f*, 193*f*
anterior talofibular ligament, 186, 187*f*
Apley's test, 193, 193*f*
apophysitis, 189, 190
  Cryo/Cuff in, 188, 189*f*
arch, painful, 196–197

arms, self-massage, 244–245
  flexor/extensor muscles of forearm
    and hand, 245
  thumb, 245, 245*f*
  Stick, The, 245, 245*f*
  flexor/extensor muscles of upper arm,
    244, 245*f*
arms, stretch, 115–116
arthrosis, 189, 191
Aston patterning, 140
autogenic inhibition, 81, 83
avulsion, 184

B

back, self-massage, 240–242
Baker's cyst, 191
balance boards, 183, 184*f*
ballistic flexibility, 77, 77*f*
barrier of resistance, 85, 86
baseball, massage for, 69
basketball, massage for, 69–70
  foot, fist compression in, 70*f*
  suggested areas, 69–70, 69*f*
benefits of massage, 2
biceps brachii, 171, 176*f*
  release, 230–231, 231*f*
  strain counterstrain, 125–126, 125*f*
  stretch of, 115, 115*f*
  tender points, 125*f*
biceps femoris muscles
  Active Isolated Stretching (AIS) of,
    88, 89, 89*f*
Bindegewebsmassage *see* connective
  tissue massage

blocks, 98–99
blood lactate, 2
BOSU training, 192
brachialis release, 231, 231f
brachioradialis release, 231, 232f
broadening, 11–15
    elbow, 12, 12f
    palm heel, 11, 12, 35
    thenar eminence, 12, 12f, 35
bucket handle injury, 193
Buddy taping, 204, 205f
bursa, acute injuries to, 188
bursitis, 190–191

C

calcaneofibular ligament, 186, 187f
calcaneus see Achilles tendon
calor, 183
capsular ligament, 186
carpal tunnel syndrome, myofascial
        release manipulation in, 140
cautions/contraindications for sports
        massage, 32
center of movement, 7f
cervicis muscles, stretch of, 112, 113f
chest, self-massage, 244
child's pose, 144, 145f
Chinese splits, 76f
chondromalacia patellae, 195
chronic compartment syndrome, 194
chronic pain, 183
chronic rotator cuff pain, Tui Na
        treatment for, 135–136
circular friction, 35
Claudius Galenus, 1
coach tape, 199
common sports injuries, 192–193
compartment syndrome, chronic, 194
compression techniques, 9–11
    elbow, 11, 11f, 35
    fist, 10, 10f, 35
    forearm, 11, 11f
    palm, 9–10, 35
        double-handed, 9–10, 10f
        single-handed, 10, 10f
    thumb, 10–11, 11f
concentric muscle contraction, 78
connective tissue, 139, 140f
    ordinary, 139
    specialized, 139
connective tissue massage
        (Bindegewebsmassage), 157–158
    anterior treatment pattern, 159f

posterior treatment pattern, 159f
reflex zones, 158f
treatment technique, 158, 158f,
        159f
contract-relax (CR), 81–82, 83f
    modified, 83
contract-relax antagonistic contract
        (CRAC), 84–85, 85f
cortisone injections, 192
coxae saltans/"snapping hip", 196
cramp release, 32, 186f
    see also muscle cramps
cross-fiber friction, 18–19, 19f
cruciate ligament, 186
Cryo/Cuff, 188, 189f
cun measurements, 127–129, 129f
    back, 127
    chest and abdomen, 127
    head, 127
    lower extremities, 128–129
    upper extremities, 127
cycling, 68
    peroneal muscle group, lock and
        stretch, 68f
    suggested areas, 68, 68f

D

dance, 65–66
    gastrocnemius muscle, broadening,
        66f
    suggested areas, 65–66, 65f
De Quervain's syndrome, 190
deep forearm extensor muscle release,
        232, 232f
deep forearm flexor muscle release, 232,
        233f
deep gliding strokes, 210–213
    elbow glide, 212–213, 216f
    fist glide, 211, 212f
    forearm glide, 212, 216f
    palm glide, 211, 212f
    planar glide/reinforced 4-finger glide,
        211, 211f
    rhythmic lock and stretch, variation,
        213, 217f
    thumb glide, 211, 211f
deep stroking massage (stripping),
        167–168, 167f
degenerative conditions, 189, 191
delayed onset muscle soreness
        (DOMS), therapeutic massage
        and, 2
deltoid muscle release, 228–229

deltoid anterior, 228, 228f
deltoid intermedius, 228–229, 228f
deltoid posterior, 228f, 229
deltoid muscle, self-massage,
        244, 244f
deltoid muscle, stretch of, 113–114, 114f
dislocations (luxations)/subluxations,
        184–185
diving, platform and springboard,
        massage for, 64
    suggested areas, 64, 64f
dolor, 183
dynamic flexibility, 76–77, 76f
dynamic neutral, 120–121

E

eccentric muscle contraction, 78
edging, 20–21
    elbow, 20–21, 21f
    palm heel, 20, 21f
    thumb, 20, 20f
effects of sports massage, 2–3
effleurage, 2, 35
effleurage strokes, 6–9
    forearm, 9, 9f
    one-sided, 7–9, 8f, 9f
    palm heel, 6, 8f
    palm heel and fingertip, 6, 8f
    regular superficial, 6, 8f
    through sheet, 6, 7f, 28, 28f
eight-finger friction, 15–16, 15f
elbow
    adductor muscle release, 220,
        221f
    compression, 11, 11f, 35
    edging, 20–21, 21f
    glide, 212–213, 216f
empty can test, 196–197, 196f
epicondylitis, lateral/medial, 197
    test for, 197f
erector spinae C-release, 223, 223f
erector spinae fasciae, 145, 145f
erector spinae muscle group, 108–109
    stretch of, 108–109, 108f
erector spinae muscle, thumb edging,
        65f
event-based massage
    differentiation, 27
    suggested items for, 29b
exercise balls in self-massage,
        235, 236f
extramuscular myofascial connections,
        141

F

fascial network, effects in, 141, 141f
fascial release, 120, 120f
feet, self-massage, 235
　dorsal aspect, 236f
　plantar aspect, 235, 236f
fencing stance, modified, 5, 5f
fibromyalgic tender points, 123
finger percussion, 169–170, 170f
fist
　adductor muscle release, 220, 220f
　compression, 10, 10f, 35
　friction, 17, 17f
　glide, 211, 212f
fixating, 98
flexibility, 75–77
　ballistic, 77, 77f
　dynamic, 76–77
　fast, 76f
　functional, 76–77
　static, 76
　static active, 76, 76f
　static passive, 76, 76f
focal stretching, 97–98, 98f
football and rugby, massage for,
　　　71–72
　gastrocnemius muscle, forearm
　　　compression, 72f
　general neck release, 72f
　lower neck release, 72f
　quadriceps femoris muscle,
　　　hypothenar rubbing, 72f
　suggested areas, 71–72, 71f
forearm
　compression, 11, 11f
　glide, 212, 216f
　superficial extensor muscles, stretch
　　　of, 115, 116f
　superficial flexor muscles, stretch of,
　　　116, 116f
four-finger friction, 16, 16f
four-finger stroke, stretch of, 169, 169f
fractures, 184, 185f
friction, 2
friction strokes, 6, 15–20
　circular, 35
　cross-fiber, 18–19, 19f
　eight-finger, 15–16, 15f
　fist, 17, 17f
　four-finger, 16, 16f
　one-finger, 16, 16f
　palm, 17, 17f
　thumb, 16, 16f, 17f

　transverse, 19, 19f, 35
　　deep, 19
　V-frictions, 17–18
　　regular, 17–18, 18f
　　reversed, 18, 18f
full can test, 196–197, 196f
functio laesa, 183
functional flexibility, 76–77
functional pain, 182
functional technique, 120–122, 121b,
　　　121f
　balance and hold, 121–122
　　in shoulder, 121–122, 121f
　dynamic functional, 122
　　in hip joint, 122, 122f

G

gastrocnemius muscle, 171, 173f
　broadening, 66f
　forearm compression, 72f
　release, 215, 215f
gate control theory mechanism, 192
gluteus maximus
　fascial structure of, 150–151, 150f
　release, 222, 222f
　stretch, 105, 106f
gluteus medius/minimus, 171, 174f
　release, 222, 222f
　stretch, 105, 106f
golf, massage for, 65
　erector spinae muscle, thumb edging,
　　　65f
　suggested areas, 65, 65f
golfer's elbow see epicondylitis, lateral/
　　　medial
Golgi tendon organ (GTO), 83b, 83f
goniometry, 75–76
gracilis muscle
　release, 220, 221f
　stretch, 102–103, 104f
greater trochanter release, 222, 222f
Greece, ancient, 1

H

hamstring muscles, 144, 144f, 171, 173f
　Active Isolated Stretching (AIS) of,
　　　89, 89f
　active stretching
　　dynamic, 80f
　　static, 80f
　ballistic stretching, 79f
　contract-relax, 84f

　dynamic stretching, 79f
　isolytic muscle energy technique,
　　　86–87, 88f
　passive stretching, 78f
　release, 219
　　elbow, 219, 220f
　　fist, 219, 220f
　stretch, 100, 102f
hand placement, 7f
hands, self-massage, 246
　ball, 246
　trigger wheel, 246, 246f
Hatha yoga, 139
Hawkins impingement test, 196–197,
　　　197f
heel pad, painful, 194, 195f
　taping, 202, 203f
Heller work, 140
hemobursitis, 188
hepatitis B, 31
hepatitis C, 31
hip joint, dynamic functional technique
　　　in, 122, 122f
Hippocrates, 1
history of massage, 1
HIV, 31
hold-relax (HR), 83
home stretching exercises, 170
horse stance, modified, 5, 5f
housemaid's knee, 191
hydraulic table, 5, 6f
hyperthermia, 31
hypothenar rubbing, 35
hypothermia, 31

I

ice and stretch, 169
ice hockey, massage in, 70
　hip joint, ROM stretch, 70f
　suggested areas, 70, 70f
iliacus release, 219, 219f
iliopsoas muscle
　release, 218–219, 219f
　stretch, 104, 105f
iliotibial band (ITB) release, 221f
iliotibial band friction syndrome
　　　(runner's knee), 122, 195–196
　Tui Na treatment for, 136–137
iliotibial tract, myofascial release, 150,
　　　150f
impingement in the shoulder, 196–197
India, wrestling in, 1
inflammations, 189

inflammatory battle, 183
inflammatory pain, 182
infraspinatus and teres minor muscles, 171, 175f
  release, 227
    alternate reinforced elbow glide, 227, 227f
    elbow glide, 227, 227f
    stretch of, 112, 112f
integrated neuromuscular inhibition technique (INIT), 170
integrated trigger point hypothesis, 162, 163f
intercostal muscles, myofascial release, 151, 152f
interevent massage, 27, 30, 44–51
  broadening
    of ischiocrural/hamstring muscle group, 47, 47f
    of left calf muscles, 48, 48f
    palm, of right thigh, 50, 50f
  edging of left calf muscle, 48, 48f
  effleurage
    of back, 49, 49f
    of gluteal area and lower back, 46, 46f
    of left leg and gluteal area, 49, 49f
    of posterior aspect of left leg, 45, 45f, 46f
    right leg, 49, 50f
  fist compressions
    of left foot, 48, 49f
    of left gluteal and lower back muscle, 47, 47f
  fist/palm compressions
    of ischiocrural/hamstring muscle group, 47, 47f
    of right thigh, 49f, 50f
  highlights, 30b
  hypothenar rubbing of right quadriceps muscle, 50, 50f
  jostling of hip and both legs, 51, 51f
  lock/stretch of soleus, tibilias, posterior and peroneal muscles, 48, 48f
  palm compressions
    of right tibialis anterior and peroneal muscles, 50, 51f
    alternating, of left calf muscles, 48, 48f
  palm heel petrissage of selected tensed areas of left leg, 46, 46f
  palm/thumb compressions of shoulder and neck area, 49, 49f

rhythmic lock and stretch of ischiocrural/hamstring muscles, 47, 47f
ROM stretch of right hip joint, 51, 51f
S-stroke petrissage of selected tensed areas of left leg, 46, 46f
stretch
  of right gastrocnemius and soleus muscles, 41f, 51
  of right ischiocrural/hamstring muscles, 51, 51f
  of right quadriceps and iliopsoas muscles, 51, 52f
  time distribution, 45
intermuscular bleeding, 185
intracapsular ligament, 186
intramuscular bleeding, 185
inverse myotactic reflex, 81, 83
ischemic muscle pressure, 23, 23f, 168, 168f
ischiocrural muscle group see hamstring muscles
isokinetic training, 183
isolytic muscle contraction, 78
isolytic muscle energy techniques (MET), 86–87
  of hamstring muscles, 86–87, 88f
isometric muscle contraction, 78
isotonic muscle contraction, 78

J

Janda's postfacilitation stretch method, 86, 87f
jostling/oscillation, 23, 23f, 35
jump sign, 167

K

knee joint, ligaments in, 187f

L

Lachman's test, 192, 193f
lacrosse and tennis balls in self-massage, 235, 236f
lateral scalp fascia, 148, 148f
latex/rubber gloves, 31
latissimus dorsi and teres major muscles
  release, 223–224, 224f
  self-massage, 242
    fingers, 242, 243f
    foam roll, 242, 243f

Stick, The, 242, 243f
  stretch of, 109, 110f
levator scapular, 171, 176f
  release, 229, 229f
  stretch of, 111–112, 112f
ligaments
  in ankle joint, 187f
  injuries, 186, 186f
  in knee joint, 187f
limitations of research, 2–3
lines of pull, 153–154
Ling, Per Henrik, 1
local twitch response (LTR), 167
long-distance runners, prevent treatment see prevent sports massage treatment
lower back, stretch, 109
lower body muscles
  anterior aspect, 99f
  posterior aspect, 99f
lower leg, fascial structures, 149–150, 150f
lower legs, self-massage, 235–237
  anterior, 235–237, 237f
    Stick, The, 237
    thumbs, 235
  posterior, 237, 238f
    Stick, The, 237
    thumbs, 237
lumbar strain, Tui Na treatment for, 135–137
luxations, 184–185
lymphatic drainage massage (LDM), 208–210, 209f
  J-stroke, 210, 210f
  long strokes, 210, 210f
  pump, 209, 210f
  stationary circles, 209, 209f

M

maintenance massage, 32, 207, 208b
Markus Aurelius, 1
McConnell taping, 217
mechanical efficiency, 27–28, 28b
medial meniscus
  strain counterstrain, 124, 124f
  tender points, 124f
medial tibial stress syndrome (periostitis), 189, 190, 190, 194–195, 190, 214–215
membranosus muscle, Active Isolated Stretching (AIS) of, 88, 89f
meniscus tear, 193

mobile point, 122, 123*f*
modified contract-relax, 83, 84*f*
muscle contraction types, 78*b*
muscle contusions, 185
muscle cramps, 185
    idiopathic cramps, 185
    paraphysiological cramps, 185–186
    symptomatic cramps, 185
muscle energy techniques (MET)
        stretching methods, 85
muscle injuries, 185–186
muscle spindle, 81, 82*b*, 82*f*
muscle strains, 185
myofascial foam roll in self-massage,
        235, 236*f*
myofascial meridians, 141
myofascial pain syndrome, 161–180
    manual massage techniques, 167–168
    muscle and connective tissue stretch
        techniques, 169–170
    treatment, 167–171
    drug treatments, 171
    dry or wet needling, 170
    herbal remedies, 171
    microcurrent therapies, 171, 171*f*
    moist heat, 170
    transcutaneous electric nerve
        stimulation, 171
    example, 171
    common MTPs of the lower body, 171
    common MTPs of the upper body,
        171
myofascial release techniques, 141–156,
        170
    arm lines, 153–155, 154*f*
    deep front line, 155, 156*f*
    functional lines, 155–156, 157*f*
    lateral line, 148–152, 149*f*
        abdominal obliques, 151, 151*f*
        external and internal intercostal
            muscles, 151, 152*f*
        gluteus maximus muscle, fascial
            structure of, 150–151, 150*f*
        iliotibial tract, 150, 150*f*
        important myofascial structures,
            148–152
        lower leg, fascial structures,
            149–150, 150*f*
        SCM, 152, 152*f*
        splenius capitis, 151, 152*f*
        superficial fasciae of lateral aspect
            of chest, 151, 151*f*
        tensor fasciae latae fascia, 150,
            150*f*

spiral line, 152, 153*f*
stroke examples, 141–142, 142*f*
superficial back line (SBL), 142–145,
        143*f*
superficial front line, 146–148, 146*f*
    deep/superficial toe extensor
        muscles and tibialis anterior, 147,
        147*f*
    important myofascial structures,
        146–148
    lateral scalp fascia, 148, 148*f*
    patellar ligament, 147, 147*f*
    quadriceps femoris, 147, 147*f*
    rectus abdominis, 147, 148*f*
    SCM, 147–148, 148*f*
    sternalis/sternochondral fascia,
        147, 148*f*
myofascial structures, 143–145,
        148–152
myofascial tender points, 123
myofascial trigger points (MTrPs),
        161–180
    classification, 164–165
        active, 164
        associated trigger points, 164
        attachment, 164
        central, 164
        key trigger points, 164
        latent, 164
        satellite, 165
    localization of, 165–166
        increased skin moisture over MTrP,
            165, 165*f*
        palpation, 165–166
        reduced skin motility over the
            MTrP, 165, 165*f*
        referred pain, 166, 167*f*
    of lower body, 171
        quadriceps femoris and adductor
            magnus, 171, 172*f*
        ischiocrural muscles, 171, 173*f*
        gastrocnemius and soleus, 171, 173*f*
        gluteus medius and minimus, 171,
            174*f*
        piriformis, 171, 174*f*
        TFL and tibialis anterior, 171, 174*f*
    pain and, 163–164
        convergence-projection, 164
        sympathetic hyperactivity, 164
    palpation, localization by, 165–166
        deep/probing, 166, 166*f*
        flat, 166, 166*f*
        locating the taut band, 165–166,
            166*f*

        pincer, 166, 166*f*
        taut band and, 161, 162*f*
        trauma and, 161–163
    of upper body, 171
        supraspinatus, infraspinatus, and
            teres minor, 171, 175*f*
        subscapularis and biceps brachii,
            171, 176*f*
        trapezius and levator scapulae, 171,
            176*f*
        rhomboids, 171, 177*f*
        pectoralis major and minor, 171,
            178*f*
        SCM and scalenus anterior, 171,
            178*f*
myositis ossificans, 185
myoskeletal approach, 140

N

naprapathy, 139–140
neck
    posterior aspect of, 145, 145*f*
    self-massage, 242
        Stick, The, 242, 243*f*
        thumbs, 242, 243*f*
    stretch, 112–115
neuropathic pain, 182
neurotendinous spindle, 83*b*, 83*f*
nociceptive pain, 182
nociceptors, 182
nonsteroid antiinflammatory drugs
        (NSAIDs), 191, 183
Nurmi, Paavo, 1–2

O

Ober's test, 196, 196*f*
olecranon bursitis (student's elbow),
        191
Olympic Games, 1924 (Paris), 1–2
one-finger friction, 16, 16*f*
oscillation/jostling, 23, 23*f*, 35
Osgood-Schlatter disease, 190
osteoarthritis, 189, 191
osteoarthrosis, 191
osteopathy, 139
overuse (overload) injuries, 189–191,
        189*f*, 194–197
    environmental factors, 190
    equipment-related factors, 190
    extrinsic factors, 189–190
    inflammation, 190–191
    intrinsic factors, 190

overuse (overload) injuries (*Continued*)
  stress fractures, 191
  training-related factors, 189
  treatment, 191–192

P

pain
  anatomy, 182–183, 182*f*
  classification, 182–183
  definition, 182
  inflammation and, 182–183
  myofascial trigger points, 163–164
    convergence-projection, 164
    sympathetic hyperactivity, 164
pain receptors, 182
painful arch, 196–197
painful heel pad, 194, 195*f*
palm compression, 9–10, 35
  double-handed, 9–10, 10*f*
  single-handed, 10, 10*f*
palm friction, 17, 17*f*
palm glide, 211, 212*f*
palm heel edging, 20, 21*f*
palm heel petrissage, 13, 13*f*
  reinforced, 13, 13*f*
palm petrissage, 35
palmar hand muscle release, 233, 233*f*
panniculosis, 168
paratendinitis, 189, 190
patellar ligament, myofascial release,
    147, 147*f*
patellofemoral pain syndrome (PFPS),
    195, 217
pectoralis major, 171, 178*f*
  release, 225, 225*f*
  self-massage, 244, 244*f*
  stretch of, 114, 114*f*
pectoralis minor, 171, 178*f*
  release, 226, 226*f*
  self-massage, 244, 244*f*
  stretch of, 114–115, 115*f*
percussion and stretch, 169–170
periostitis *see* medial tibial stress
    syndrome
peritendinitis, 190
peroneal muscle
  release, 216, 216*f*
  stretch, 100, 100*f*
peroneus longus and brevis, 216
petrissage, 12–15
  cycle ergometer pedaling and, 2
  forearm, 13, 14*f*
  lifting, 13, 13*f*

palm, 35
palm heel, 13, 13*f*
  reinforced, 13, 13*f*
S-stroke, 14–15
  modified, 14, 14*f*
  modified S-stroke/elbow, 15, 15*f*
  regular, 14, 14*f*
forearm, 13, 14*f*
lifting, 13, 13*f*
Pilates, 192
pirisiformis muscle, 98, 171, 174*f*
  strain counterstrain, 123–124,
    123*f*
  stretch, 105–106, 107*f*
  tender points, 123*f*
planar glide/reinforced 4-finger glide,
    211, 211*f*
plantar aponeurosis
  fist glide of, 143–144, 144*f*
  focal stretch and thumb glide of, 214,
    214*f*
plantar fasciitis, 194, 214
  taping, 201, 202*f*
point of light irritation, 88
portable massage table, 5, 6*f*, 30*f*
position of ease, 119, 120
positional release techniques (PRT),
    119–126, 170
post isometric relaxation (PIR)
    technique (Karel Lewit's
    modification), 85–86, 85*f*
posterior talofibular ligament, 187*f*
posterior tibial syndrome (periostitis),
    190
postevent massage, 27, 30–32, 52–58
  broadening of right calf muscles, 55,
    55*f*
  circular finger frictions and mild
    traction of neck area, 58, 59*f*
  coherency, 31
  effleurage
    of back of right leg, 53, 54*f*
    of right gluteal and lower back area,
    53, 54*f*
    of right leg and gluteal area, 56, 56*f*
    of right leg, 57, 57*f*
  fist compressions, 56, 56*f*
    of right gluteal and lower back
    muscle, 53, 54*f*
  fist/palm compressions
    of right thigh, 57, 57*f*
    on ischiocrural/hamstring muscle
    group, 53, 54*f*
  highlights, 31*b*

jostling
  of both legs, 53, 53*f*
  of shoulders, pelvis, hips and legs,
    58, 58*f*
observation, 53
palm broadening
  of ischiocrural/hamstring muscle
    group, 53, 55*f*
  of right thigh, 57, 57*f*
palm compressions
  alternate, of right calf muscles, 55,
    55*f*
  of lower leg, 57, 58*f*
  of shoulder area, 58, 59*f*
palm scrubbing
  alternate, 53, 53*f*
  of right leg, 57, 57*f*
right ischiocrural/hamstring muscle
    group suddenly cramps, 55, 56*f*
ROM stretch of right hip joint, 58,
    58*f*
stretch
  of right gastrocnemius and soleus
    muscles, 58, 59*f*
  of right ischiocrural/hamstring
    muscles, 58, 59*f*
  of right quadriceps and iliopsoas,
    58, 59*f*
thumb compressions, 56, 56*f*
time distribution, 52
treatment, 30–32
postural integration, 140
preevent massage, 27–30, 35–43
  broadening
    of ischiocrural/hamstring muscle
    group, 38, 38*f*
    of right calf, 38, 38*f*
    palm, of right thigh, 40, 41*f*
  circular finger frictions of neck area,
    43, 45*f*
  edging of right calf muscle,
    39, 39*f*
  effleurage
    of back, 39, 40*f*
    of back of right leg, 37, 37*f*
    of gluteal area and lower back, 37,
    37*f*
    of right leg, 40, 41*f*
    of right leg and gluteal area, 39, 40*f*
  fist compressions of right gluteal and
    lower back muscles, 38, 38*f*
  fist/palm compressions
    of ischiocrural/hamstring muscle
    group, 38, 38*f*

of right thigh, 40, 41f
fist/thumb compression of right foot, 39, 40f
highlights, 28b
hypothenar rubbing of right quadriceps, 41, 42f
jostling
of both legs, 36, 37f
of hip and both legs, 42, 42f
muscle stretching, 29–30
pace, 29
palm compression
of right tibialis anterior and peroneal muscles, 41, 41f
of shoulder area, 43, 44f
palm scrubbing, 36, 37f
palm/thumb compressions of shoulder/neck area, 39, 40f
primary massaged areas, 36f
rhythmic lock/stretch
of peroneal muscles, 39, 39f
of soleus and tibialis posterior muscles, 38, 39f
ROM stretch
of left hip joint, 42, 43f
of right hip joint, 42, 42f
scrubbing of right leg, 40, 41f
stretch
of left gastrocnemius and soleus muscles, 43, 44f
of left hamstring/ischiocrural muscles, 43, 44f
of left quadriceps and iliopsoas muscles, 43, 44f
of right gastrocnemius and soleus muscles, 42, 43f
of right ischiocrural/hamstring muscles, 42, 43f
of right quadriceps and iliopsoas muscles, 42, 43f
strokes used in, 35
time distribution, 36
prepatellar bursitis (housemaid's knee), 191
PRICE mnemonic, 188, 192f
proprioceptive dysfunction, 120f
proprioceptive neuromuscular facilitation (PNF), 80–81
irradiation, 81
reciprocal inhibition/innervation, 81
successive induction, 80–81
psychological value, 3
pulsed muscle energy techniques (MET), 86, 86f

Q

quadratus lumborum
release, 223, 223f
stretch, 109, 109f
quadriceps femoris, 171, 172f
hypothenar rubbing, 72f
myofascial release, 147, 147f
stretch, 101, 103f

R

reciprocal inhibition, 77–78, 77b, 83–84, 84f, 86, 98
rectus abdominis, myofascial release, 147, 148f
rectus femoris C-release, 217–218
elbow C-release, athlete supine, 218, 218f
palm C-release, athlete supine, 218, 218f
pulling, 217f, 218
pushing, 217–218, 217f
referred autonomic phenomena, 166–167
rehabilitation, principles of, 183
remedial massage, 32, 207–233, 208b
restorative massage, 207, 208b
rhomboids, 171, 177f
release, 224, 224f
stretch of, 110, 110f
rhythmic lock and stretch, variation, 213, 217f
rhythmic stabilization (RS), 81
Rolfing, 140
rolling, 35
rotator cuff pain, chronic, Tui Na treatment for, 135–136
rubber gloves, 31
rubor, 183
Ruddy's rapid pulsing duction, 86, 86f
runner's knee see iliotibial band syndrome
runners, massage in, 61
suggested areas, 61, 62f
tibialis anterior muscles, compression with mild lock and stretch, 61, 62f
see also prevent sports massage treatment

S

sartorius muscle, stretch, 103–104, 104f
scalenus anterior, 171, 178f

scaphoid bone fracture, 193
scrubbing, 35
self-massage, 235–246
abdominal area, 242–243, 244f
arms, 244–245
flexor/extensor muscles of forearm and hand, 245, 245f
flexor/extensor muscles of upper arm, 244, 245f
back, 240–242
latissimus dorsi/teres major muscles, 242, 243f
lower back, 240–242, 241f
mid and upper back with tennis/lacrosse balls, 242, 242f
chest, 244, 244f
feet, 235
dorsal aspect, 236f
plantar aspect, 235, 236f
hands, 246, 246f
lower legs, 235–237
anterior, 235–237, 237f
posterior, 237, 238f
neck, 242
upper neck muscles, anterior aspect, 242, 243f
shoulders, 244, 244f
thighs, 237–240
anterior aspect, 237–238, 238f
medial aspect, 240, 240f
posterior aspect, 238–239, 239f
thigh, hips and gluteal area, lateral aspect of, 240, 241f
tools, 235
exercise balls, 235, 236f
lacrosse and tennis balls, 235, 236f
myofascial foam roll, 235, 236f
Stick, The, 235, 236f
semitendinosus muscle
Active Isolated Stretching (AIS) of, 88, 89f
Sen lines, 89–90
Sen Sib, 89–90, 90f
serratus anterior release, 226, 226f
Sever-Haglund disease, 190
Shiatsu, 128–129
shin splints syndrome (periostitis), 190
shoulder
balance and hold in, 121–122, 121f
impingement in, 196–197
self-massage, 244
stretch, 112
Simmond's calf squeeze test, 186–187, 187f

Sinding-Larsen's disease, 190
skiing, massage for, 67–68
  cross-country, 67–68, 67f
  downhill/snowboarding, suggested
    areas, 67, 67f
  soleus muscle, lock and stretch, 68f
skin bend, 24, 24f
skin lift, 25, 25f
skin push, 24–25, 24f
skin rolling, 24, 24f, 168, 168f
skin strokes, 24–25
slow rehearsal (SR), 81
snapping hip, 196
  myofascial release manipulation in, 140
soccer, massage for, 71
  hamstring stretch, 71f
  suggested areas, 71
soft tissue manipulation, 140
soft tissue release
  arms, 229–232
  chest region, 225–226
  feet and ankles, 214
  feet and lower legs, 214–216
  hands, 233
  hips and gluteal area, 222–223
  lower and upper back, 223–224
  neck area, 229, 230f
  shoulders, 226–229
  thighs, groin and knees, 217–222
soleus muscle, 171, 173f
  lock and stretch, 68f
  release, 215, 215f
soleus syndrome (periostitis), 190
splenius capitis
  myofascial release, 151, 152f
  stretch of, 112, 113f
sprain, 186
spray and stretch, 169
S-stroke petrissage, 14–15
  modified, 14, 14f
  modified S-stroke/elbow, 15, 15f
  regular, 14, 14f
static active flexibility, 76, 76f
static flexibility, 76
static passive flexibility, 76, 76f
static stretching, 75
sternalis, myofascial release, 147, 148f
sternochondral fascia, 147, 148f
Stick, The, in self-massage, 235, 236f
strain counterstrain (SCS), 122–126
  calcaneus, 124–125, 124f, 125f
  examples, 123–126
  long head of biceps brachii muscle,
    125–126, 125f

medial meniscus, 124, 124f
mobile point, 122, 123f
piriformis muscle, 123–124, 123f
subdeltoid bursa, 126, 126f
tender points (TPs), 122–123, 125f,
  126f
straps, stretch, 98–99, 99f
stress fractures, 189, 191
stretch
  active, 80
  dynamic, 80f
  gluteal area and hips, 104–106
  lower body, 99–104
  static, 80f
  upper body, 106–116, 107f, 108f
stretch techniques, muscle and
    connective tissue, 169–170
  finger percussion, 169–170, 170f
  home stretching exercises, 170
  integrated neuromuscular inhibition
    technique (INIT), 170
  myofascial release, 170
  percussion and stretch, 169–170
  positional release, 170
  range of motion, 170
  spray and stretch/ice and stretch, 169
  stretch with '4-finger stroke', 169, 169f
  trigger point pressure release, 169,
    169f
  voluntary contraction and release
    methods, 170
stretch/myotatic reflex, 77f, 78b
stretching, 77–80
  ballistic, 79–80, 79f
  dynamic, 78–79, 79f
  passive, 78, 78f
  static (yoga type), 77–78, 77f
stretchments, 139–140
stripping, 35, 167–168, 167f
strokes, basic, 6–25, 7f
structural integration, 140
strumming, 168, 168f
student's elbow, 191
subdeltoid bursa
  strain counterstrain, 126, 126f
  tender points, 126f
subluxations, 184–185
subscapularis, 171, 176f
  release, 228, 228f
  stretch of, 112, 113f
superficial forearm extensor muscle
    release, 232, 232f
superficial forearm flexor muscle
    release, 232, 233f

supraspinatus, 171, 175f
  release, 227–228, 227f
  stretch of, 112, 113f
supraspinatus tendinitis, 122
Swedish Movement Cure, 1, 139
swimming, massage for, 61–62
  ankles, alternate bilateral palm
    frictions, 62f
  suggested areas, 62, 62f

T
talofibular ligaments, taping, 201, 201f
taping, 199–206
  basic rules, 199
  finger stabilization/Buddy taping, 204,
    205f
  to lateral ligaments, 200–201, 200f
  painful heel pad, 202, 203f
  plantar fasciitis, 201, 202f
  prevention of thumb hyperextension,
    204, 204f
  to talofibular ligaments, 201, 201f
  thumb stabilization, 202–204,
    203f
tapotement, 21–22, 35
  cupping, 22, 22f
  hacking, 21–22
    double-handed, 21–22, 22f
  pounding, 22, 22f
  slapping, 22, 22f
tender points (TPs), 119, 122–123
  of calcaneus, 125f
  of long head of biceps brachii muscle,
    125f
  of medial meniscus, 124f
  of piriformis muscle, 123f
  of subdeltoid bursa, 126f
tendinitis, 189, 190
tendinopathy, 189, 190, 191
tendinosis, 189, 190, 191
tendon injuries, acute, 186–188
  hamstring muscles, palm broadening,
    69f
  suggested areas, 69, 69f
tennis elbow see epicondylitis,
    lateral/medial
tennis, massage for, 66–67
  gluteal muscle, fist compression, 67f
  suggested areas, 66–67, 66f
  triceps surae group, fist frictions, 66f
tenovaginitis, 190
tensor fasciae latae, stretch, 104, 105f
tensor fasciae latae fascia

myofascial release, 150, 150f
release, 222–223, 223f
teres major muscles *see* latissimus dorsi
and teres major muscles
teres minor muscles *see* infraspinatus
and teres minor muscles
thenar rubbing, 35
therapeutic stretching, 98
thighs, self-massage, 237–240
anterior aspect, 237–238, 238f
foam roll, 237
hands, 237
reinforce thumb cross frictions,
237
Stick, The, 237
lateral aspect of thigh, hips and gluteal
area, 240
fingertips, 240, 241f
foam roll, 240, 241f
palm heel, 240, 241f
medial aspect, 240
hands, 240, 240f
Stick, The, 240, 240f
posterior aspect, 238–239
fingertips, 238, 239f
foam roll, 238, 239f
Stick, The, 239, 239f
Thompson's test, 186–187, 187f
thoracolumbar fascia, 144, 145f
thumb
compression, 10–11, 11f
edging, 20, 20f
friction, 16, 16f, 17f
glide, 211, 211f
hyperextension prevention, taping
and, 204, 204f
stabilization, taping, 202–204, 203f
tibial stress syndrome(periostitis),
190
tibialis anterior, 147, 147f, 171, 174f,
216
stretch, 99, 100f
tibialis anterior release, 216, 216f
tibialis posterior muscle, stretch, 100,
100f
toe extensor muscles, deep/superficial,
147, 147f
traditional Thai massage-influenced
stretching techniques, 89–93,
90f
adductor massage and hip stretch, 91,
91f
rectus femoris massage with hip
stretch, 91, 91f

palm compression with hip stretch,
91, 92f
gluteus medius and minimus muscles
and lateral thigh stretch, 91, 92f
hip extensor stretch, 92, 92f
enhanced hip adductor stretch,
92–93, 93f
stretch of medial aspect of thigh,
including gracilis muscle, 93, 93f
stretch of ischiocrural muscle group/
hamstring muscles, 93, 93f
transverse friction, 19, 19f, 35
deep, 19
trapezius muscle
release, 224, 225f
stretch of, 111, 111f
trapezius scapulae, 171, 176f
triceps brachii
release, 231, 231f
stretch of, 115, 115f
triceps surae muscle
fist glide/ thumb glide on, 144,
144f
stretch, 100, 101f
trigger point pressure release, 169,
169f
true lines of stretch, 98, 98f
Tui Na, 128–129, 130–135
in chronic rotator cuff pain, 135–136
arm movement, 136
digital pressing, 135
grasping and forearm rolling of
muscles in lower back, 135
palm pressing and grasping, 135,
136f
treated acupoints, 135, 136f
grasping, 134, 134f
kneading, 134, 134f
lateral knee pain/'runner's knee',
136–137
leg movement, 137
pressing, 137
rolling, 137
treated acupoints, 136–137, 137f
in lumbar strain, 135–137
elbow pressing, 135
grasping and forearm rolling of
muscles in lower back, 135
palm pressing, 135
treated acupoints, 135, 135f
pressing, 131
digital pressing, 131, 132f
elbow pressing, 131, 132f
palm pressing, 131, 132f

rolling, 133–134
forearm rolling, 134f
rolling finish, 134f
rolling start, 133f
rubbing, 132
thumb, 132, 133f
thenar, 132, 133f
hypothenar, 132, 133f
scrubbing, 131
palm scrubbing, 131, 131f
tumor, 183

U

United States, massage in, 2
upper back, stretch, 109–112
upper body, muscles of
anterior aspect, 107f
posterior aspect, 108f

V

V-frictions, 17–18
regular, 17–18, 18f
reversed, 18, 18f
vastus lateralis release, 218, 218f
vibrations, 24
Virén, Lars, 1–2
voluntary contraction and release
methods, 170

W

wedges, 98–99
weight lifting, massage for, 63–64,
64f
quadriceps femoris muscle, fist
compression, 64f
suggested areas, 64
wrestling, massage for, 63
levator scapulae muscle, braced
thumb compression, 63f
suggested areas, 63, 63f
vastus lateralis muscle, lock and
stretch massage, 63f

Y

Yin-yang, 129–130, 130f
yoga, 77–78, 192

Z

Zen bodytherapy, 140
zinc oxide tape, 199